The Practice of Clinical and Counselling Supervision

Quality supervision assists in quality service provision. *The Practice of Clinical and Counselling Supervision: Australian and International Applications* is the third edition of the leading Australian state-of-the-art text for supervision training applicable to a vast range of applied therapists. Counsellors, psychologists, psychotherapists, social workers, and clinical nurse supervisors will all find the presentation of supervision approaches, methods, and applications helpful.

From introductory conceptualisations of counselling to ethical applications, and from interacting with suicidality to addressing supervisee fears, this book has what supervisors need to know about supervision. Specialty areas including domestic violence, Christian counselling, and the status of supervision research are also covered. This third edition uniquely details information on supervision and counselling in various countries, and thus honours the diversity of applied supervision globally.

With an impressive list of contributors from Australia and the broader region, this book provides a wealth of practical information, advice, theory, research evidence, and essential training for supervisors.

Nadine Pelling is a clinical psychologist, member of the Australian Psychological Society and the APS College of Clinical Psychologists, and an approved supervisor with the Psychology Board of Australia. She is a senior lecturer in clinical psychology and counselling at the University of South Australia and maintains a private practice in the southern suburbs of Adelaide.

Philip Armstrong is the past CEO of the Australian Counselling Association (April 2000 to October 2023), current executive director of Optimise Potential, and the founder of the RISE UP Supervision program. Philip also held an adjunct senior industry fellow position at the University of South Australia from 2000 to October 2023.

The Practice of Clinical and Counselling Supervision

Australian and International Applications

Third Edition

Edited by Nadine Pelling and Philip Armstrong

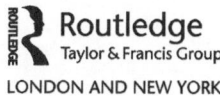

Routledge
Taylor & Francis Group

LONDON AND NEW YORK

Third edition published 2025
by Routledge
4 Park Square, Milton Park, Abingdon, Oxon, OX14 4RN

and by Routledge
605 Third Avenue, New York, NY 10158

Routledge is an imprint of the Taylor & Francis Group, an informa business

First edition published by Australian Academic Press 2009
Second edition published by Australian Academic Press 2017

British Library Cataloguing-in-Publication Data
A catalogue record for this book is available from the British Library

ISBN: 9781032785271 (hbk)
ISBN: 9781032785264 (pbk)
ISBN: 9781003490067 (ebk)

DOI: 10.4324/9781003490067

Typeset in Galliard
by Newgen Publishing UK

Nadine Pelling – For L.G. Pelling. Your daughters, Natalie and Nadine, loved you and will forever remember you as a beer drinking, salmon fishing, carpenter with a creative streak. For my daughter, Jasmine, who continues to provide me with new memories of joy and connection. Finally, for Shelley Rogers for her workplace support over many years and her wife, Leonie McKeon who recently passed, two women whose kindness is memorable.

Philip Armstrong – For Phillip, Kataryna, Alyciana and Kiernan my four wonderful children and my ever-suffering wife, Alison, you continue to ensure my life remains challenging with never a dull moment. Nadine, the lead editor who has spent significant time on this project. I thank her for the dedication of her talents and time towards the completion of this text. To all the members of the Australian Counselling Association who allowed me to represent and advocate for them for over two decades.

Contents

Figures

Tables

Chapter Authors

Deah Abbott, MA, earned her Bachelor's in Psychology from the University of Oklahoma and her Master's in Experimental Psychology from the University of Central Oklahoma. Her research interests include treatment process and outcomes for anxiety-related disorders and the impact of vicarious trauma on therapists and advocates. Ms Abbott has published research on vicarious resilience, mindfulness, and anxiety disorders, as well as presenting at numerous national-level conferences.

Elisa Agostinelli, PhD, is currently the program director of the postgraduate counselling programs in UniSQ. Elisa had studied and trained as a clinical psychologist in Rome, Italy. She has a Bachelor's and Master's in Psychology and a Master's in family therapy. She obtained her PhD from the University of Toledo, Ohio, in counselling and mental health. She is currently registered as a clinical family therapist and clinical counsellor. Her counselling experience had been with families, couples, children, and adults, running individual and group sessions. She has extensive counselling experience in the area of trauma, domestic and family violence, palliative care, terminal illness, and bereavement. Elisa also worked with clients with schizophrenia and children in a neurological and psychiatric hospital in Italy. She has trained counsellors at the University of Toledo; the University of New England, NSW; the Australian Catholic University, QLD; and the Domestic Violence Prevention Service, Gold Coast. In the past ten years she has supervised students, professional counsellors, and psychologists. She has presented in several national and international conferences and run workshops on trauma, DFV, and grief and loss. Her research interests are personal and professional development of counsellors and psychologists, supervision, multicultural counselling, trauma diagnosis and treatment, and bereavement counselling. She is passionate about creating a new generation of counsellors and psychologists that are trauma informed, culturally sensitive, and curious about new developments in the area of neuroscience.

Margaret Helen Alvarez, PhD, is Dean for Graduate Programs at Silliman University, Philippines. She completed her Master's at the University of the Philippines and her PhD in clinical psychology at the Ateneo de Manila University. A licensed psychologist, her practice and research focus have primarily been in family systems and dynamics.

Jessica Ariela, S.Psi., MA, earned her graduate degree in clinical and mental health counseling from Wheaton College, IL, USA, and her undergraduate in Psychology from Universitas Pelita Harapan. Besides her counselling activities, she enjoys her role as a lecturer at the Psychology Department at Universitas Pelita Harapan, Tangerang, since 2015, teaching counselling courses, and actively engages in both national and international events. Jessica was licensed as a professional counselor in Illinois, USA, and is a certified Master Facilitator in Trauma Healing, by Trauma Healing Institute.

Philip Armstrong is the past CEO of the Australian Counselling Association (April 2000 to October 2023), current executive director of Optimise Potential, and the founder of the RISE UP Supervision program. Philip also held an adjunct senior industry fellow position at the University of South Australia from 2000 to October 2023.

Nancy Arthur, PhD, is currently appointed as professor and Dean Research for UniSA Business. She previously held the role of Dean: Research & Innovation, in the Division of Education Arts & Social Sciences. Prof Arthur holds a BA (Hons) majoring in sociology (Waterloo), a Master's in sociology (Alberta), and MSc and PhD degrees in educational psychology (Calgary). She is a Professor Emeritus from the University of Calgary, where she was awarded a Canada Research Chair in professional education for diversity and social justice. Professor Arthur's current research programme focuses on career development and the international transitions of students and workers. She is a registered psychologist (AB Canada) and elected fellow of the Canadian Psychological Association. Her recent edited books include *Counseling in Context: Identities and Social Justice* (Springer) and *Contemporary Theories of Career Development: International Perspectives* (Routledge).

Dini Farhana Baharudin, is a senior lecturer at the Faculty of Leadership and Management, Universiti Sains Islam Malaysia. She holds a Master's in community counseling from Western Michigan University and a doctoral degree in counseling from the National University of Malaysia. She is also a registered counselor.

Matthew Bambling, PhD, holds adjunct professorial positions at ACAP-Navitas and University of Queensland. Matt has been credited with the first randomised trial that tested the impact of supervision on client outcome in the treatment of depression and he has published several articles and book chapters on supervision. He has broad research interests and has published in the areas of telemental health, behaviour management in schools, behavioural health, the microbiome and treatment response to depression.

John Barletta, PhD, is a counselling and clinical psychologist who has provided education and psychological services since 1984. He began his career as a teacher, then guidance counsellor, relationship educator, and a tenured and adjunct university senior academic, including extended studies and work in the USA and Italy. He trained at Queensland University of Technology (DipT, GradDipCouns), Australian Catholic University (BEd), University of Queensland (MEdSt), Ohio University (PhD), and Accademia di Psicoterapia della Famiglia (Rome). Ohio University flattered him with the prestigious distinguished alumni honour, the George Hill Memorial Award which recognises outstanding scholarship, service, and leadership. A member of the Australian Psychology Society, a fellow of the College of Counselling Psychologists and the College of Clinical Psychologists, John is an approved clinical supervisor with the Psychology Board of Australia. He has a passion for helping adults and organisations flourish in their wellbeing, relationships, and performance using integrated positive psychology principles. An energetic, down-to-earth professional, he bases all his work on scientific research, clinical expertise, and lived experience. John is responsible for over 500 publications and presentations, is co-editor of *The Home Therapist*, co-editor of *The Practice of Clinical Supervision* (1st ed.), is the long-standing expert psychology columnist for *Style* magazine, and is an occasional ABC-Radio commentator on psychological issues.

Herbert Biggs, PhD, is a former professor and current adjunct professor in the School of Psychology and Counselling at the Queensland University of Technology. He is a psychologist and certified rehabilitation counsellor in Australia. He earned his doctorate from Massey University in New Zealand, and subsequently has taken academic positions at Southern Cross University and Griffith University. Herbert was a founding member of the Australian Society of Rehabilitation Counsellors and is a member of the Rehabilitation Counsellors Association of Australasia and the Australian Psychological Society. He serves on several editorial boards, is a member of the Australian Psychological Society National Ethics Committee, and a board member of the combined Departments of Defence and Veterans' Affairs Human Research Ethics Committee. He has recently been appointed to the Academic Council of the Pacific Coast University for Workplace Health Sciences, British Columbia, Canada. He teaches in the Master's and is the University Manager for Flexible Admissions.

Rebecca Braid, PhD, owns and practices at Eden Therapy Services Pty Ltd in Sydney, Australia. Dr. Braid's original degree is in social work from the University of NSW. After holding health management positions, Dr. Braid gained a graduate diploma in couples and family therapy and a Master's in couples and family therapy. Dr. Braid researched "Our Healing: An empirical study of the interrelationship between therapeutic intervention and spiritual intervention in a social work private practice" to honour spiritual interventions for healing. Dr. Braid's publication such as "How to run groups for complex trauma survivors" documented her unique group work service to trauma victims which has been acknowledge and recognised by Victim Services, part of the Attorney Generals Department for Victims of Crime.

Thomas E. Davis, PhD, was trained in counselor education at the Ohio State University and Miami University, Master's in counselor education from Marshall University, and earned a Bachelor's in general studies from Ohio University. His major research interests include counselor education and supervision, legal and ethical issues, and clinical mental health and school counseling. He has directed 56 doctoral dissertations, and has authored numerous pieces of scholarly work and professional presentations. He has held many professional leadership positions, including vice chairperson for the Council for the Accreditation of Counseling and Related Educational Programs (CACREP), and chaired the 2009 Standards Revision Committee for CACREP. He also served as president of the Ohio Counseling Association, president of the Ohio Association for Counselor Education and Supervision, served on the board of directors for the Ohio School Counselors Association, served as chair of the Ohio Counselor and Social Worker Board Counselor Professional Standards Committee, and president of the American Association for State Counseling Boards. Within Ohio University he has served as the program coordinator of the Counselor Education Program, chair of the Department of Counseling and Higher Education, Associate Dean for Graduate Studies, and a one-year appointment as Interim Dean of the College of Education. He was also asked by the president and trustees to serve (for six years) as the secretary to the Ohio University Board of Trustees.

Jason Dixon, PhD, has been a research consultant, interpreter, and counsellor educator who provided clinical supervision to counsellors, psychologists, and social workers. He holds a doctorate from The Ohio University and a Master's in counselling from Australian Catholic University. He taught clinical and research courses at universities in the USA and Australia, was senior research fellow in mental health at the Queensland University of Technology, and served on the board of directors of the Australian Counselling Association. Jason specialised in the treatment of alcohol and other drug use issues. His research pursuits were psychometrics, online survey design and deployment, cross-cultural psychology, and counselling culturally and linguistically diverse populations. Jason now spends his days in the pursuit of a range of creative endeavours, particularly documentary filmmaking.

Nicola Gazzola, is Professor of Counselling Psychology at the University of Ottawa. He is a licensed psychologist (Quebec) and has 25 years of clinical experience. His research interests are in the area of professional issues in counselling and psychotherapy and include professional identity of counselling and clinical supervision. His research team is currently investigating the therapist use-of-self in counselling and psychotherapy.

Kate Gignac, PhD, trained at the University of Ottawa and is a Canadian Certified Counsellor (CCC) and a Certified Counsellor Supervisor (CCC-S). Her research centres on professional identity formation, clinical supervision, the articulation of identity work, place of values and religiosity in identity narratives, and the nexus of exogenous events with professional becoming.

J. Kyle Haws, PhD, is a postdoctoral fellow in the Department of Family Medicine and the Adult & Child Center for Outcomes Research & Delivery Science (ACCORDS) at the University of Colorado Anschutz Medical Campus. He completed his doctoral training in clinical psychology at the University of Nebraska-Lincoln with concentrations in child/family and quantitative methodology after finishing his Master's in experimental psychology at the University of Central Oklahoma. Operating within integrated behavioural health in primary care, Dr. Haws provides assessment and treatment to children, adolescents, adults, and their families with a special focus on providing services to historically underserved and marginalised communities. The overarching goal of his line of research inquiry is to optimise the delivery of evidence-based interventions to improve care for posttraumatic stress disorder and other trauma-related conditions and to adapt those interventions for delivery in real-world primary care or community-based settings.

Zoë Hazelwood, PhD, is a clinical psychologist, clinical program coordinator and senior lecturer in the School of Psychology and Counselling, Queensland University of Technology. Zoë is Director of the Communication, Attachment and Relationship Experiences (CARE) Research Laboratory. She completed her doctorate at Griffith University in attachment and communication in relationships and has conducted extensive research in intimate relationships and the factors that influence the development of healthy, happy coupling. Her areas of special interest include adult attachment and bonding in relationships, communication in relationships, family relationships, and the influence of child behaviour on adult relationships. Zoë is an accredited supervisor with the AHPRA and the Psychology Board of Australia and has an area of practice endorsement in clinical psychology. She conducts clinical supervision at QUT, and supervises psychology registrars for their area of practice endorsement registrar program. Zoë also carries a small case load in a part-time private practice. She is a fellow of the Australian Psychological Society, a fellow of the APS College of Clinical Psychology, and a committee member for the International Association for Relationship Research.

Eunike M. Himawan, MPsi, is a registered clinical psychologist from Indonesia, and is currently undertaking a PhD in social psychology at the University of Queensland, Australia. She earned her Master's from the University of Indonesia in 2013, and has been practising as a psychologist since then at Experiencing Life Foundation, a private clinic in Gading Serpong, Tangerang. Besides practising as a professional, Eunike is also a part-time lecturer at the Faculty of Psychology, Universitas Pelita Harapan, Tangerang. Eunike is currently a treasurer of Indonesian Counselling Association.

Karel K. Himawan, PhD, clinical psychologist, obtained his doctorate in clinical/social psychology from faculty of medicine, the University of Queensland, Australia. He actively engages in the academic profession as a head of department at the Faculty of Psychology, Universitas Pelita Harapan, and a course coordinator for Master of Mental Health Program, the University of Queensland. He currently serves as vice president of Indonesian Counselling Association. He has over seven years of professional practice as a clinical psychologist at Experiencing Life Foundation (www.experiencing-life.com), a private clinic located in Gading Serpong, that he co-founded with his colleagues.

Shannon Hood, is Dean of Counselling and Chaplaincy at Perth Bible College (PBC). He holds Master's in Commerce, as well as in Education and Counselling. He is a clinical counsellor and supervisor with the Australian Counselling Association. He completed a year of his Bachelor of Theology under full scholarship at the University of Cambridge. His PhD focused on the use of spiritual and religious interventions by professional counsellors. Prior to joining PBC Shannon supervised the practice of over 100 mental health professionals as a clinical manager at Converge Interventional. He has published and presented in Australia and internationally and is on the editorial board of the *Waverley Journal*. He sustains a part-time private counselling and supervision practice.

Norfaezah Md Khalid is a senior lecturer at the Department of Educational Psychology and Counselling, Faculty of Education, University of Malaya, Kuala Lumpur, Malaysia. She is also a registered counsellor with the Malaysian Board of Counsellors. Dr. Md Khalid holds a Bachelor's and Doctoral degree in counselling from the University of Malaya, Kuala Lumpur.

Caleb W. Lack, PhD, is Professor of Psychology and the Counseling Psychology MA Program Coordinator in the Department of Psychology at the University of Central Oklahoma. A specialist in evidence-based psychological practice, he completed a predoctoral internship at the University of Florida and earned his doctorate from Oklahoma State University in 2006. A licensed clinical psychologist, Dr. Lack is the best-selling author or editor of six books, most recently *Critical Thinking, Science, & Pseudoscience: Why*

You Can't Trust Your Brain (Springer). He has also authored more than 60 scientific publications relating to the assessment and treatment of psychological problems such as Obsessive-Compulsive Disorder, Tourette's Syndrome, pediatric mood disorders, and post-traumatic stress, and frequently presents nationally and internationally on a variety of topics, in addition to consulting for national and international companies. Learn more online at www.caleblack.com.

Fran Lane, M.Couns, worked as an Abuse & Trauma Counsellor in the NGO sector. She worked with clients who had experienced FDV, sexual assault, childhood abuse, and war trauma. Whilst studying for her PhD from the University of Notre Dame she was diagnosed with vicarious trauma. On recovery she utilised her visual journals and completed an auto-ethnographic study on recovery from vicarious trauma. Now working as a clinical supervisor and sessional lecturer, Fran is most interested in the emergence of compassion in theoretical models and as a protective factor for counsellors.

Tiffany Lee, PhD, is the program director of the Specialty Program in Alcohol and Drug Abuse at Western Michigan University. She has a PhD in counsellor education and is a licensed professional counselor and certified advanced alcohol and drug counselor. Her research and grant activities primarily focus on addictions training in counselor education.

Alf Lizzio, PhD, is Professor of Psychology and Dean (Learning Futures) at Griffith University. As a counselling and consulting psychologist, he has extensive experience in both the public sector and private practice in areas related to the development of people in organisations, the effective functioning of teams and the management of change. Alf has a particular interest in processes related to the support and development of professionals and leaders.

Tracey Milson, lives on the Gold Coast in Queensland, Australia, where she conducts a successful private practice. She has over 20 years' experience as a counsellor and family therapist specialising in faith-based practice. She is a counselling and supervisor trainer. She has worked for the Australian College of Ministry (ACOM) in the higher education sector and the Australian Institute of Family Counselling (AIFC) in the vocational sector. For ACOM she is Manager of Professional Supervision and facilitates a graduate certificate in professional supervision. Her specialty area is supervision, and supervision of supervision (SoS). Supervision of Supervision is also one of the supervision training courses she delivers for the Clinical Counselling Centre (CCC) where she is the Director of Training and delivers and manages the CCC *Rise Up* supervision training courses. Tracey completed a diploma in counselling in 2001, an advanced diploma of counselling and family therapy in 2002, a bachelor of social science (counselling) in 2008, a graduate certificate in human behaviour in 2011, a graduate diploma of counselling and integrated psychotherapy in 2015, and a master of counselling in 2016. She is registered with the ACA (level 4/supervisor) and a member of the ACA College of Supervisors.

Ann Moir-Bussy, PhD, is currently an adjunct associate professor in the College of Indigenous Futures, Education and the Arts at Charles Darwin University supervising students in counselling and mental health. Ann has been a counsellor and psychotherapist for over 27 years and is a fellow of the Australian Counselling Association. She has previously worked at the University of New England, Hong Kong Shue Yan University, and the University of Sunshine Coast. Ann is the editor of the *Australian Counselling Research Journal.* She was the Founder, and for 7 years the editor, of the *Asia Pacific Journal of Counselling and Psychotherapy.*

Stephen O'Kane, PhD, is a specialist family violence counsellor at the EACH Family Relationship Centre and a counselling supervisor in private practice with experience in working with clients who have experienced trauma, violence, and related issues. He is based in the Eastern suburbs of Melbourne, Australia, and has worked extensively with clients in crisis and clients experiencing homelessness; within the Magistrates Court assisting men with Intervention orders; and in a community counselling agency supporting women and children fleeing violent situations. He has facilitated parenting orders programs and men's behaviour change programs, and assisted with engaging men in fathering programs. He has previously worked as a senior leader in several government organisations and was a private consultant specialising in mentoring and coaching. Stephen is a member of the Australian Counselling Association College of Supervisors, a member of Counsellors Victoria and is an alumnus of the Williamson Community Leadership Program.

Cynthia J. Osborn, PhD, is Professor of Counselor Education and Supervision at Kent State University, Ohio, where she has supervised Master's and doctoral students in their counseling practicum and supervision of counseling experiences. She coordinates the addictions counseling certificate programme and is the PI/PD of two federal awards focused on addictions counseling curriculum development and training. She is a licensed professional clinical counselor (with supervisory endorsement) and a licensed chemical dependency counselor. Publications, research activities, and trainings are in the areas of addictions counseling, motivational interviewing, and counselor supervision. She has served as president of Chi Sigma Iota International, the counseling academic and professional honour society, and she is the 2022 recipient of Kent State University's Distinguished Teaching Award.

Nadine Pelling is a clinical psychologist, member of the Australian Psychological Society and the APS College of Clinical Psychologists, and an approved supervisor with the Psychology Board of Australia. She is a senior lecturer in clinical psychology and counselling at the University of South Australia and maintains a private practice in the southern suburbs of Adelaide.

Jeffrey Po, PhD, is a counselling psychotherapist in private practice in Singapore. He holds his doctorate in counselling psychology and has academic qualifications in counselling and telecommunication engineering. Jeffrey is also an AIHCP certified meditation instructor and spiritual counsellor. Additionally, he holds a diploma in Buddhist studies and a post graduate diploma in counselling supervision. Jeffrey has authored three books: *The Buddhist Companion*, *Buddhist Snippets,* and *Meditative Flow-Psychotherapy.* Jeffrey is the founding president of the Association of Psychotherapists and Counsellors (Singapore).

Hartini Abdul Rahman, was a licensed psychologist and was a senior staff clinician at Counseling & Psychological Services, Oregon State University, Oregon, USA, during the development of this chapter. She holds a Master's and Doctoral degree in Counseling Psychology from Western Michigan University.

Marina Salmond, earned her Master's in pastoral counselling from Singapore Bible College, and in clinical mental health counseling from Wheaton College, USA. She has been practising counselling in various settings in Indonesia for 15 years. She currently has her own practice and practises at the psychology clinic Experiencing Life Foundation (ELF), in which she works with individual clients as well as couples. She also gives lectures on counselling and conducts counselling training. She is a member of the Indonesian Counselling Association (ICA), an associate member of Singapore Association for Counselling (SAC), and a Prepare-Enrich Facilitator.

Yasmin Shirali, MA, is a program specialist for the Health and Human Services Commission for the State of Texas, where she focuses on improving employee outcomes via quantitative research and effective means of storytelling through data. She completed her Bachelor's and Master's in Experimental Psychology at the University of Central Oklahoma.

Bridget Rose Stanton, MS, Bridget is a registered mental health counselor. She completed a Master's of Science in clinical mental health counseling at the University of North Florida in 2020. Currently working with adolescents, she strives to celebrate her clients individual strengths with wonder and admiration every day.

Helen Stallman, PhD, is a highly regarded clinical psychologist, visionary innovator, and trailblazer in the field of health and wellbeing. With a career spanning over two decades, she has wholeheartedly dedicated herself to developing groundbreaking solutions that empower individuals, families, and communities to overcome challenges that impact their overall wellbeing. As the esteemed founder and CEO of Care Collaborate Connect Pty Ltd, as well as a former academic, including the role of Professor of Suicide Prevention, Dr. Stallman has led transformative initiatives that have earned international acclaim. Her visionary programs, such as Family Transitions Triple P, Care Collaborate Connect: Suicide Prevention, Psychological First Aid, Bereavement Resilience Program, thedesk, and The Learning Thermometer, have revolutionised the field. Dr. Stallman's exceptional contributions have been recognised with a remarkable 11 prestigious awards and accolades. These include the esteemed Healthy Development Adelaide Women's Excellence in Research Award, multiple Uniquest Trailblazer awards, acceptance into the renowned CSIRO ON Prime national innovation program, and the recognition of Triple P as one of the Top 10 Australian Inventions by The Brilliant. Her unwavering commitment to innovation and compassionate care has had a profound impact on countless individuals, transforming their lives for the better. Through her expert consultation, extensive publications, and engaging speaking engagements, Dr. Stallman has firmly established herself as a respected thought leader and a catalyst for positive change.

Janeé Steele, PhD, is a core faculty member in the School of Counseling at Walden University. She is also the co-owner and clinical director of Kalamazoo Cognitive and Behavioral Therapy, PLLC, where she provides therapy, supervision, and training in CBT. Janeé has a PhD in counselor education and is a licensed professional counselor and diplomate of the Academy of Cognitive and Behavioral Therapies. Her research interests primarily include pedagogy, supervision, and diversity in counsellor education.

Brian Sullivan completed advanced counsellor training in the USA and completed his doctorate in counseling and mental health at the College of Health and Human Services, University of Toledo, Ohio, in 2000, where he researched readiness for change of court-mandated male perpetrators of domestic violence (DV). While studying for his PhD in the USA, Brian also trained in the Duluth Model of Domestic Violence Intervention. He worked intensively with court ordered men in Ohio, using the Duluth programme. Brian was instrumental in designing and developing the Master of Counselling Program at the University of Queensland, where he coordinated a course in violence issues in counselling. He has also provided training for professionals in DV intervention regularly working with police, correctional officers, DV services, men's programme facilitators, and with communities organising coordinated community responses to domestic violence.

In 2022, Brian launched SICURA (www.sicura-dv.com.au), a training initiative to support professional development for practitioners who work with DV victims/survivors and perpetrators. His understanding of DV is not only as a legal issue, but also urgent public health and human rights issues where the safety, freedom, and dignity of women and children are under threat, now and into the future.

Melati Sumari is an associate professor at the Department of Educational Psychology and Counselling, Faculty of Education, University of Malaya, Kuala Lumpur, Malaysia. She holds a doctoral degree in counselor education from Western Michigan University. She is also a registered counsellor.

Pui Chi, TSE, is an assistant professor and program director of the Department of Counselling and Psychology at Hong Kong Shue Yan University, as well as the founder of the Asian Professional Counselling and Psychology Association.

Ma. Teresa G. Tuason, PhD, is a professor and the clinical director of the CMHC program and also a licensed psychologist. She completed her doctorate at the University at Albany and her postdoc at the University of Utah. Born and raised in the Philippines, she learned resilience of spirit and using one's personal power for transformative teaching and social justice research.

Keithia Wilson, PhD, is a professor of psychology at Griffith University, and currently the Academic Leader for Student Success and Retention at Griffith. Professor Wilson has extensive experience in the development and implementation of innovative learning, teaching and assessment practices. She has published widely in higher education around issues of teaching quality and learning design. She has been recognised both for her effectiveness as an educator and for her scholarship in learning and teaching, receiving the Australian Learning and Teaching Council (ALTC) Prime Minister's Award for the 2007 Australian University Teacher of the Year, and recently completed an ALTC National Senior Teaching Fellowship on the First Year Experience (2010-2012). She has worked for over 30 years as a consultant, educator and counsellor in organisational and community settings. Her organisational work with clients focuses, in particular, on improving interpersonal and team effectiveness. Her individual work with clients focuses on issues of loss and grief, and personal and spiritual development. She is active in the supervision, mentoring, and training of novice and experienced practitioners, and is a consultant on the implementation of a range of supervisory systems in the community and public sectors.

Foreword to the Third Edition

Allen E. Ivey, EdD, ABPP
Board Certified in Counseling Psychology
Distinguished University Professor (Emeritus)
University of Massachusetts, Amherst
Past President Society for Counseling Psychology and Fellow, American Psychological Association

In 2017 I wrote the forward for the second edition of Nadine Pelling and Philip Armstrong's book on counselling supervision. Since then, several changes have occurred in the fields of counselling and supervision, both in Australia and internationally. This third edition of Pelling & Armstrong's counselling supervision book is titled *The Practice of Clinical and Counselling Supervision: Australian and International Applications.* This third edition has been developed in acknowledgment of many of the changes we have all experienced over the last few years.

This third edition maintains the core chapters and sections that have made this text the most popular counselling supervision text in Australia. It is Australian Counselling Association approved for supervisor status training. Additional international perspectives relevant to the Australasia region have been included, acknowledging the development of professional counselling in the region.

The comprehensiveness of this book is illustrated through an array of chapters covering vital topics in detail. This third edition is organised into seven sections: Introduction; Professional Issues; Approaches; People; Evaluation; Research; and International Variations.

The introductory section includes the first two chapters by John Barletta and Philip Armstrong, which provide a solid introductory foundation to supervision, well referenced and thorough. Armstrong's inclusion of the administrative and business aspects of counselling supervision in the third chapter continues to be unique.

It is increasingly clear that counsellors are facing a highly competitive environment and that other helping professions are constantly challenging us. There is a need to market our unique services to communities and to show what we can deliver. At the state and national level, political action will be necessary to ensure our inclusion in the provision of mental health services. Counselling, of course, needs to be a central focus in many areas and especially in schools.

The section on professional issues has been expanded and now includes addressing suicidality, vicarious trauma, and family violence by including work by Helen Stallman, Fran Lane, and Stephen O'Kane. Similarly, the section on approaches to supervision now includes information on Christian counselling supervision and social work supervision provided by Shannon Hood, Tracey Milson, and Rebecca Braid.

The section on people continues to describe those typically involved in counselling supervision in Australia as well as an encouragement to adjust one's approach based on individual differences. This includes a chapter on strengthening learning and practice via multicultural supervision written by Nancy Arthur. Sections exploring the often-difficult subjects of evaluation and research are also included. Reviews of research literature and alternative practices are informative.

Completely new is the section on international variations. Counselling and counselling supervision in Canada, Hong Kong, Indonesia, and the Philippines has been added. I am pleased to see emphasis given to international aspects of supervision in which we see the need to respect alternative frames of reference.

This third edition contains many chapters designed to address the worldwide challenge faced by counselling. Namely how the counselling profession and supervision in counselling is distinct from psychology, social work, and other applied professions with its central emphasis on respect for the uniqueness of the individual and the belief in movement toward the good. We need to maintain our integrity and commitments as we face these challenges.

The unique voices in each chapter provide a whole that is larger than the sum of its parts and encourage the reader to move into more depth in supervision with confidence. The tone of the book balances a scholarly research voice with practitioner views, honouring individual choice by the supervisor with the need for professional awareness and the inevitable differences among our supervisees and their working context.

Supervision is our opportunity to provide a lasting legacy. Those of us selected as supervisors are counselling's link to the future. Enjoy this opportunity for both your own growth and the development of your supervisees and indeed the profession.

Acknowledgments

The authors, editors and publisher would like to gratefully credit or acknowledge the following:

The Practice of Clinical and Counselling Supervision: International Applications is the 3rd updated, retitled, and revised edition of *The Practice of Counselling and Clinical Supervision* (2nd Edition) (Pelling & Armstrong Eds.) which itself was an update of the original *Practice of Clinical Supervision* (Pelling, Barletta, & Armstrong Editors) published in 2009. The text has been expanded to encompass international counselling supervision and select speciality supervision areas.

Chapter 1, by Dr. John Barletta, is based upon Barletta, J. (2007). Clinical supervision (Chapter 6). In N. Pelling, R. Bowers, & P. Armstrong (Eds.), *The practice of counselling* (pp. 118–135). Melbourne: Thomson.

Some of the information contained in Chapter 17, by Dr. Nadine Pelling and Dr. Elisa Agostinelli, originates from the following previously published items and originally Dr. Pelling's doctoral dissertation from Western Michigan University (2000).

Pelling, N. (2008). The relationship of supervisory experience, counselling experience, and training in supervision to supervisory identity development. *International Journal for the Advancement of Counselling, 30*(4), 235–248.

Schofield, M. & Pelling, N. (2002). Supervision of counsellors. In M. McMahon & W. Patton (Eds.), *Supervision in the helping professions: A practical approach* (pp. 211–222). NSW: Prentice Hall.

Chapter 20, by Dr. Nadine Pelling, was originally published as follows and is reprinted here with permission:

Pelling, N. (2006). Counsellor competence: A survey of Australian counsellor self perceived competence, *Counselling Australia, 6*(1), 3–14.

Pelling, N. (2007). Counsellor competence (Chapter 2). In N. Pelling, R. Bowers, & P. Armstrong (Eds.), *The practice of counselling* (pp. 36-45). Melbourne: Thomson.

Chapters 26, 27, 29, 30, and 32, were originally published in a Special Winter Issue (Volume 15, 2021) of the *Australian Counselling Research Journal*, edited by Dr. Nadine Pelling. They are reproduced with permission.

Chapters 7, 8, 13, 14, and family violence supervision were originally published in a Special Spring Issue (Volume 15, 2021) of the *Australian Counselling Research Journal*, edited by Dr. Nadine Pelling. They are reproduced with permission.

Part 1

The Introduction

Part 1, The **Introduction**, is a section comprised of three chapters that encourage the reader to reflect on the major issues associated with counsellors accessing and providing professional clinical and counselling supervision. Chapter 1 essentially establishes the domain of clinical supervision and generally sets the scope for the remainder of the textbook. It surveys the literature to provide an informative snapshot that will encourage greater reflection of processes which have often become mindlessly habitual. Chapter 2 further explores how counselling supervision is conceptualised and defined. The historically evolving definition of counselling supervision and its various components are identified. Chapter 3 then examines what is involved in considering the option of establishing clinical supervision as a regular service, within the scope of their practice, to helping professionals.

Chapter overview

Chapter 1, **Introduction to Clinical Supervision**, by John Barletta, sets the context for supervision and clearly establishes supervision as an integral part of clinical practice for all of the helping professions. The chapter methodically works its way through introducing the goals, roles, and models in supervision, so the reader quickly develops a framework for understanding the specialty, and also to anticipate what will be explored in greater depth in later chapters. Given the anxiety and misperceptions some practitioners have about supervision, this chapter clearly articulates the opportunities people have available to them as they receive and/or provide clinical supervision via respectful consultation. The supportive and challenging nature of the supervisory relationship is possibly best highlighted through Barletta's presentation of the mentor role, with the hope and optimism embedded in such a caring model.

Chapter themes

In this chapter you will explore the following themes:

- Clinical supervision
- Administrative supervision
- Aims of clinical supervision
- Need for clinical supervision
- Roles of the clinical supervisor
- Methods in clinical supervision
- Process of clinical supervision

DOI: 10.4324/9781003490067-1

- Techniques in clinical supervision
- Beneficiaries of supervision
- Maximizing supervision
- Current practices

Chapter 2, **Conceptualising Counselling Supervision**, by Philip Armstrong, offers insight into the evolving definition of counselling supervision. The various components of supervision are then explored. Specifically, the issues of supervisory responsibility, relationship, and the realities of providing and engaging in both peer and professional supervision are illuminated.

Chapter themes

In this chapter you will explore the following themes:

- The complexity involved in the evolving definition of supervision
- How experience as a counsellor is not sufficient for providing competent supervision
- Some main problems in supervisory relationships

Chapter 3, **Administration and Marketing of Supervision**, by Philip Armstrong, offers the reader a pragmatic view of the considerations that need to be addressed as one establishes oneself as a provider of supervision to the professional counselling community. His experience as a businessman shines through. Although the international market of this text means that individuals will still need to explore their local laws and regulations, it provides a useful sense of what questions to ask and which areas to explore to ensure a legal and ethical supervision practice is maintained. The sample client and supervision contracts provided in this book's appendixes are useful models to copy until one develops their preferred and individualised style and format for such documents.

Chapter themes

In this chapter you will explore the following themes:

- Supervision as a paid professional activity
- Administration is not a dirty word
- Sample clinical supervision contract
- Sample counselling contract

1 Introduction to Clinical Supervision

John Barletta

Introduction

The professional tasks of those who provide therapy are multidimensional and complex, just as those who conduct therapy come from multiple disciplines. Counsellors, psychologists, social workers, psychiatrists and, in some instances, nurses, educators, clergy, coaches, and pastoral carers all engage in psychologically therapeutic activities. There is a view that those who provide counselling simply attend to *worried well* middle-class clients with change and success being the common outcome from the process. This is only a small part of the reality. Indeed, those who counsel, in general, have a broad range of clients from differing backgrounds, with a complexity of issues, varying levels of capacity and motivation, and sometimes inconsistent or unknown outcomes. This is coupled with an ever-increasing demand for paperwork, accountability, effectiveness, efficiency, and productivity.

Typically, a counsellor's tasks include:

1. individual, couple, and family therapy
2. group sessions
3. intake appraisals and assessment
4. programme development and evaluation
5. resource coordination
6. consultation and report-writing
7. professional development
8. mediation and workshops
9. referral management
10. administration, financial, and clerical responsibilities

These tasks include involvement with clients' family members, administrative personnel, managers, bureaucrats, and professionals external to their own system. Such a demanding role necessitates counsellors to monitor their personal functioning, professional practice, and to review their effectiveness. One reality, constant over time, has been that counsellors regularly practise in isolation from professional peers. Counsellors without the support and encouragement of colleagues run the risk of stagnating relative to their growth and development. Thus, the need to be involved with a relevant professional association, and ongoing supervision, is essential as these can minimise the sense of isolation, increase self-care, and enhance the development of expertise.

Counsellors have become increasingly aware of risks such as compassion fatigue, vicarious traumatisation, burnout, and legal action related to professional malpractice. These

DOI: 10.4324/9781003490067-2

issues are increasing in the helping professions. Counsellors need to have access to a range of professional supports, including peer consultation, managerial considerations, counselling, and increasingly, clinical supervision. A huge amount of writing and research on the topic of supervision for counsellors exists and includes the specialty journals *Counselor Education and Supervision* (American Counseling Association) and *The Clinical Supervisor* (Taylor and Francis).

Various types of supervision have been described in the literature, and the commonality existing in descriptions centres around the name and function of two types: clinical supervision and administrative supervision. To continue the discussion of supervision, it is imperative that a definition of the specialty activity be established. I will then examine clinical supervision broadly, outline the aims, needs, and benefits of supervision, and examine the applied aspects of supervision.

Clinical supervision

Although each scholarly writing on clinical supervision offers a different characterisation of the specialty, numerous elements remain common. For the purpose of clarity, clinical supervision is considered to be a process whereby colleagues of a similar profession regularly engage in a prepared meeting for the intention of developing understanding, skills and a professional orientation, while concurrently focusing on enhancing client wellbeing. Such supervision has both a preventative and corrective function.

The clinical supervisor monitors the appropriateness of the individual counsellor's practice, while also serving as a preceptor of the profession. The dual role of ensuring the quality of services, as well as the development of the counsellor is indeed a challenging task for the clinical supervisor. Essentially, this form of supervision enables a practitioner to have a supportive colleague help them to examine their clinical interventions and effectiveness. Due to the significance and magnitude of the role, and the reality that supervision is often recognised as a professional specialisation, clinical supervision is now usually only carried out by an accredited individual, or a senior professional, who has recognised training and expertise in supervision theory and techniques. This chapter serves as an introduction to this specialty.

Administrative supervision

The second type of supervision for counsellors is administrative supervision. Whereas the focus of clinical supervision is concerned with counselling and aims to be educational, the focus of administrative supervision is involved with organisational, managerial, and procedural issues. Administrative supervision includes the managing of areas such as service evaluation, financial issues, time considerations, record keeping, role and function, professional development, policy and procedures, resource allocation, information technology and organisational issues.

In a work environment, it is probably not imperative that administrative supervision be managed by another counsellor, but could be better handled by a manager or member of an administrative team. The purpose of administrative supervision relates to organisational issues; hence an administrator might realistically be the preferred choice for this role as they would be capable of attending to the issues raised during the process.

The focus of this opening chapter is on clinical rather than administrative supervision, as the practical issues related to administrative supervision require a discussion

Table 1.1 Ways counsellors are supervised, managed, and evaluated (Barletta, 1996)

Clinical supervision	*Administrative supervision*
Techniques and methods:	Organisational and management issues:
- *self-report*	- *in-service training*
- *log review*	- *professional development*
- *audio file*	- *program development*
- *visual recording*	- *attendance*
- *live observation*	- *role statement*
- *role-playing*	- *progress notes*
- *sitting-in*	- *record keeping*
- *co-counselling*	- *caseload*
	- *fiscal issues*
	- *resource allocation*

more from a management perspective rather than a counselling viewpoint. This is quite different to that taken when considering clinical matters, and outside the scope of this text's discourse.

Table 1.1 provides a snapshot of these two categories of supervision and identifies a range of methods reviewed briefly in this chapter and explored in more detail later in the text. It serves to provide the reader with a snapshot from which supervision may be examined with counselling and perhaps even non-counselling professionals.

Overview of clinical supervision

Clinical supervision stimulates and challenges the practitioner to examine their professional decisions, and explore practice issues in a methodical way. As this chapter provides an overview of the roles and processes in supervision, it becomes apparent the activity is invaluable for all stakeholders, particularly in nurturing the supervisee to examine the interface between theory and professional practice.

Professionals in all cultures are held to extraordinary standards by the public. The community expectation is for professionals to be trained to superior standards, and to behave in exemplary ways. Hence professionals need to engage in processes that ensure they continue to grow in knowledge and competence. This has seen professionals routinely attending training, participating in scholarly conferences, reading peer-reviewed journals, affiliating with professional associations, and consulting with expert colleagues. Increasingly, practitioners have found an effective way to foster their lifelong learning is by formalising a supervisory relationship with a practitioner who has more and different experiences from them, and is also aptly qualified in the specialty of supervision.

Although counselling is a well-established independent profession in the USA, and accordingly produces a plethora of resources, it has only been in recent years that other countries, including Australia, have experienced the steady growth of the profession (Pelling, 2006; Schofield, Grant, Holmes, & Barletta, 2006). This development has seen an explosion of counselling programmes aimed at preparing competently trained practitioners. In these programmes, fieldwork is an opportunity for reappraisal of career choice, development of key competencies, learning the culture of the profession, and exploration of practical interest areas. In conjunction with the training institution's fieldwork handbook, both this initial and final chapter will help guide the trainee counsellor, hereafter referred to as supervisee, on the path to their development as a safe and helpful entry-level professional.

Within the context of the supervisory relationship, the supervisee in the clinical environment presents cases, explores their treatment modalities, reviews sessions, presents assessments, examines psychopathology issues, and explores a mixture of personal and professional challenges raised by their work. These broad topics will arise for discussion with supervisees in a range of settings such as community agencies, hospitals, government departments, schools, and private practice.

As trainees move through their counselling studies, they are regularly exposed to an assortment of educative and evaluative processes and procedures aimed at ensuring they have requisite knowledge and skills to practice safely and effectively. Although writing essays, presenting seminars, and taking examinations are methods typically used by counsellor educators to assess learning outcomes, processes to enhance learning about clinical issues and to augment the professional orientation of supervisees vary enormously. When supervisees are involved in practical experiences (e.g., communication skills sessions, clinical placement, fieldwork practicum, counselling internship) techniques such as analysing learning journals, reviewing recorded sessions, discussing client cases, and examining critical incidents are commonly well employed. It is in these applied areas that emerging professionals are introduced to the aims and methods of clinical supervision.

In these practical endeavours, the clinical practicum supervisor, usually a senior counsellor with considerable applied experience and supervision training, is responsible for the supervisee. The supervisor ensures the supervisee is involved with an array of activities, increasing in complexity. These are processed in ways that enhance the supervisee's learning. These early supervisory experiences are an amalgam of education and evaluation and are intended to be supportive as well as challenging.

With appropriate consultation and well-planned feedback, the supervisee is fostered in developmental growth and professional awareness. This progression occurs by way of various modes such as individual supervision, within a group forum session, and in conversation with peers.

Aims of clinical supervision

Some supervisees and practitioners hold concerns about supervision worrying that it will be offered as a predominantly evaluative process. These anxieties rapidly dissipate when supervisees experience a quality supervisory relationship and are able to negotiate clear goals for their sessions. The mistaken belief that supervision is focused on evaluative judgements, which may impact on identity, relationships, duties, tenure, salary and promotion may be minimised by clinical supervisors being accessed from outside the agency. In this situation supervisees can benefit significantly from a greater sense of confidentiality and privacy. Generally, the purpose of evaluation is to confer opinions of value and is limited in its utility. Conversely, supervision aims to increase self-awareness and enhance professional competence. The aspiration for supervision is ongoing development of capabilities in an environment of honesty and trust in a close relationship where the focus is on professional experiences.

With regard to the specific goals of supervision, irrespective of location or specialty of the professional (e.g., addictions, community, corrections, education, health, mental health, private practice, rehabilitation), the focus to enhance, extend and develop remains similar. The aims of supervision include:

1. Monitoring client safety and enhancing outcomes
2. Developing realistic self-evaluation
3. Integrating research, theory and skills
4. Increasing scope of practice
5. Exploring values, beliefs and creativity
6. Encouraging and ensuring legal and ethical practices
7. Developing a sense of collegial and professional support
8. Updating innovative, current perspectives and best practice
9. Improving perception and developing clinical wisdom
10. Observing agency policies and procedures
11. Facilitating and increasing self-awareness
12. Promoting team perspective and multidisciplinary orientation
13. Encouraging a feedback-informed approach
14. Identifying strengths and barriers to development
15. Developing critical reflection skills
16. Clarifying work preferences and personal priorities
17. Developing and managing short, intermediate and long-term goals
18. Monitoring lifelong learning
19. Promoting an orientation to the profession
20. Supporting self-care and ensuring wellbeing

The above aims will serve as the basis for discussions between the supervisor and supervisee as they consult and negotiate to develop the practicalities (e.g., goals, context, methods, duties, procedures, scope) contained within a *supervision contract* (Osborn & Davis, 1996). Educational institutions may label a supervision contract a *learning covenant* or *agreement of understanding*. If a third party is involved or interested in the supervisory process, that is, employer, training provider, registration body or professional association, additional input into the development of the aims for the contract must be considered. Additional contributors frequently encourage or direct the supervisor to ensure the supervisee is developing the knowledge, skills and dispositional qualities that are representative of what is required to operate independently in the profession.

Need for clinical supervision

The variety of responsibilities required of counsellors makes it essential for the provision of appropriate support to be provided by the employer or educational institution, or if in private practice, is organised by the practitioner. Training, consultation, professional development, counselling, and clinical supervision aim to offer support to the counsellor while also developing professional competencies. There is a chance that supervision may increase stress due to the time commitment which takes the counsellor away from an already busy schedule. Typically, this is merely a short-lived concern as the benefits of supervision are experienced.

Receiving clinical supervision facilitates more effective service delivery for the practitioner while simultaneously ensuring some quality control for the employer or institution, and the public. The counsellor may be in a situation of having to provide services in a field in which they have little experience. In such cases, the counsellor can call on the assistance of a colleague who has such experience to offer consultation through supervision until an acceptable level of ability is developed. The employer or institution takes responsibility for providing supervision for the counsellor, since it is from required activities the need for supervision arises and high standards of professional practice are expected. Most associations in Australia (e.g., Australian Psychological Society, Australian Counselling Association, Psychotherapy and Counselling Federation of Australia) mandate that those providing therapy engage in regular clinical supervision by an appropriately trained practitioner.

Roles of the clinical supervisor

To enable the aims of supervision to be realised for the supervisee and the full range of benefits to emerge, the supervisor employs a multitude of positions or roles, namely:

- educator
- evaluator
- consultant
- facilitator
- coach
- counsellor
- mentor

Clinical supervisors must be experienced practitioners who have the ability to connect with a diversity of people quickly and with relative ease. They create a congenial and safe environment in which supervisees can explore and learn. That is not to suggest supervision is only characterised by care and support. Without challenging and appropriately provoking supervisees, learning and development will be constrained. Effective supervisors make efforts to understand how the supervisee learns, how they like to work in professional contexts, where they are situated developmentally, and what they want and need from supervision at this time of their career. This invariably means in the first session, or at initial phone contact, the supervisor spends time gaining a sense of the identity of the supervisee, their experience, what their broad goals are, and where it is that they would like to journey professionally. This clarifying process is invaluable in starting the supervisory relationship in an appropriate and sustainable way.

Supervisors use a variety of roles in supervision, but typically the educator and evaluator roles come to the fore with supervisees who developmentally have much to learn and are dependent, for example, students and novice practitioners. These roles need to be carried out sensitively, so supervisees feel supported, relaxed, empowered, and extended, and develop the critical habit of self-reflection. As clinical cases and critical incidents for the supervisee are being explored, the supervisor spends a lot of time allaying the supervisee's anxieties while simultaneously being instructive and clear in their directions for subsequent client contact. At this stage, supervisees need considerable structure and unambiguous plans to implement. Supervisors cannot risk being viewed as condescending as there is a critical need to ensure supervisees connect with them, so they carry out what is negotiated.

With supervisees who are practitioners with extensive training, significant experience, exceptional insight, and justified confidence, supervisors are more typically a consultant, facilitator, or coach to these autonomous individuals. Such clinical supervision is challenging to provide and engage with, but the collegial nature of these sessions is invigorating for all involved. As a consultant, facilitator, or coach the supervisor provides less structure and prescriptions, rather the competence of the supervisee is validated and integrated as they discover new insights into cases and their own development and awareness. In this scenario supervision is less hierarchical and more companionate.

Given that most clinical supervisors of counsellors are, or have been, a practising counsellor, this brings the potential of overusing or inappropriately employing the counsellor role in supervision. Supervisors must be mindful of this possible dilemma and remember supervisees are not their counselling clients and going deeply and intrusively into their personal history or issues is neither ethical nor appropriate. However, during supervision, if there develops an awareness that a supervisee's personal issues are a significant part of the impasse or learning, a supervisor may address the issue in a cursory fashion, and encourage the supervisee to seek counselling for themselves, before moving on with supervision. It is the supervisor's responsibility, as a quality assurer and gatekeeper to the profession, to develop the supervisee while showing respect and privacy.

Although the counsellor role is minimised when providing supervision, having advanced training in counselling theories and skills adds enormously to interactions with supervisees. Supervisors draw on communication and helping skills, the use of which ensures supervisees feel heard and understood. It is important for novice and experienced practitioners alike, that personal feelings as well as professional concerns are addressed. It is by acknowledging and working through a supervisee's apprehensions that they openly offer and explore the genuine issues that need to be scrutinised. Using specific praise, targeted reinforcement and constructive feedback, supervisees are encouraged in their development and movement toward established goals.

The final supervisor role is based on Greek mythology. When Odysseus, the King of Ithaca, went to fight with the alliance in the Trojan War, he left his son Telemachus with Mentor, an older wise man who acted as teacher and personal friend to provide guidance in developing values and education in the ways of the world. In an analogous style, people at various stages of their professional career can work closely with someone in a supervisory, mentoring relationship for the purposes of being guided, comforted, supported and sustained. In these ways, the mentor role serves psychosocial, role-modelling, and vocational functions.

Irrespective of whether the role being performed is that of teacher, evaluator, consultant, facilitator, coach, counsellor or mentor, for the supervisory relationship to be useful specific factors are essential. The supervisor must be able to listen and encourage, occasionally nudge, appropriately disclose, provide opportunities for learning, and examine and modify the supervisory programme as needed. There are also responsibilities for the supervisee to maximise the benefits of the supervisory process. It is imperative the supervisee set measurable goals and be willing to review and adjust them, pledge time and motivation, reflect on practice, dedicate themselves to self-assessment, and explore possibilities. It is by each individual involved in supervision taking shared responsibility that greatest benefit is reaped.

Methods in clinical supervision

Although clinical supervision is typically offered on an individual basis, it can be arranged with peers or conducted in small groups (e.g., five supervisees). The advantages of peer and group supervision are the containment of costs, a convenient supportive context, and the vicarious learning that emerges as members observe others and interact with discussions.

The disadvantages include that the presence of peers may inhibit sharing, individuals have less time available for their own concerns, and mediocre group dynamics will be counter-productive. Regardless of how many supervisees are present, the supervisor will promote experiential learning, so supervisees have a life-changing, affirming experience.

Self-report, as unpredictable as it may be, remains the standard method used in sessions. The supervisee starts a conversation regarding cases, critical events, the impact of practice on themselves, and recurring themes. Supervisors using a case management approach suggest or require supervisees bring to sessions case annotations, process notes, reports, and client files for review. Although this indirect approach to supervision is fraught with difficulties, with regard to taking agency files and supervisees distorting information, it remains a pragmatic and realistic mode for professional exploration. As the supervisory relationship flourishes, the supervisee invariably becomes more open and honest as they realise these behaviours hold them in good stead.

As part of training supervision, the review of an audio file or visual recording of supervisees' sessions is customary. Supervisors processing sessions using this technology can use a sensitive inquiring method where the supervisee listens to, or watches, the recording of their clinical work with the supervisor observing. Either person stops the recording at various points to encourage reflection on what the supervisee recollects experiencing during the session. Supervisees speculate about what was occurring and explore how they were functioning. With a positive supervisory alliance established, this method of interpersonal process recall (Kagan, 1980) can use discovery learning to excellent effect.

For numerous years, mail, telephone, facsimile, text-messages, email, and the Internet have been used routinely to communicate interpersonally and transmit professional information. In the context of supervision methods, these systems are used for the supervisee and supervisor to stay in contact and convey records and requests, which now requires being very mindful of confidentiality and privacy issues. If significant issues arise between sessions, telephone, and email contact specifically ensures support and guidance can be dispensed swiftly and efficiently.

Direct methods of supervision are strongly encouraged but are often difficult to arrange for a host of reasons. Live observation by the supervisor in the session, co-counselling with the supervisor and live observation (e.g., two-way mirror, walk-in, phone-in, consultation breaks) are the classic ways supervisors get an authentic impression of how the supervisee is performing and progressing. Although there are issues of cost, resources, confidentiality, and time to perform direct methods, it is critical supervisees have at least some experience of these approaches.

Finally, and possibly most importantly, client feedback provides the most accurate information about the impact, skills, and disposition of the clinician. Given that counselling is a process that seeks to help clients change, it follows that experiences from the recipients of the service are highly useful. Although there was a routine to have clients complete questionnaires at the cessation of the therapy and/or at a follow-up time, there is an increasing trend for counsellors to be seeking feedback on alliance and outcomes at every session (see the routine outcome monitoring and feedback-informed research of Michael Lambert and Scott Miller, see Lambert, 2013; Miller, Hubble, & Chow, 2020). This process additionally helps with knowing what (failing) cases to bring to supervision. Finally, feedback from the supervisee's trusted colleagues, collected with caution, is useful as they observe the supervisee engage in activities in the workplace.

Process of clinical supervision

The customary procedure for supervision is to initially develop a positive working alliance between supervisee and supervisor, being clear about what each expects and prefers in supervision, and then engage with clinical material to increase capability, awareness, and self-assurance. Although many people do not like to admit experiencing difficulties, supervisors expect supervisees to volunteer cases where they are most stuck as this is when greatest learning will transpire. Supervisees will realise that struggles simply highlight what they need to learn, and it does not suggest they are fundamentally inadequate. To increase the likelihood of staying focused during supervision sessions to ensure supervisees' needs are met, a supervisor clarifies what the supervisee has done in the past with regard to practice and supervision, and asks where they would like help. After learning about what their practice consists of, and what they want from supervision, and if it is reasonable in terms of their development and professional requirements, working with clinical cases and applied issues commences. Issues discussed in supervision predictably include:

- client issues and goal-setting
- case conceptualisation and progress
- intervention strategies and future plans
- supervisee–client alliance and boundaries
- ethical and legal issues
- counsellor professional development
- supervisor–supervisee relationship

In processing practical cases, the supervisor avoids moving too quickly toward solutions, but rather acts simply as a guide on the path of learning. A series of basic structured questions can be helpful for supervisees (and novice supervisors) to consider as they prepare for and conduct supervision. Initially seeking responses to the following questions will be helpful:

1. What are the significant details I need to know about the case?
2. Where do you feel most trapped?
3. What are you thinking and feeling about these issues?
4. What assistance would you like?

Toward the end of the supervision session, seeking reactions to the following queries will be valuable:

1. What new understanding and ideas have been helpful?
2. What patterns have emerged for yourself and your clinical practice?
3. What obstacles may you encounter as you take the next steps?
4. What will you do now given this additional learning?

It is beneficial and appropriate for the supervisee and supervisor to take notes during sessions to have an ongoing record of clients discussed, issues, plans, themes, struggles, learning, and progress. These notes will be invaluable as the supervisory relationship continues over an extended period of time. Throughout the supervision process, the supervisee is encouraged in seeking to:

- Understand the dilemma and its complexities.
- Find connections among the information.
- Formulate a working hypothesis (to avoid an explanatory fiction).
- Develop a reasonable treatment plan to implement.

It is an important part for the development of a supervisor to regularly gain feedback on the impact and quality of their supervision. Expert supervisors develop the habit of asking supervisees to at least give verbal feedback at end of each session (i.e., How useful was the session for you today?), and also use specialised supervision inventories at regular intervals (e.g., annual reviews). Although more so early in their career, supervisors prefer to avoid considering negative feedback about their efforts. After sincere reflection, and with additional training and reading, experienced supervisors become committed to continuing education in this specialty so they can improve their style of relating, and enhance their roles in supervision.

Techniques in clinical supervision

Within a nurturing supervisory environment founded on a bond of trust, the supervisor debriefs the supervisee's issues and responds in ways that are supportive and educational. The supervisor uses various techniques aimed at encouraging reflection, and increasing the usefulness of the processing of material. Despite some people's erroneous beliefs that supervisors provide a lot of advice, in reality advice is provided only sparingly. This is usually reserved for significant issues of almost life- or career-threatening magnitude with the supervisee clearly unaware of what action to take. More often a supervisor will use subtle influencing techniques such as explorative questioning, encouraging statements, clarification skills, empathic confrontation, self-disclosure, observations, and interpretations. These interventions convey to the supervisee the nature of the supervisor's concerns, and potential areas for exploration.

When the characteristics of a case presentation are such that the supervisee has something clinical they need to learn, the supervisor may use modelling and role-play to show the supervisee what could be attempted. In addition to information and skills being reviewed via a didactic approach, the supervisor's challenges and confrontations will facilitate the supervisee's critical reflection and learning. It is this area of augmentation of critical reflection that promotes the supervisee to see themself developing as an autonomous professional.

Irrespective of the developmental stage of the supervisee and the type of issues or themes being explored in sessions, the setting of and agreeing to between-session activities (i.e., homework) is common and valuable. Given that supervision is only part of lifelong learning and self-improvement, homework tasks such as research, reading, reflection, and writing are critical supplements. Supervisees engaging with between-session tasks is parallel to what they routinely suggest to clients.

Beneficiaries of supervision

There are a multitude of individuals and organisations that profit from the provision of quality clinical supervision. Given that the heart of supervision focuses on ensuring the client is not being harmed and is, additionally, helped to achieve established goals in professionally appropriate ways, the recipient of counselling services is the first to benefit. Most discussions in supervisory sessions focus on interventions being used for the client and advance to how the supervisee is struggling with some aspect of the case.

As the supervisor interacts to clarify the situation and explore potential explanations and interventions to consider, another person is being supported – the supervisee. This is where the supervisee's scope of practice, expertise and insight is being deliberately and incrementally (often exponentially) expanded. Engaging supervisees in the desire for understanding is valuable for deep learning to occur. In this sense it is the clinical material that is the teacher, not just the supervisor themself. Supervision can insulate the supervisee from work-related stress, variously referred to as burn-out, rust-out, compassion fatigue, emotional exhaustion or vicarious trauma.

Furthermore, if the supervisee is a trainee at an educational institution, or if they are an employee at an agency, the organisation itself benefits with the development of a more expert and safer practitioner. This has the potential to decrease the likelihood of the organisation being involved in accusations of not supporting or appropriately training the people in their charge, and maintains their collective reputations.

With supervision providing clear benefits to the client, practitioner, educational institution and employer, the positive impact will also be more broadly experienced by the profession, its members and the community generally. There is, however, one often forgotten individual who profits from supervision: the clinical supervisor themself. Although it is seldom mentioned for fear of being misconstrued, the supervisor benefits enormously from offering supervision. As they support supervisees, their understanding of clinical work, human nature, and themselves improves enormously, and the sense of satisfaction of being additive to so many is indeed gratifying and fulfilling. It must be reiterated, however, that it is the needs of the client and supervisee that are always the primary focus in supervision.

Maximising supervision

There are a few requirements for supervisees to increase the likelihood of supervision being genuinely beneficial to personal and professional growth. Supervisees need to gain an awareness of where they are developmentally, be as open as possible in sessions, and understand what supervision can and cannot provide. Being prepared for sessions with material and reflections, being committed to regular supervision (e.g., a weekly or monthly session), and reading before and after sessions is highly desirable. During their formal studies, supervisees have little or no choice of supervisor. After graduation, the emerging professional can find a supervisor by asking colleagues who they respect for guidance, or search databases of professional associations that maintain lists of accredited supervisors.

Having an effective supervisor who is optimistic, caring, curious, self-evaluative, and self-aware, and who can develop and maintain trust, provide clear and useful feedback, set and monitor realistic goals, and use power appropriately, is indeed a blessing for any supervisee. The supervisor needs to ensure the practice of supervision is not seen as part of a paternalistic guild ritual, rather a collegial initiative to develop quality clinical practice. Supervisors need to be competent in many areas, that is, professional content and the learning process, but also know the limits of their expertise, and consult appropriate people when the supervisee or they are in difficulty.

Current practices

Although increasing numbers of counsellors are participating in clinical supervision, many report they receive more supervision which is administrative rather than clinical in nature. This situation is usually not the preferred position. Counsellors indicate they find clinical supervision revitalising as they review and discuss clinical practice. If supervisory provisions fall short of desirable standards and best practice, this raises a host of legal, ethical, and professional concerns in an increasingly litigious and demanding cultural context. If counsellors are to receive professional support, appropriately qualified personnel must be provided by the employer or accessed externally.

Concluding thoughts

Every piece of scholarly work has limits to its scope and this chapter is no different. A range of issues that have not been covered in a significant way, or at all, include diversity (e.g., age, culture, gender, religion); power; conflict; learning styles; therapeutic schools; contexts of practice; conflict; and legal and ethical issues. Some of these issues are addressed in other chapters in this text. Supervisees with a significant interest in any of these topics are also encouraged to review the plethora of theory and research in the professional literature.

For many years, supervision for counsellors was on the periphery of professional discussion. A structured and well-thought-out approach to both clinical and administrative supervision is imperative to facilitate the process of increased professional credibility. Counsellors should be highly trained professionals who are competent in dealing with the range of psychological issues impacting clients. Professional competence is developed initially through formal academic or in-service training. All counsellors need to broaden their expertise, and in the work setting, newly acquired skills can be nurtured and developed by a supervisor who has a broad education and diverse clinical history. In this scenario, the supervisor performs the role of teacher, consultant, and mentor.

Quality supervision seldom occurs by chance, accident, or miracle. Rather it is the result of strategic planning by counsellors, administrators, and supervisors working in partnership. The aim of such collaboration is to find a practical and appropriate process of supporting the counsellor in the workplace. Without a precise approach to supervision, counselling services are destined to remain out-of-step with best practice. Counsellors need support services commensurate with their training and responsibilities, hence supervision must be seen as an integral component of their practice. Regardless of setting, counselling issues remain similar and the majority of counsellors desire, and benefit from, clinical supervision. Considerations of time, personnel, and cost should be the responsibility of the employer or training provider.

I have had a number of supervisors during my career, including professionals in different countries (i.e., Australia, USA, Italy), a variety of disciplines, and assorted models (e.g., Psychiatry – systemic-relational; Social Work – contextual; Counselling – psychodynamic, humanistic, solution-focused; Psychology – psychoanalytic, social constructivism, cognitive-behavioural therapies), and modes (i.e., individual, peer, group). These diverse people and approaches have profoundly impacted me, and positively influenced my professional awareness and clinical work. Learning from supervisors' stories was enhanced through their authenticity and the relationship.

Socrates wondered if learning was analogous to kindling a fire or filling a bucket. The following comments that supervisees have made in reference to their experiences in supervision, indicates their fires have been kindled. One supervisee suggested supervision was *a great discussion about a good conversation*. Another said it was *a robust challenge toward integration*, while one supervisee said it was *the place for true growth, the only safe space to share mistakes* and *a time when play is encouraged*.

Supervision is not an add-on service nor is it a luxury that can be neglected. Rather it is a necessity to ensure that a responsive and comprehensive counselling service is offered to the public. To ensure optimal client care, the focus for supervision must be on counsellor growth. Counsellors choose the profession because they have a desire to help others as well as aiming to stay mentally stimulated. They gain a lot of meaning and satisfaction from being in the service of others. As a profession, if client welfare is kept foremost in deliberations, it follows that the need for supervision will be high on the professional agenda. Counsellors and professional associations should take responsibility for communicating supervision needs to the appropriate people as there should not be practitioners providing any mental health services without receiving guidance. With attention to quality supervision, the emerging professional can be protected from their euphoria of a grand vocational adventure dissolving into the despair of a fading dream.

Educational questions & activities

After reviewing this chapter and additional readings on the topic, respond to the following questions based on your experiences of, or plans for, clinical supervision. When you have developed some notes on each of the questions, share and discuss your reflections with a colleague.

1. Where and with whom did you experience supervision?
2. What were the stated and implicit aims?
3. What was the focus of the interaction?
4. What was the frequency, intensity, duration, and location of the supervision?
5. What format, style, or model did the supervisor use?
6. What material was discussed and how?
7. What was the fee and who paid for the sessions?
8. What were the beneficial aspects of the experience?
9. What were the unhelpful aspects of the experience?
10. What are some of the lasting effects of the encounters?
11. If you have never received supervision, what do you think you need for it to be additive to your personal and professional growth?

Selected references for further reading

Australian Psychological Society. (2020). *Ethical guidelines on supervision*. Melbourne, VIC: Author.

Barletta, J. (1995). *Legal and ethical issues for school counselors: Supervision as a safeguard*. Athens, OH: Ohio University, Department of Counselor Education (ERIC Document ED379577).

Barletta, J. (2001). An uncommon family therapist: A conversation with Maurizio Andolfi. *Contemporary Family Therapy, 23*(2), 241–258.

Barletta, J. (2006). An exceptional psychotherapy researcher: A conversation with Michael Lambert. *Psychotherapy in Australia, 12*(2), 66–70.

Barletta, J. (2007). Clinical supervision. In N. Pelling, R. Bowers, & P. Armstrong (Eds.), *The practice of counselling* (pp. 118–135). Melbourne: Thomson.

Barletta, J. (2012). Work-life balance (Chapter 1.1). In J. Barletta, & J. Bond (Eds.), *The home therapist: A practical, self-help guide for everyday psychological problems* (pp. 3–7). Brisbane, Australia: Australian Academic Press.

Barletta, J., & Vecchione, T. P. (2004). Enhancing the training of counselling professionals: A process approach. *Australian Journal of Guidance and Counselling, 14*(2), 186–194.

Bernard, J. M., & Goodyear, R. K. (2018). *Fundamentals of clinical supervision* (6th ed.). Upper Saddle River, NJ: Pearson.

Borders, L. D., & Leddick, G. R. (1987). *Handbook of counseling supervision*. Alexandria, VA: American Counseling Association.

Carroll, M. (2014). *Effective supervision for the helping professions* (2nd ed.). London: Sage.

Falender, C. A., & Shafranske, E. P. (2012). *Getting the most out of clinical supervision and training: A guide for practicum students and interns*. Washington, DC: American Psychological Association.

Gonsalvez, C. J., & Calvert, F. L. (2014). Competency-based models of supervision: Principles and applications, promises and challenges. *Australian Psychologist, 49*, 200–208.

Haber, R. (1990). From handicap to handy capable: Training systemic therapists in use of self. *Family Process, 29*, 375–384.

Holloway, E. L. (1995). *Clinical supervision: A systems approach*. Thousand Oaks, CA: Sage.

Loganbill, C., Hardy, E., & Delworth, U. (1982). Supervision: A conceptual model. *The Counseling Psychologist, 10*, 3–42.

McMahon, M., & Patton, W. (Eds.) (2002). *Supervision in the helping professions: A practical approach*. Frenchs Forest, NSW: Prentice Hall.

Ronnestad, M. H., & Skovholt, T. M. (1993). Supervision of beginning and advanced graduate students of counseling and psychotherapy. *Journal of Counseling and Development, 71*, 396–405.

Spence, S., Wilson, J., Kavanagh, D., Strong, J., & Worrall, L. (2001). Clinical supervision in four mental health professions: A review of the evidence. *Behaviour Change, 18*, 135–155.

Stoltenberg, C. D., & Delworth, U. (1987). *Supervising counselors and therapists: A developmental approach*. San Francisco: Jossey-Bass.

Stoltenberg, C. D., McNeill, B., & Delworth, U. (1998). *IDM supervision: An integrated model for supervising counselors and therapists*. San Francisco: Jossey-Bass.

Watkins, C. E., & Milne, D. L. (Eds.) (2014). *The Wiley international handbook of clinical supervision*. Oxford: Wiley-Blackwell.

References

Barletta, J. (1996). Supervision for school counsellors: When will we get what we really need? *Australian Journal of Guidance and Counselling, 6*, 1–7.

Kagan, N. (1980). *Interpersonal process recall: A method of influencing human interaction*. Houston, TX: Mason.

Lambert, M. (2013). *Bergin and Garfield's handbook of psychotherapy and behavior change* (6th ed.). Upper Saddle River, NJ: Wiley.

Miller, S., Hubble, M., & Chow, D. (2020). *Better results: Using deliberate practice to improve therapeutic effectiveness*. Washington, DC: American Psychological Association.

Osborn, C. J., & Davis T. E. (1996). The supervision contract: Making it perfectly clear. *The Clinical Supervisor, 14*, 121–134.

Pelling, N. (2006). Introduction to the special issue on counselling in Australia. *International Journal of Psychology, 41*(3), 153–155.

Schofield, M., Grant, J., Holmes, S., & Barletta, J. (2006). The Psychotherapy and Counselling Federation of Australia: How the federation model contributes to the field. *International Journal of Psychology, 41*(3), 163–169.

2 Conceptualising Counselling Supervision

Philip Armstrong

Defining supervision

For simplicity purposes, this chapter will refer generically to the person receiving supervision as 'supervisee' and the person providing supervision as 'supervisor.' We use the terms generally in this way with the understanding that these terms are used in various professions and not just those related to counselling. Likewise, the term therapist in this paper refers to counsellors, psychotherapists, social workers, psychologists, and mental health workers who are qualified and registered to practise counselling. The interaction between a supervisee and a supervisor is in essence supervision. Supervision involving counselling is the focus of this chapter.

The requirement for supervision exists to support therapists who work in areas where they are regularly exposed to people in crisis (West, 2010). Professional supervision is also now a mandatory membership requirement of most professional counselling associations, such as the Australian Counselling Association (ACA, 2019). Other professionals such as social workers and psychologists who practise counselling are also required to undergo regular supervision in Australia (Johnson, 2007; Pelling, 2017).

A review of the relevant supervision literature produces several definitions and lists numerous aims of supervision from a variety of experts over many decades. It is interesting to note the evolution of definitions and identified skills and how they become more specific over time. In particular, how the definitions become more complex and multi-faceted over time. The following are examples of this in chronological order:

1. Bartlett (1983, p. 9) defines counselling professional supervision as "an experienced counsellor helping a beginning student or less experienced therapist learn counselling by various means."

   Bartlett's definition is an early one and is simplistic in its meaning as it does not define experience. The primary issue and danger with this definition is it assumes that simply by being experienced the counsellor has the knowledge and ability to help a more junior counsellor. The assumption of knowledge, competency, ethics, and practice based on survival within a profession is dangerous.
2. Stoltenberg and Delworth (1987, p. 34) define professional supervision as "an intensive interpersonally focused, one-to-one relationship in which one person is designated to facilitate the development of therapeutic competence in the other person."

   This definition is slightly more complex than our first as it is defining the elements of supervision. It is restrictive in nature by defining supervision as a one-to-one experience.

DOI: 10.4324/9781003490067-3

3. Lane (1990, p. 10) defines professional supervision as "a therapeutic process focusing on the intra- and interpersonal dynamics of the counselor [sic] and their relationship with clients, colleagues, professional supervisors and significant others."

   Lane's definition is now starting to reflect an understanding that supervision is not singularly focussed but incorporates many elements. Unfortunately, these elements are primarily focused on the relationship aspects of supervision and ignores learning.

4. McMahon (2002) describes the three conceptualisations of the practicalities of professional supervision, these being:

   • professional supervision as a relationship,
   • professional supervision as a developmental process, and
   • professional supervision as a learning environment.

   In this definition, McMahon is expanding on Lane's definition by breaking supervision down to individual components which adds structure to the process and moves beyond relationships. The supervisee now has an idea as to what supervision will cover and what comprises the supervisor's responsibilities.

5. Armstrong (2006) defines professional supervision as a process whereby a professional can discuss various items including:

   • Personal (where appropriate and impacts on work),
   • Professional/clinical,
   • Business, and
   • Industry/work-related issues,

   with a qualified professional supervisor, who is usually more experienced than the supervisee, with a view to resolving professionally orientated issues and with the intention of helping the supervisee to further evolve professionally in a positive manner as well as identifying any emotional issues.

   Armstrong's definition covers a full array of supervision elements by including business skills as a separate element. Although his definition is not as comprehensive as some, it is unique in including the standard of the supervisor being required to be qualified specifically as a supervisor. This is a shift from Bartlett's 1983 definition of a supervisor being an experienced counsellor.

6. Falender and Shafranske (2010, p. 3) in their book *Clinical Supervision* define Supervision as "Supervision is a distinct professional activity in which education and training aimed at developing science-informed practice are facilitated through a collaborative interpersonal process. It involves observation, evaluation, feedback, the facilitation of supervisee self-assessment, and the acquisition of knowledge and skills by instruction, modelling, and mutual problem solving."

7. Carroll (2014, p. 18) when discussing "What is Supervision" states "In a nutshell, supervision is a relational conversation where supervisees reflect on their work and their work experiences in order to learn how to practice better."

Collectively these definitions cover the many aspects of professional supervision and reflect many different expectations. The Armstrong definition is the only one to consider business issues separately identified from clinical issues. All these definitions infer the supervisory process is itself a therapeutical process. Unfortunately, this is not the case when the supervisor does not have extensive experience and qualifications as a supervisor, in the first instance, and a therapist, in the second instance.

Supervisory components

There are a variety of opinions as to how many aspects there are to professional supervision as a process. This is particularly so when clinical supervision is specifically focused upon. Perhaps it is better to take our supervisory definitions a bit further. One possible way of doing this is to section supervision definitions into their core components. Additionally, one extra dimension that is rarely discussed – business building – needs to be included. What follows is an outline of some important components of supervision.

Giving advice is distinct to providing guidance or options to a supervisee. Counsellors are in many cases reticent to give advice, much preferring to explore options and guiding clients through leverage. We are warned, whilst still students, to in general, not give advice (Corey, 1996) as it may be considered unethical and could lead to litigation. Most counsellors are apprehensive or even fearful of giving advice (Silver, 1991). This fear generally comes from the indoctrination that many of us receive as students, that as therapists we should not give advice. This fear is often embedded in the fear of litigation and having a professional complaint made against us (Couture & Sutherland, 2006). Ironically this belief can lead to supervisors or their employers away from giving advice when needed and subsequently being more exposed to litigation and/or complaints from supervisees. To put it simply, a supervisor does not wish to leave themselves open ethically and legally to criticism due to a lack of affirmative and clear direction when this is needed. Supervisors are required to be directive sometimes to the point of being authoritarian. This is a significant and challenging thought and indeed paradigm shift for many therapists who wish to train as supervisors. The following are some examples of when advice is necessary:

- To militate against litigation
- To protect against ethical complaints
- To ensure supervisees follow the correct ethical, professional and/or workplace policies
- Occupational Health Safety issues
- Legislation such as mandatory reporting

Therefore, the guidance offered to supervisees should not be vague, non-committal, or non-directional, as this can lead to confusion and potentially the dangerous implementation of poorly thought-out strategies. Adopting a non-directional and non-advice giving policy can lead to confusion in supervisees who when left to their own devices in regard to policy and procedures may make a wrong decision (Lizzio, Wilson, & Que, 2009). There will be times when supervisees will need specific direction to ensure their practice is effective. Indeed, giving this guidance or advice is the job of the professional supervisor (Shaw & Williams, 1994).

Professional supervisors can address supervisees' need for clarity as well as maintain the edict to 'not personally resolve supervisee's issues' or deliver therapy 'through' the supervisee via supervision (Corey, 1996). Obviously, the learning process is more valuable if the supervisee is able to resolve their own professional issues through supervision. However, there are times when they need to be told of an appropriate action. This is another reason why professional supervisors need specific training in professional supervision; it is a skill to know when to challenge and when to tell or direct. Unlike a counsellor, a professional supervisor is sought out not just for professional and personal growth but actually for answers and professional direction.

There is a school of thought that would suggest that some supervisors do not take to this more directive model very well (Bannink, 2014). This is despite the fact that there is a place for the clear, overt, and at times direct model of support proposed in this chapter (which is loosely based on problem focused supervision). Positive Supervision (Bannink, 2014) suggests that a stance of not knowing may be less directive, and therefore a more collegial relationship is developed in supervision. Supervisors work more as facilitators than directive supervisors in this positive conceptualisation. The problem with this line of thinking is that it doesn't take into account real world ethical and legal issues or duty of care by third party issues which are items so very present in this day and age.

According to the supervision training model developed by the present author, the RISE UP (Relationship based Integrated Supervision and Education to Unlock Potential) model, supervisors need to cover four specific areas in supervision. The professional supervisor is required to help the supervisee investigate and self-reflect on four important areas:

1. Identifying any possible mental or emotional health issues. This is not inferring the supervisor needs to counsel the supervisee. These skills are primarily observational and take an early intervention perspective.
2. Challenging the supervisee's use of theories, modalities, and ethics in relationship to the client and workplace.
3. Helping the counsellor to further develop themselves as a professional within accepted guidelines.
4. Helping the supervisee with business-building skills or career development.

What supervision is not

Before we can confidently apply supervision we need to be fully aware of what supervision is not. Supervision is not personal therapy (Falender & Shafranske, 2010), case management, or a performance review. Rather, it is a forum in which professional issues that the supervisee might need to address, clarify or seek guidance in, can be identified (Lizzio, Wilson, & Que, 2009). Professional supervision may identify personal and/or mental health issues that may require therapeutic intervention (Sumerel & Borders, 1996). The professional supervisor, if local, may be able to refer appropriately for such help, but in the context of professional supervision, should not take steps that would be seen as providing such a service themselves. Supervision is not therapy in and of itself.

Professional supervision is not the appropriate time to go through a training process, which is best done in a professional workshop or course. Professional supervisors may recommend such workshops or courses where they note a deficiency in performance by the supervisee (Hird, Cavalieri, Dulko, Felice, & Ho, 2001). They may even offer such workshops that the supervisee can attend, although dual relationships, conflicts of interest, and ethical issues need to be considered. Professional supervision needs to identify such needs and how to address them. Of course, professional supervisors will be painfully aware of the potential for conflict of interest in promoting their own workshops.

This last point also covers the issue that professional supervision is not about promulgating the professional supervisor's vision/belief of what a profession or job should be, without regard to the industry standards, and best practice guidelines. I will cover how cult-like groups form later on, and you are warned to watch for such developments, as they may be attractive at first glance but are eventually toxic. For this reason, it is also important to note that professional supervision is not about bullying the supervisee, being a friend, offering religious or spiritual guidance (in isolation), nor is it about being just a sounding board that merely reflects without amplifying and elaborating on issues (Muratori, 2001).

Professional supervision also is not a forum for providing legal advice. That is the domain of the supervisee's lawyer. However, that is not to say that legal matters are not to be discussed. Indeed, identification of legal issues that may be lurking in the background is of essential importance (Smith, Riva, & Cornish, 2012). But again, the professional supervision session is a time to identify what those issues might be so that steps can be taken – with a lawyer as necessary – to resolve or mitigate (so as not to litigate) them.

Professional supervision is not about performance reviews or case management, the professional supervision process requires a safe place where the balance of power is as even as possible and not fully one-sided in favour of the professional supervisor (Pearson & Piazza, 1997). Therefore, it is not recommended that managers and team leaders offer professional supervision to workers who answer to them.

A professional supervisor needs to ensure that their professional relationship with the supervisee does not morph into a personal or social relationship (Pearson & Piazza, 1997). The relationship needs to maintain an appropriate balance of power. However, it cannot be equal in all aspects (Carroll, 2014) or in supervisees' favour as this would reflect peer supervision as opposed to professional supervision. This balance becomes redundant if the supervisor transforms the relationship with the supervisee into one where an emotional, financial or physical commitment is required (Pearson & Piazza, 1997). The types of relationships professional supervisors should avoid with supervisees are covered by the following areas:

- being a personal therapist
- being in a personal relationship be it emotional and/or physical
- being related
- being the boss or a superior within the same workplace
- teacher or lecturer
- having a joint business relationship or interest
- loaning or borrowing money
- going into business

Lastly, professional supervision does not exclusively focus on mental health. A good professional supervisor will balance issues that have been raised in the session and not focus on one or two to the exclusion of others. Professional supervision, applied competently, can help ensure one does not become an impaired professional.

The supervisory relationship

The relationship between the Supervisor and Supervisee needs to be respectful, constructive, productive, and critical (Lizzio, Wilson, & Que, 2009). As with all relationships, there are times when the relationship can become unhealthy and toxic. To ensure this does not happen to you as a supervisor you need to be aware of the dangers of relationship issues. The dangers or pitfalls in the supervisor-supervisee relationship are very similar to those of the counsellor – client relationship (Grant, Schofield, & Crawford, 2012). Again, it is difficult for a supervisor without counselling experience to apply this knowledge as it is skill based. The shadow side to competent supervisors and functional relationships are impaired and dysfunctional supervisors. These shadow difficulties will be discussed later on in this chapter.

Supervisory requirements

Although professional supervision in the therapeutic area has been around since Freud, it is only recently that it has become mandatory by some professional bodies and through legislation for others. The requirement for supervision of mental health professionals has been recognised for some time, as we can see from the documented history of professional supervision. Professional supervision had originally established itself in social work as a therapeutic process in the 1930s (Grauel, 2002). It has now become a mandatory component of other allied health professions outside of social work. In the United States of America, mandatory professional supervision for members of the American Association for Marriage and Family Therapy was established in the 1980s (Powel, 1993). Professional supervision became a mandatory component of the membership criteria for full practising members of the Australian Counselling Association in 1999 and, of course, continues today (ACA, 2019). Professional supervision is now being identified as appropriate and necessary outside of the helping professions.

The need for regular on-going professional supervision has been a contentious issue, causing much debate, since the 1980s (Grauel, 2002; Grant & Schofield, 2007). Evidence-based research has been slow in coming, and there is no definitive evidence-based research that we can draw on at the moment to show conclusively the efficacy of supervision. However, the current author's own experience as a member of a national complaints mechanism regarding counselling activities does provide some evidence. Specifically, the vast majority of complaints that have been submitted to the Australian Counselling Association for review have involved therapists who have either ignored their supervisors or had not undertaken supervision. Experience indicates that out of over 100 transcripts of complaints over a 10-year period that the vast majority of responses by counsellors who have had complaints levelled against them have not undergone proper supervision and have demonstrated an inability to personally and professionally reflect on their questionable behaviour. Instead, such counsellors focus on defending and justifying poor behaviour as opposed to being objective and introspective. Supervision could assist with the need to reflect on one's behaviour.

Professional supervision requires specialist training just as does any other professionally based role (Dye & Borders, 1990). Supervisors of supervisees who are self-employed or subcontracted also require knowledge of business, marketing, and management techniques.

Advanced counselling skills, over and above those learned in initial qualification courses, are also required (Dye & Borders, 1990) for ongoing work. Being an experienced professional counsellor is not sufficient to make one a professional supervisor (Powell, 1993), just as being a good nurse does not qualify one to be a doctor. The old adage that doctors make the worst patients is also valid for supervisees. As specialists in communication, counsellors are able to effectively mask or fail to disclose their own issues. Therefore, a professional supervisor needs to be able to observe the image management engaged in by a supervisee who may be having problems in need of addressing. Unfortunately, supervisees are often the last to acknowledge that they are having problems and need to discuss certain items with a supervisor.

Professional supervisors who are not appropriately qualified or have not completed any specific training in supervision are prone to demonstrating weaknesses in their provision of supervision. According to Powell and Brodsky (1998) untrained and poorly trained professional supervisors are prone to certain characteristic errors. These include

- Confusing clinical professional supervision with case management, thereby attending inappropriately to the client's rather than the supervisee's needs.
- Falling back on what they know – their counselling skills – so that they become counsellors to the supervisees, a form of role confusion that may give rise to boundary issues.
- Taking a laissez-faire attitude, even to the point of excessive familiarity or other serious boundary violations.
- Becoming judgemental, authoritarian, demanding, to the edge of sadism.

Unfortunately, many good potential professional supervisors are put in the position whereby they are expected to perform the duties of a professional supervisor without the appropriate support or training (Hadjistavropoulos, Kehler, & Hadjistavropoulos, 2010). The end result for most is a reputation of being inept or professional burnout, caused by feelings of inadequacy and the knowledge of not being able to dispense professional supervision competently. Supervisors who are put in this position owe it to themselves to demand that they attend an appropriate professional supervisory training course (Hadjistavropoulos, Kehler, & Hadjistavropoulos, 2010). Supervisees who use their experience of professional supervision as a basis for practising as a supervisor themselves can also suffer from similar issues (Hadjistavropoulos, Kehler, & Hadjistavropoulos, 2010). Models of behaviour are only helpful when they are appropriate models of behaviour.

Supervisory sessions

A session of professional supervision will usually cover most aspects of the supervisee's therapeutic practice, duty of care, if appropriate legal issues, practice into theory – theory into practice issues, stress and crisis-related issues, and ethical issues. A professional supervisor will discuss recent negative and positive work experiences that a supervisee may have been confronted with as well as pay attention to how and why the supervisee used particular theories (Mills & Chasler, 2012).

The professional supervisor has to respect supervisee-client confidentiality and adhere to the same ethical conditions as a supervisee. A professional supervisor must respect the personal integrity of the supervisee particularly if the professional supervisor is also responsible for performance reports regarding the supervisee. In addition, the professional supervisor may also be just as open to litigation (Mc Bride & Tunnecliffe, 2002) from the supervisee's clients as the supervisee. Good professional supervisors require the added experience and knowledge of working in the field in which their supervisees operate.

Professional and peer supervision

Professional supervision should be on a contractual basis regardless of context, even in a work situation. Professional supervision does not need to be face-to-face (Gibson & Miller, 2003); it can be conducted over the phone, zoom, video, or webcam just as effectively. If using the Internet one needs to ensure they have a secure line with appropriate encryption (or better) to protect your information as it passes over many machines between your system and that of your professional contact (Robson & Whelan, 2006).

Choosing a professional supervisor is similar to choosing a supervisee, in that you need to be comfortable with the professional supervisor and be able to work collaboratively with them. The professional supervisor needs to be familiar with the field in which he or she works and should have a history of working with similar clients (Gunn & Pistole, 2012). The supervisor needs to be capable of challenging and confronting in a positive and constructive manner. Some therapists may have more than one professional supervisor, according to their needs, such as those who work part-time in a specialist area and part-time in more a general field (Johnson & Stewart, 2008).

Professional supervisors should also have professional supervisors. We do not know yet if there comes a time when therapists don't need further supervision. The RISE UP model proposes that time and experience do not necessarily make you an expert, and therefore we all need to continue professional supervision as long as we work in a profession where we are exposed to humans in crisis (Johnson & Stewart, 2008). However, experience and training are necessary, simply not sufficient, for effective supervision (Pelling, 2008, 2021).

Professional supervision can be conducted in many different settings. Supervision does not need to be undertaken in an office. Creative art therapists may choose to use a studio, and some supervisors may prefer a quiet park (Newsome, Henderson, & Veach, 2005). At the end of the day as long as the supervisee is comfortable and the setting has been agreed upon settings can vary just so long as privacy and confidentiality are maintained.

Supervision can be professional or peer in nature. Peer supervision is technically not professional supervision as there is no individual leader who has been identified to accept responsibility. Peer supervision is very popular among workers who meet with peers on a regular basis and has value in that each person brings new experiences to the mix. However, peer supervision can at times be directionless. Peer supervision is common within agencies and organisations and usually, involves a time and place being set where once a week all the workers will meet and discuss work-related issues. This is a form of peer supervision unless a nominated leader takes on the responsible supervisor role. Peer supervision is generally conducted, as the word suggests, by a gathering of peers. There is generally no identified leader who is solely responsible or accountable for the facilitation or clarification of issues or has authority over the group even if it is only for the period of supervision (Crutchfield & Borders, 1997).

Peer supervision allows for each member of the group to have the opportunity to learn from their colleagues' experiences and discuss their experiences with their colleagues. The setting is usually informal within the workplace or an agreed upon venue. With peer supervision, a resulting lack of knowledge or skill can occur. Put colloquially, there is the chance that the blind will be leading the blind. This can be especially dangerous and insidious when a charismatic supervisee convinces a peer supervision group of something that is incorrect that can then influence members of the group to perpetuate poor practice. Without a good leader, groups can quickly become toxic and political and cease to be a positive learning experience (Crutchfield & Borders, 1997).

Professional supervision often occurs one-to-one and face-to-face. This is possibly the most popular known and sought after form of professional supervision and the setting for this is generally at the professional supervisor's office or other agreed venue. The advantage of face-to-face professional supervision is that each person is able to not only hear what is said but observe nonverbal communication as well. The professional supervisor can also introduce tools such as whiteboards and paper to visually demonstrate processes. Face-to-face supervision also has the advantage that it allows for professional rapport to be built upon with someone who you are looking at whilst undergoing professional supervision. The most common negative comment in relation to face-to-face supervision is the time spent in travelling to and from the professional supervisor's office if the professional supervision is external (Stafford & Henderson, 2008).

Professional group supervision occurs when two or more supervisees are present with an identified responsible supervisor. There is an identified leader who is acknowledged as the professional supervisor for the group. There are a set of rules that each member of the group adheres to and are policed by the supervisor, allowing for a safe space in which supervision is to occur. Group supervision can be a wonderful learning experience. It is very refreshing and comforting to hear that other supervisees are confronted with similar issues and have the same doubts and fears. It is also a good learning experience to hear how other supervisees handle difficult clients or issues. The advantage of group sessions over peer supervision is that the professional supervisor can challenge members of the group who may be making statements that hold no credence (Smith, Riva, & Cornish, 2012) and learning can be both direct as well as observational.

Group supervisors must have sound knowledge of group dynamics and experience regarding how to work with both introverts and extroverts. The safety of the group is paramount as is confidentiality. Therefore group supervisors need to be strong individuals who can bring balance to a group and ensure all are heard and respected (Smith, Riva, & Cornish, 2012).

A downside to group sessions is that they are not practical for those who are not comfortable in group settings and prefer to focus on their own work issues as opposed to others. Weak or non-directive group supervisors can easily allow the meeting to fall into a chat session where group dynamics dominate and little if any learning is accomplished and individual members may feel unsafe to speak. The other danger, although rare, is that groups can be turned into cults by manipulative and charismatic leaders (Smith, Riva, & Cornish, 2012). In such cases, participants are generally indoctrinated into a specific way of thinking and behaving which is not challenged or examined appropriately.

Technology and supervision

Supervisory activities can occur using technology. The telehealth is a handy mode of providing supervisory interactions particularly for those who are isolated or in regional areas. There is also the added advantage of not needing to travel, and therefore sessions can be conducted in the comfort of a location of the supervisee's own choosing (Robson & Whelan, 2006). The COVID-19 pandemic has introduced many to the use of Zoom, Microsoft Teams, and other ways of connecting using telehealth. Supervision can use phone and video for interactions.

A drawback to phone professional supervision is that the professional supervisor cannot see the supervisee and therefore may miss out on any important non-verbal cues. In spite of this, experienced phone professional supervisors can pick up changes in vocal qualities, which can mitigate for a loss of visual signs (Robson & Whelan, 2006).

The internet has made professional supervision available via the use of various communication mediums. Supervision facilitated via technology, such as webcams, Skype, Zoom, and Microsoft Teams and generally the internet are now all possible. With the advent of webcams, body language may be discernible to a greater or lesser degree, depending on bandwidth and camera positioning. Efficacy in using the web is still being researched and therefore there is little evidence available as to effectiveness but with many using such telehealth connections during and following the COVID-19 pandemic such media appear to be here to stay. Conceptually, it is likely it will be found to be as good as traditional face-to-face supervision. If you wish to read more about these, I suggest you get a copy of Technologies in Counselling and Psychotherapy available through Palgrave

Macmillan edited by Goss and Anthony (2003). A copy of the Australian Counselling Association ethics for the use of the internet is also available to interested readers via the ACA website (Smith, Amrhein, Brooks, Kenneth, Carpenter, Levin, Schreiber, Travaglini, & Nunes, 2007).

Of course, when providing supervision via the internet or other technologies, the usual principles involving technologies apply. For example, if any information goes out over the Internet, you have a responsibility to ensure that it is secure by using software that supports appropriate levels of encryption. The use of the computer also has privacy implications because of the way data are stored (Litz, Williams, Wang, Bryant, & Engel, 2004).

Issues in supervision

Unfortunately, being a professional supervisor does not necessarily mean a person is ethical or even functional. Some supervisors can abuse their position of relative power. Being a supervisee can put you in a vulnerable situation. There have been cases where impaired professional supervisors have justified improper practices by colluding with supervisees and passing on those improper practices to spawn similar practitioners (Muratori, 2001). By building a group of impaired practitioners, the professional supervisor can justify improper practices and, by numbers, convince others that they are appropriate. In some ways, this is similar to forming a cult.

The majority of people who form cult-like groups are usually motivated by money, power, sex, self-idealisation, or any combination of these things. They perpetuate their groups through persuasive arguments and justifying their practices by numbers. These types of professional supervisors are generally very charismatic and intelligent. The justification of having physical relationships with counselling clients and/or supervisees is a common thread to these groups. A tell-tale common denominator with cult-like groups is the acceptance of abuse as a form of punishment for any member who goes outside the group or who threatens its integrity. Groups such as these generally will isolate themselves so that there can be no influence or questioning from outside. The group leader (professional supervisor) will generally build an aura of being special or of holding a position that has been sanctified by a higher power (Tourish & Irving, 1995).

Some supervisors are or can become impaired. Impaired supervisors are different from the cult-like professional supervisors. They may not be aware of their poor practices, and they do not intentionally pass on poor practices to their supervisees. In many cases, these supervisors have not undergone any formal training and have not received appropriate supervision themselves. Their legacy can be to pass poor practices from one generation of professional supervisors and supervisees to another (Worthington, 1987).

A special type of impaired professional supervisors is one who uses a personal experience usually based on a trauma as their basis of expertise. They will use the coping mechanisms they used to overcome their traumatic experience and believe these are the answers for everyone who is experiencing the same trauma. These types of professional supervisors generally will attract supervisees who have similar experiences such as supervisees who have suffered from depression or have a disease such as cancer. Their only point of reference in relation to expertise is recovery and they use a one size fits all model that is usually inflexible and flawed (Muratori, 2001).

Of all improper practices conducted by cult-like or impaired professional supervisors, sexual exploitation is the most prevalent (McBride & Tunecliffe, 2002). Sexual relationships between professional supervisors, supervisees, or current and past clients are not acceptable and can lead to legal action and de-registration from professional bodies (Thoreson, Shaughnessy, & Frazier, 1995). The Australian Psychological Society, its North American counterparts, and the Australian Counselling Association all prohibit sexual relationships with former clients for at least two years after the last session of therapy. Grooming (maintaining contact) an ex-client over this period to enter into a sexual relationship after the two-year period is also unethical (Pelling, 2019).

It is the possibility of crossing boundaries that makes certain supervisees off limits for professional supervisors. A professional supervisor should not supervise any person with whom they have or have had an emotional or physical relationship currently or prior to a contract of professional supervision, or any member of their immediate family. The reason for this is that, in any relationship, a power base is established by those involved. This power base is generally functional for the personal relationship and is part of the dynamics of the decision-making processes within the relationship. It would be realistic to expect these dynamics to be carried across into a business/professional relationship, whether consciously or unconsciously. These dynamics would in most cases not be conducive to an objective and fair relationship between a professional supervisor and supervisee (Cobia & Boes, 2000).

Similarly, professional supervisors of supervisees in organisations or businesses that also hold a management position need to carefully consider their roles (Carroll, 2014). It would be unrealistic to expect supervisees to be open and honest with regard to workplace issues if their advancement within the organisation was reliant on their professional supervisors work performance reviews. How can a supervisee openly criticise or question a workplace policy or superior in supervision safely if the supervisor is that superior or was responsible for the workplace policy? Supervisees may also try to dissuade the professional supervisor from other staff members who may pose a threat to the supervisee's advancement. There are many conflicting issues a professional supervisor in this type of dual relationship must consider.

Gender can be an issue in supervision (Nelson & Holloway, 1990). A woman who has been brought up with an overbearing father may seek approval from a male professional supervisor. A male who has been brought up with an unemotional father may seek a male professional supervisor, assuming they will be unemotional as well. A supervisee needs to reflect on why they may have a preference for a gender in supervision because they may be going into professional supervision with a hidden agenda.

Supervisees who find they have a preference for a gender due to a previous unpleasant experience may need to consider whether they have dealt with the issue satisfactorily. For instance, a female supervisee who has been a victim of domestic violence and therefore seeks out a female professional supervisor because of power issues with males would need to consider whether she takes these issues into her practice. In this scenario, the supervisee needs to consider counselling in relation to this issue. Similarly, a male supervisee who has been brought up by an abusive stepmother may seek a male professional supervisor so as not to put himself in the position of being subordinate to a female. Again, this supervisee needs to consider his agendas and dealing with the issue. A well-balanced professional would in most cases seek out the most experienced and qualified professional supervisor who also has an understanding of the supervisee's field; gender would be a minor consideration. Supervisors need to ensure they are not enabling their supervisee to perpetuate poor practices by agreeing to be a supervisor for the wrong reasons. It is not the supervisor's role to counsel these supervisees through their issues but it is their role to identify such issues and refer the supervisee for therapy.

Gender can be an issue for supervisors just as it can for supervisees (Nelson & Holloway, 1990). Professional supervisors may use the professional supervisor/supervisee relationship to play out unresolved issues. A female professional supervisor from a feminist background may use the relationship to cause change in male clients that she believes are necessary to meet her beliefs. A male professional supervisor may have traditional ideas as to the roles of the sexes and use the relationship to thwart the careers of female supervisees. Female professional supervisors may over-identify with female supervisees emotionally. Male professional supervisors may encourage male supervisees to deal primarily cognitively with cases. All of these examples are inappropriate for professional supervisors. Early conditioning of the professional supervisor may see supervisors employing tactics to subvert supervisees without being conscious of their agendas. Professional supervisors need to be aware of their own broader issues.

Conclusion

Supervision is a complex activity involving various components, settings, professional, as well as personal aspects. Being experienced as a counsellor does not simply translate to being a competent supervisor. Competent supervision takes clarity in role, professional or peer, and skill in application. Competent supervision also mandates self and other awareness and the courage to address issues as they arise for the benefit of all involved in supervisory processes … including eventually clients.

Those interested in the RISE UP model of supervision and training mentioned in this chapter may contact the author Philip Armstrong via email prwarmstrong@gmail.com for details.

Educational questions & activities

1. True or False. Definitions of supervision have become more complex and multi-faceted over time.
2. According to the author supervision is a process in which all but the following can be discussed:
   a. Personal issues (where they impact on work)
   b. Professional or clinical issues
   c. Business and
   d. Industry/work-related issues
   e. All of the above
3. Ponder and discuss in a group your feelings about having a male, female, or gender diverse supervisor and how your past personal and professional have influenced your feelings about same.

References

Armstrong, P. (2006). *Establishing an allied health service*. Victoria, Australia: Cengage Learning Australia.

Australian Counselling Association (2019). Australian Counselling Association: Supervision Policy. Available www.theaca.net.au/documents/ACA%20Supervision%20Policy%20V12.2019.pdf.

Bannink, F. (2014). *Handbook of positive supervision for supervisors, facilitators, and peer groups* (p. 139). Boston: Hogrefe Publishing.

Bartlett, W. E. (1983). A multidimensional framework for the analysis of professional supervision of counseling. *The Counseling Psychologist, 11*, 9–17. doi:10.1177/0011000083111003

Carroll, M. (2014). *Effective supervision for the helping professions* (2nd Ed.). London: Sage.

Cobia, D. C., & Boes, S. R. (2000). Professional disclosure statements and formal plans for supervision: Two strategies for minimizing the risk of ethical conflicts in post-masters supervision. *Journal of Counseling & Development, 78*(3), 293–296.

Corey, G. (1996). *Theory and practice of counseling and psychotherapy* (5th Ed.). Pacific Grove: Brooks and Cole.

Couture, S. J., & Sutherland, O. (2006). Giving advice on advice-giving: A conversation analysis of Karl Tomm's practice. *Journal of Marital and Family Therapy, 32*, 329–344. doi:10.1111/j.1752-0606.2006.tb01610.x

Crutchfield, L. B., & Borders, L. D. (1997). Impact of two clinical peer supervision models on practicing school counselors. *Journal of Counseling & Development, 75*(3), 219–230.

Dye, H. A., & Borders, L. D. (1990). Counseling supervisors: Standards for preparation and practice. *Journal of Counseling and Development: JCD, 69*, 27–29. doi:10.1002/j.1556-6676.1990.tb01449.x

Falender, C. A., & Shafranske, E. P. (2010). *Clinical supervision: A competency-based approach.* Washington D.C, USA: American Psychological Association.

Gibson, A., & Miller, R. (2003). Relationships: On-screen supervision relationships versus face-to-face. *Australian Journal of Psychology, 55*(1), 1–4.

Goss, S., & Anthony, K. (2003). *Technology in counselling and psychotherapy: A Practitioner's guide.* Basingstoke: Palgrave Macmillan.

Grant, J., & Schofield, M. (2007). Career-long supervision: Patterns and perspectives. *Counselling and Psychotherapy Research, 7*, 3–11. doi:10.1080/14733140601140899

Grant, J., Schofield, M. J., & Crawford, S. (2012). Managing difficulties in supervision: Supervisors' perspectives. *Journal of Counselling Psychology, 59*, 528–541. doi:10.1037/a0024863

Grauel, T. (2002). Professional oversight: The neglected histories of professional supervision. In M. McMahon, & W. Patton (Eds.), *Supervision in the helping professions: A practical approach* (pp. 3–16). Frenchs Forest: Pearson Education.

Gunn, J. E., & Pistole, M. C. (2012). Trainee supervisor attachment: Explaining the alliance and disclosure in supervision. *Training and Education in Professional Psychology, 6*, 229–237. doi:10.1037/a0030805

Hadjistavropoulos, H., Kehler, M., & Hadjistavropoulos, T. (2010). Training graduate students to be clinical supervisors: A survey of Canadian professional psychology programmes. *Canadian Psychology, 51*, 206–212. doi:10.1037/a0020197

Hird, J. S., Cavalieri, C. E., Dulko, J. P., Felice, A. A. D., & Ho, T. A. (2001). Visions and realities: Supervisee perspectives of multicultural supervision. *Journal of Multicultural Counseling and Development, 29*, 114–130. doi:10.1002/j.2161-1912.2001.tb00509.x

Johnson, B. (2007). Transformational supervision: When supervisors mentor. *Professional Psychology: Research and Practice, 38*(3), 259–267.

Johnson, E. A., & Stewart, D. W. (2008). Perceived competence in supervisory roles: A social cognitive analysis. *Training and Education in Professional Psychology, 2*, 229–256. doi:10.1037/1931-3918.2.4.229

Lane, R. C. (1990). *Psychoanalytic approaches to professional supervision.* New York, NY: Brunner/Mazel.

Litz, B. T., Williams, L., Wang, J., Bryant, R., & Engel, C. C. (2004). A therapist-assisted internet self-help program for traumatic stress. *Professional Psychology Research and Practice, 35*, 628–634. doi:10.1037/0735-7028.35.6.628

Lizzio, A., Wilson, K., & Que. J. (2009). Relationship dimensions in the professional supervision of psychology graduates: Supervisee perceptions of process and outcome. *Studies in Continuing Education, 31*(2), 127–140.

McBride, N., & Tunnecliffe, M. (2002). *Risky practices: A counsellor's guide to risk management in private practice* (2nd Ed.). Palmyra, WA: Bayside Books.

McMahon, M. (2002). Some supervision practicalities. In M. McMahon, W. Patton., & M. Carroll (Eds.), *Supervision in the helping professions: A practical approach* (pp. 17–26). Frenchs Forest: Pearson Education.

Mills, J. A., & Chasler, J. K. (2012). Establishing priories in the supervision hour. *Training and Education in Professional Psychology*, *6*, 160–166. doi:10.1037/a0029548

Muratori, M. C. (2001). Examining supervisor impairment from the counselor trainee's perspective. *Counselor Education & Supervision*, *41*, 41–56. doi:10.1002/j.1556-6978.2001.tb01267.x

Nelson, M. L., & Holloway, E. L. (1990). Relation of gender and involvement in supervision. *Journal of Counseling Psychology*, *37*(4), 473–481.

Newsome, D. W., Henderson, D. A., & Veach, L. J. (2005). Using expressive arts in group supervision to enhance awareness and foster cohesion. *Journal of Humanistic Counseling, Education and Development*, *44*(2), 145–157.

Pearson, B., & Piazza, N. (1997). Classification of dual relationships in the helping professions. *Counselor Education & Supervision*, *37*, 89–99. doi:10.1002/j.1556-6978.1997.tb00535.x

Pelling, N. (2021). Singaporean supervisory identity development and its relationship to supervisory experience, counselling experience, and training in supervision. *Asia Pacific Journal of Counselling and Psychotherapy*, *12*(2), 186–204. doi:10.1080/21507686.2021.1960400

Pelling, N. J. (2008). The relationship of supervisory experience, counselling experience, and training in supervision to supervisory identity development. *International Journal for the Advancement of Counselling*, *30*(4), 235–248.

Pelling, N. J. (2017). Ethics. In N. Pelling & L. Burton (Eds.), *The elements of applied psychological practice in Australia: Preparing for the National Psychology Exam* (pp. 17–39). Abingdon, Oxon: Routledge.

Pelling, N. J. (2019). Overview of ethics in Australian psychology. In N. Pelling & L. Burton (Eds.), *The elements of ethical practice: Applied psychology ethics in Australia* (pp. 12–38). Abingdon, Oxon: Routledge.

Powell, D. J. (1993). *Clinical supervision in alcohol and drug abuse counseling*. New York, NY: Lexington Books.

Powell, D. J., & Brodsky, A. (1998). *Clinical supervision in alcohol and drug abuse counseling: Principles, models, methods*. San Francisco, CA: Jossey-Bass.

Robson, M., & Whelan, L. (2006). Virtue out of necessity? Reflections on a telephone supervision relationship. *Counselling and Psychotherapy Research*, *6*, 202–208. doi:10.1080/14733140600857576

Shaw, K., & Williams, A. S. (1994). Supervision: The trainee's perspective and a proposed curriculum. *Australian Psychiatry*, *2*, 49–54. doi:10.3109/10398569409082045

Silver, E. (1991). Should I give advice? A systemic view. *Journal of Family Therapy*, *13*, 295–309. doi:10.1046/j..1991.00429.x

Smith, J. L., Amrhein, P. C., Brooks, A. C., Carpenter, K. M., Levin, D., Schreiber, E. A., Travaglini, L. A., & Nunes, E. V. (2007). Providing live supervision via teleconferencing improves acquisition of motivational interviewing skills after workshop attendance. *The American Journal of Drug and Alcohol Abuse*, *33*, 163–168. doi:10.1080/00952990601091150

Smith, R. D., Riva, M. T., & Cornish, J. A. E. (2012). The ethical practice of group supervision: A national survey. *Training and Education in Professional Psychology*, *6*, 238–248. doi:10.1037/a0030806

Stafford, D. E., & Henderson, P. (2008). Supervision – the grown-up relationship?. *Therapy Today*, *19*(9), 38–40.

Stoltenberg, C. D., & Delworth, U. (1987). *Supervising counselors and therapists: A developmental approach* (1st Ed.). San Francisco, CA: Jossey-Bass.

Sumerel, M. B., & Borders, D. L. (1996). Addressing personal issues in supervision: Impact of counselors' experience level on various aspects of the supervisory relationship. *Counselor Education and Supervision, 35*(4), 268–286.

Thoreson, R. W., Shaughnessy, P., & Frazier, P. A. (1995). Sexual contact during and after professional relationships: Practices and attitudes of female counselors. *Journal of Counseling & Development, 74*(1), 84–89.

Tourish, D., & Irving, P. (1995). Group influence and the psychology of cultism within re-evaluation counselling: A critique. *Counselling Psychology Quarterly, 8*(1), 34–49.

West, A. (2010). Supervising counselors and psychotherapists who work with trauma: A Delphi study. *British Journal of Guidance & Counselling, 4*, 409–430. doi:10.1080/03069885.2010.503696

Worthington, E. L. (1987). Changes in professional supervision as counselors and professional supervisors gain experience: A review. *Professional Psychology: Research and Practice, 18*(3), 189–208.

3 Administration and Marketing of Supervision

Philip Armstrong

Introduction

There is a common agreement in the provision of supervision that there are two components to, or types of, supervision, these being clinical and administrative (Barletta, 2006; Bernard & Goodyear, 2004). The primary difference between the two is that clinical supervision refers to working with the supervisee in relation to client issues, therapy, and self, whereas administrative supervision refers to working primarily with practice/organisational issues centred around paperwork, accounts, policy, and procedures, administration, organisation, and the employee's role (Haynes, Corey, & Moulton, 2003). The two overlap in many cases and are not distinct from each other. Having said that, it is important that a supervisor has a sound working knowledge of the differences and can separate the two and articulate to a supervisee which component is being addressed. Or in some cases which component is being offered as supervision as some supervisors may not be able to focus on both.

A supervisor whose whole experience lies within the realms of academia may struggle to understand competently the administrative needs of a supervisee whose primary work is undertaken in private practice. Indeed, one of the editors of this book has worked primarily in an academic setting for the last 20 years and notes an ongoing concern that many who teach applied counselling and psychological skills in academe tend not to practice said skills after their initial training and registration. This is why they maintain an ongoing private practice to keep current their applied skills and experience of the private practice world as this is where most psychologists, in the main, are a clinical psychologist, are employed (Australian Institute of Health and Welfare, 2022). Maintaining currency in applied work with clients is no simple feat in academe because often such applied work is excluded from academic workload models and applied academic practitioners can be prohibited from engaging in private practice during their regular working hours and such work is generally kept separate from academic work to limit related liability. This thus can necessitate taking a fractional appointment in academe or conducting such work out of regular university hours, such as on a Saturday, as well as obtaining one's own professional indemnity insurance as their practice is not likely covered by the university employer (Pelling, personal communication, October 20, 2022; Pelling & Proeve, 2006).

When I consult with a supervisor I see a professional mental health worker who has worked intensely, gained significant experience and qualifications, and also carries the scars of battles. Supervisors come from varying backgrounds, disciplines and deliver supervision from different perspectives but in the main, they are veterans of the mental health sector. Veterans can distinguish between the romantic notions of being pro-active, making

DOI: 10.4324/9781003490067-4

a difference, helping others with the necessary reality of paperwork, and threading their way delicately through protocols and politics. Most clinicians maintain the status quo, survive, and practice somewhere between the two, helping others while enduring the accompanying paperwork. Supervisors can help make the journey for most as painless as possible as clinicians learn from their own experiences. As a supervisor, and also one who undergoes regular supervision, I look forward to the interactions of supervision and the intellectual and emotional challenges it provides. However, I have also learnt that what some may see as being the 'dark side,' administration within the supervisory process, can be as challenging and important as clinical supervision.

There is common agreement that for supervision to be effective there needs to be a level of training in supervision theory and models, and assessed competence (Haynes, Corey, & Moulton, 2003). Incompetent supervisors may not be aware of their poor practices, and therefore supervisees learn poor practices themselves, which can be passed on from one generation of professional supervisors and supervisees to another (Worthington, 1987). A lack of experience and poor training in administrative tasks and protocols is one area in which an incompetent supervisor could unintentionally sabotage the futures of many highly skilled supervisees. This is why training in administrative skills needs to be a core subject in the training of supervisors. The challenge of keeping students awake while spending time discussing what many possibly see as a very boring subject certainly exists. It is difficult to compete and deliver a lecture on administration when the previous lecture was on 'theories in action' or on ethical dilemmas.

There is one definite strategy that I find works to capture and maintain students' attention and that is to focus first on what the potential outcomes might be for a clinician or supervisor who does not keep on top of administrative tasks. One of the leading causes of bankruptcy for small businesses in Australia according to the Australian Bureau of Statistics is a combination of lack of business ability, lack of capital, and personal reasons (Charleston, 2016). All these issues should be comprehensively covered through supervision. No-one is suggesting a supervisor should become a financial adviser. However, directing a supervisee who wishes to go into private practice to seek the advice of a financial adviser regarding capital and financial issues would fall under the duties of supervision. Bankruptcy due to poor skill levels by tradespeople or professionals is uncommon. Regardless in which sector you work, the worst case scenarios are the same: loss of your job and income if employed, loss of your business if self-employed, and potential action by the tax office, involvement of a government watchdog such as Australian Securities and Investment Commission, legal action (civil or criminal), and potential deregistration by your professional body or licensing board. Many of these actions can lead to penalties that can impact on you for years as well as the potential loss of any assets such as your home. Supervisors and supervisees need to understand competent administration is a business, professional and ethical requirement, and supports the provision of clinical work. It is also in the financial interest of the supervisor to ensure their supervisees remain financially solid.

Graduates rarely have any real notion of administrative responsibilities when first employed as counsellors. Many experienced therapists who come from noncommercial sectors also lack the appropriate administrative and marketing knowledge required to set up and maintain a private practice. The reliance on supervision at this stage of career development or change in career direction is critical and for good reason. However, what happens if your supervisor is not well versed in administrative requirements or does not include this in their educational support? A therapist whose family is dependent on their income is generally not in a position to forgo large amounts of monies due to a poor direction from their supervisor. The developing focus of supervision definitions to include the administrative aspects of supervision illustrates the growing importance of administration. The following definitions are provided to illustrate this point.

Supervision definitions

Bartlett's (1983) definition of counselling supervision discusses the mentoring aspect of supervision in which experienced individuals help more beginning level practitioners. In contrast, the definition proposed by Stoltenberg and Delworth (1987) focuses on the interpersonal aspect of supervision to facilitate development and competence. McMahon's (2002) definition describes three aspects including relational, developmental, and learning environment. Bernard and Goodyear (2004) discuss supervision as an intervention provided by a more senior member of a profession to a more junior member or members of that same profession which is evaluative, extends over time, and enhances both professional functioning and monitors the quality of professional service provided to clients. Barletta (2006) echoes this multitasking nature of supervision and outlines no less than 20 aspects, including encouraging to ensure legal and ethical practices, and promoting an orientation to the profession – items which clearly address administrative components. Thus, from the above definitions, we can see that definitions of counselling supervision over time have begun to incorporate administrative aspects.

Supervision as a paid professional activity

Many experienced practitioners add the provision of supervision to their professional services during their career. Before actually engaging in supervision as a paid professional activity, there are some considerations one must address. Assuming that the individual who is contemplating adding supervision to their repertoire of professional activities is experienced and trained to be sufficiently competent as a supervisor, these considerations tend to be related to the business aspects of providing supervision. This section will review several considerations:

1. Reality: The provision of supervision services as a full time paid professional activity is generally not viable as a replacement for clinical practice in countries such as Australia or New Zealand. Primarily due to their small populations only small market demand exists in Australia and New Zealand. The profession is underdeveloped in most countries within our region. Therefore, a lack of demand as a full fee-paying service is a real consideration for any supervisor within the region. In many developed countries the reliance on voluntary and para-counsellors inhibits the development of supervision as a potential full-time paying profession. There are a few exceptions to this consideration however these are professionals who have spent much of their life building their creditability through research and publishing. In general, the demand for clinical services by the public far outweighs the demand for supervision by clinicians. Your target market, clinicians, is not only smaller but limited further by your own skill levels. It would be inappropriate for a supervisor who has worked primarily in the field of drug and alcohol dependency to offer supervisory services to therapists who work primarily with children with autism.
2. Credibility: A supervisor's credibility can be the difference between success and failure financially, especially for a new supervisor starting out providing supervision. Credibility

is especially important regarding supervision as the target group to whom the supervisor is marketing themselves is comprised of colleagues and peers. Initial credibility, before a reputation is established, can be helped via listing on an appropriate supervisor register (or certification or licensure depending on the region and professional speciality to which the supervisor belongs). A register itself can be a strong marketing tool. Of course supervision registration necessitates that the supervisor holds appropriate credentials in their area of practice.

3. Supply and Demand: Engaging in supervision as a paid professional activity is only likely to be successful if there is a viable supply of professionals that create a demand for such services. Supply is not necessarily the real issue as counselling is a developing profession in many regions, and growth is ongoing. Demand as a full fee-paying service is possibly the real issue, it is the burden of cost for many clinicians that is the real issue. Particularly for those who work with clients from low socio-economic communities or in low paid community not for profit organisations. Many large suppliers of counselling services (predominantly crisis lines) in Australia use volunteer counsellors who are unable to pay for professional clinical supervision and rely on in-house supervision. It is well known that counsellors are not the best paid of the helping professions (see Chapter 22 in this book for details). Yet registered counsellors in the main have an ongoing requirement to maintain annual supervision requirements. On the other hand fully registered psychologists in Australia only need to engage in peer supervision to maintain their registration status which is generally reciprocal and thus at no monetary cost (Pelling, 2016). Arguably the greatest demand within psychology for supervision comes from interns and psychologists in training. Again, this group is made up of low-paid, or in the case of many students, unpaid workers. Demand is not on its own a good indicator of potential income. It is important to ensure any identified group in need of service can pay for said service. Professional organisations, or your own market research, can help determine if supervisors are needed where you intend to provide services. Being accessible via phone, internet, as well as in person (individual and group) is likely to widen your potential target market and prove more popular than having limited availability. If one chooses to limit their provision of supervision to one mode of delivery, such as face-to-face, they are likely to limit their supervisees to those living within a relatively short geographical area. In contrast, a supervisor willing to deliver services via the phone, Zoom, or Microsoft Teams is likely to gain a greater number of supervisees from a wider geographical area.

4. Marketing: Due to the limited demand of supervision as discussed previously many traditional marketing strategies are of minimal value and generally not cost effective. Strategies such as advertising in the local paper are not a viable option and could also be seen as being unprofessional. Additionally, certain professions in various locations have legislative restrictions placed upon them regarding the type of marketing in which they can engage. Thus, the best way to market yourself as a clinical supervisor is to raise your profile within your professional community. Such a profile can be developed via contributing to newsletters or journals, engaging in research, contributing to scholarship such as textbook publications, presenting at conferences as well as conducting professional workshops. If you deliver supervision using modern technology your potential market is not limited by geography. However, if you cross borders you do need to be aware of any legislative, legal, and reporting requirements within different regions. You will also need to check with your insurers any limitations in this regard to your professional indemnity cover.

Once a professional has reviewed their position, competence, the above considerations, and any other factors that are relevant to their profession and location, and has decided to add supervision to their suite of professional services, there are a few significant decisions to be made. How much to charge a supervisee needs to be based on the needs of the supervisor as well as the resources of the supervisee. For example, is the supervision to benefit a volunteer counsellor or one providing services to a low socioeconomic group or to very affluent clients? You may also consider charging a one-off annual fee to an organisation that employs multiple clinicians as opposed to individual hourly rates. Contracting supervision services to organisations that specialise in working in disaster zones and/or critical incidences can lead to a steady flow of reasonably paid work. Once a fee rate has been determined, and you may have several rates for different groups, one needs to consider how they are going to collect the fee, especially when services are rendered over the phone, in the field, or on the internet. Fees can also reflect the type of supervision offered. Obviously, field work will attract a higher fee than services offered from a clinic where the client comes to you. Of course, one can decide to offer supervision services pro bono or to organise group supervision sessions via a professional organisation for the benefit of the emerging professionals. One must remember that 'time is money' and an hour conducting supervision for free or a lower rate than one would charge a client is actually lost money for the supervisor. Whereas volunteering can be beneficial in many aspects, professional supervisors have to determine for themselves the financial logistics of same.

Administration is not a dirty word

I suggest that administration is not a four-letter word, but rather a necessary part of any supervision, and it is now prudent to outline some of the more common, important, and necessary administrative facets encountered in any counselling or psychological practice:

1. Contracts: There are two contracts needed in a supervisory interaction. First, a Supervision Contract, which outlines the requirements and responsibilities of both the supervisor and supervisee. Secondly, a Counselling Contract between supervisee and their client which needs to be reviewed by the supervisor to ensure it meets professional requirements and adequately protects the supervisee and consumer. A standard supervision contract has six main components, yet additional components can be added to personalise them. These six components can be found in the sample supervision contract included in Appendix A. A Counselling Contract also contains six main components and an example of such a contract is located in Appendix B.

> HINT: Ensure any provisions you place in a contract are appropriate to your jurisdiction and do not breach the rights of your supervisee/client.

2. Invoicing and Receipting: Providing professional counselling or psychological services is a business, and as such one needs to be aware of the importance of invoicing and bookkeeping. Not only does accurate invoicing and receipting assist clients in gaining possible refunds for the expense incurred but also assists the professional in preparing their mandatory business assessment statements (a tax office requirement in Australia)

and end of year tax assessments. Although specific requirements vary by region and country, in the Australian context an invoice must include an Australian Business/ Company Number (ABN or ACN) issued by the Australian Tax Office and include the phrase "Tax Invoice," or "Tax Invoice/Receipt" if used in the dual role of being both an invoice and a receipt. This helps to minimise paperwork by using the one document for two purposes. It is an invoice when given to the client and then becomes a receipt when payment is made and saves the need to generate a separate proof of payment. Within Australia, Goods and Services Tax (GST) may be paid on certain professional services and, if applicable, must be shown on related invoices often with the phrase "*GST Included.*" If a therapist delivers services that do not attract GST then "*GST Exempt*" should be notated on the invoice. Regular payment of invoices is also important as not only does this mean the electricity will not be unexpectedly cut off, but you can keep an eye on your incoming and outgoing costs. Without this information, you will not be able to maintain an up-to-date balance sheet, an essential piece of paperwork if you are to keep the wolves from baying at your front door. A good balance sheet will ensure you are aware at all times of your financial position, good or bad. Readers are specifically referred to a professional accountant for relevant local details and more detailed accounting information, as these guidelines are provided for basic informational purposes only.

HINT: To maximise cash flow and keep balance sheets relevant:

a. Dispatch and pay invoices on a weekly basis.
b. Sent invoices should notate payment is on a 14-day basis.
c. If you are a procrastinator in regard to maintaining your books, engage a Bookkeeper.

---

3. Record Keeping: There are many issues that need to be considered regarding how you write up your case notes and keep client records (for additional information, see Armstrong, 2006 and/or Bond & Mitchels, 2008). Regarding administration, however, there are certain considerations of which one should be aware. Additionally, different geographical regions and insurance companies may limit or require certain specific practices. For tax and auditing purposes, notes should be kept for between five to seven years in Australia. Your professional indemnity insurance provider may also have a requirement that supervision records be kept for a certain period of time. Professionals registered with various health authorities and/or professional bodies should check with same regarding paperwork related regulations. Professional indemnity coverage may need to be maintained for a certain period after ceasing practice which will also require your records to be kept. In the case of clients who are minors, there may be a need to keep records for an extended period. Such a time lag needs to take into consideration minors who reach adulthood may seek some form of legal action against others which could necessitate access to clinical records. A therapist's duty of care does not necessarily cease when therapy has terminated. The Australian Psychological Society Code of Ethics (2007) under Record Keeping, B.2.2 states 'Psychologists keep records for a minimum of seven years since last client contact unless legal or their organisational

requirements specify otherwise' and code B.2.3 covers in further detail that 'In the case of records collected while the client was less than 18 years old, psychologists retain the records at least until the client attains the age of 25 years of age.' This is probably a good rule of thumb for supervisors as well whose supervisees discuss issues related to clients under 18 years of age.

A court of law requesting or demanding notes from therapists is not rare. Individuals who have participated in past couple/relationship/family therapy may also request copies of notes many years after they have ceased therapy. It is also possible that a past difficult client who has experienced a recent negative event may look to apportion blame for their predicament onto their past therapist. I am personally aware of several therapists who have had complaints made against them by past clients. These complaints may be obviously misdirected and dated, but they still have to be processed. In Australia, the majority of professional associations for counsellors and psychotherapists do not have time limits imposed for complaints against their members. Again, a supervisor may need to keep notes on supervisees for an extended period of time to cover such occasions. Professionals need to be aware of such record keeping requirements. Another aspect of record keeping includes the long-term archiving of client notes off-site and provisions to be made for their holding and/or disposal upon the death of the professional or cessation of practice. Disposal in this case does not necessarily mean the destruction of records but their movement so that they are under the care of another professional until they can be appropriately destroyed. For space savings, one can have records electronically stored on electronic disks. However, one should note that the saving of notes to hard drive disks could have privacy and confidentiality implications and, of course, disk storage can fail. Similarly, paper records can also be accidentally destroyed by flood or fire and if such destruction occurs practitioners and supervisors should make their insurance company aware of such loss. No hard and fast rules can be made regarding such record keeping as such matters will depend on legal and insurance requirements, as well as the client base involved. However, I highly recommend that client notes not be destroyed, but rather archived. Notes, electronic or paper, should only ever be destroyed securely and after the appropriate amount of time in your region relating to your professional obligations.

HINT: Always date entries and never delete entries, as you may leave yourself open to claims of falsifying or redacting records.

---

4. Confidentiality and its Exceptions: Confidentiality is often taken for granted by clients and new practitioners. However, there are many limits to confidentiality, and these can vary according to the profession (e.g., counselling, psychology, and social work) as well as the region. First, legislative limits to confidentiality include state or federal requirements, particularly regarding Privacy laws. A good example of this is in Australia there exists legislation that many clinicians are unaware of that states the Australian Bureau of Statistics can access notes for statistical purposes. Second, the policies and procedures of the specific organisation for which one is working will have its own written requirements within their policy and procedures manuals. Clinicians need to be aware these do not subordinate legal and legislative requirements. Third, each professional

body or registration/licensure board may also have requirements, and when one is a member, they agree to abide by these requirements. A dilemma exists when two or more of these requirements conflict. This is a very common dilemma particularly in community not for profit organisations whose policies and procedures are written by volunteer management committees who may not have a solid understanding of legal and professional requirements. I have also seen government department policies that are in contradiction with legislative requirements, so it is very important supervisors are *au fait* with their regional requirements. It is only with skilful negotiation and interpretation that such conflicts are resolved. Such difficulties should be recorded in writing, so too the process used to resolve difficulties. Confidentiality for supervisees is an important issue that needs to be discussed in detail and agreements documented. This is especially the case if a supervisee works in an area where there is more grey than black and white in regard to legislative guidelines. Supervisees need strong direction by their supervisors in this regard. A supervisor needs to document for the supervisee and make clear any cases where confidentiality may be breached, just as one would for a client.

HINT: Never dispose of any document that may contain information on supervisees or clients in a general waste bin, always shred documents or place in a specially provided secure confidential document receptacle. Consider making provisions for records in your will.

---

5. Insurance: This information is a guide only and is not intended as advice. All insurance issues should be directed to your insurer in the first instance. If a supervisor operates in a country where insurance is not a requirement legally or by their professional body, they need to ensure they are aware of potential legal issues if they offer supervision services via the net or phone to supervisees in other regions. For supervisors who do carry insurance, it is in the supervisor's best interest to ensure that they notate they are practicing supervisors on their insurance policy to ensure their insurance coverage includes the provision of supervision as a separate service to counselling. The two primary types of insurance required in most countries for therapists are professional indemnity insurance and public liability insurance. Some insurers may not automatically include supervision in their policies. Professional indemnity covers the professional and provides recourse for clients harmed by the actions of the professional relationship. It is important to note that professional indemnity insurance provided by an employer may not cover an employee for practice outside of the employment situation. For example, a therapist employed within an agency will be covered by the agency for work within the agency but will not be covered for work in another sector or setting outside the agency such as a part-time practice.

Public liability insurance protects the public from harm due to property of the owner and should be held by anyone working in private practice. If a professional also lends materials, books or recordings, they should also be covered by a product liability policy, should harm result from the use of a product (i.e., a computer disk containing a virus destroys a client's computer). Finally, run-off insurance is required. Specifically, if you change your insurance company and/or policy, you need to be certain that new policies cover past actions. Similarly, professionals need to investigate their retrospective coverage once they cease to practice as professionals, often based on a statute of limitations for various issues, and you do not want to leave any part of your professional practice not covered. Not only do supervisors need insurance (various types) but they also need to ensure that their supervisees are adequately insured. Often the best place to gain your professional insurance policies is via professional associations that have usually negotiated policies to cover their members' needs at a reasonable price.

HINT: If you are self-employed ensure you consider salary protection insurance and work cover.

6. Professional Associations: From an administrative perspective, once a therapist has joined a professional association they need to do two things to maintain membership. First, one must pay an annual membership fee. Second, one must generally engage in continuing professional development, sometimes including clinical supervision. These activities need to be recorded for later reporting purposes. The simplest way to keep professional development and supervision records is to gain from your professional body, or develop one yourself, a logbook to note such activities. Such a logbook can help a professional avoid having to laboriously reconstruct their professional training and supervision if audited by their professional body. Unfortunately, it is common for busy professionals to fail to keep records of their professional development and not pay the membership fees on time.

HINT: Always ensure you receive a certificate of attendance when you engage in any professional development activity for your records, regardless of whether it is web based or in person.

7. Professional Diary: Professionals should keep a diary/calendar/agenda for work related appointments which include with whom they meet and a contact telephone number. Diary entries should include a short description regarding the nature of the meeting (e.g., supervision, counselling, professional development training). Diaries must be kept for record and auditing purposes and need to be archived. Past diaries can be important supporting documentation regarding tax audits or complaint procedures. Due to confidentiality and privacy issues, a professional diary used by a group of practitioners in a clinic setting must be protected from unauthorised access. For instance, clients/supervisees should not be able to see other client/supervisees names in the diary when the professional is making an appointment. Moreover, if a diary is used by multiple private practitioners in a private practice setting, using only first names in the group diary should be considered. Furthermore, if one is using an electronic diary (e.g., Personal Digital Assistant) one should be aware that saving material to the hard drive could pose a potential threat to confidentiality if the computer is linked to the internet or if the computer is accessible to another person (there are limits to the protection offered by computer security programs).

HINT: At the end of the year add up your client contact and supervision hours and note the totals on the last page. This will help in regard to data collection for possible future needs.

Conclusion

Although often overlooked, the administrative aspects of professional supervision are critical. While complaints and legal action are generally the result of harmful clinical practice, which can be addressed via supervision, training, and experience, haphazard administration practices can also result in difficulties and similarly need to be addressed in supervision. Indeed, administration practices can have an impact on the disposition of a complaint or legal action as good practices in this area can support a clinician's actions. Again, an example supervision contract can be found in Appendix A. Please note that this contract is based upon one presented by Osborn and Davis (1996). A sample counselling contract can be found in Appendix B.

Educational questions & activities

1. List 3 types of insurance that may be needed for a private practitioner.
2. True or false? Providing coverage for Clinical Supervision is automatically covered in all Professional Liability insurance policies.
3. Name 2 items that by law in Australia (or in your region) that must be included on an invoice for professional services.
4. In relation to keeping clinical notes and records, what is a major consideration in regard to keeping notes if your client base includes minors?

References

Armstrong, P. (2006) *Establishing an allied health service*. South Melbourne: Cengage.

Australian Institute of Health and Welfare. (2022). *Mental health services in Australia*. www.aihw.gov.au/reports/mental-health-services/mental-health-services-in-australia

Australian Psychological Society (2007). *Code of ethics*. Melbourne, Vic: Author.

Barletta, J. (2006). Clinical supervision (Chapter 6). In N. Pelling, R. Bowers, & P. Armstrong (Eds.), *The practice of counselling* (pp. 118–135). Melbourne, Australia: Thomson.

Bartlett, W. E. (1983). A multidimensional framework for the analysis of supervision of counseling. *Counselling Psychologist, 11*, 9–17.doi: 10.1177?0011000083111003

Bernard, J. M., & Goodyear, R. K. (2004). *Fundamentals of clinical supervision* (3rd ed.). Upper Saddle River, NJ: Merrill.

Bond, T. & Mitchels, B. (2008). *Confidentiality and record keeping in counselling and psychotherapy*. Los Angeles: Sage Publishers.

Charleston, L. (2016). Why small businesses fail in Australia. *HuffPost*, 14 July 2016. www.huffpost.com/archive/au/entry/why-small-businesses-fail-in-australia_n_8187166

Haynes, Corey, & Moulton (2003). *Clinical supervision in the helping professions: A practical guide*. Pacific Grove, CA: Brookes/Cole–Thomson Learning.

McMahon, M. (2002). Some supervision practicalities. In M. McMahon, W. Patton, & M. Carroll (Eds.), *Supervision in the helping professions: A practical approach* (pp. 17–26). Frenchs Forest: Pearson Education.

Osborn, C. J., & Davis T. E. (1996). The supervision contract: Making it perfectly clear. *The Clinical Supervisor, 14*, 121–134.

Pelling, N., & Proeve, M. (2006). Australian and New Zealand university clinical and cousnelling psychology staff: Maintaining practice in academe. *Australian Psychologist, 41*(2), 112–119.

Pelling, N. J. (2016). Ethics. In N. J. Pelling & L. J. Burton (Eds.), *The elements of applied psychological practice in Australia: Preparing for the National Psychology Exam*. London: Taylor & Francis Publishers.

Stoltenberg, C. D., & Delworth, U. (1987). *Supervising counselors and therapists: A developmental approach*. San Francisco: Jossey-Bass.

Worthington, E. L. (1987). Changes in supervision as counselors and supervisors gain experience: A review. *Professional Psychology: Research and Practice, 18*(3), 189–208.

Part 2

Professional Issues

Part 2, **Professional Issues**, is a section comprised of five chapters each with a unique professional focus but with all presenting supervision-related domains in our contemporary context. Chapter 4 presents the ethics relating to clinically supervising the use of the popular and timely evidence-based practices. This ethical examination is in-depth and includes a case study application. Chapter 5 explores how to cope when psychotherapy becomes a matter of life and death via the use of coping planning. Thus, the significant issue of suicidality and suicide prevention is explored directly. Chapter 6 outlines the main fears and interest areas presented in counselling supervision by novice counsellors. Chapter 7 deals with the issue of vicarious trauma, an occupational hazard in the helping professions. Finally, Chapter 8 discusses the role of hope, compassion, and justice when supervising family violence counsellors.

Chapter overview

Chapter 4, **Ethical Issues in the Clinical Supervision of Evidence-Based Practices**, by Cynthia J. Osborn and Tom Davis, delivers a timely and provocative chapter that steps up to the challenge of professionals needing to empirically validate the services they provide. The chapter offers a wonderfully applied case study approach that brings to life clinical imperatives and research-informed challenges in a charming way. Although they are best known to many for their seminal work on the supervision contract (and some of that area is thankfully explored in this chapter), this particular writing explores the nexus between practitioners and researchers. The reader will find the clinical case, and the questions that are provided to explore it, an invaluable resource, so too the comprehensive references to quality research literature.

Chapter themes

In this chapter you will explore the following themes:

- Types of supervision
- Training supervision
- Remedial supervision
- Ongoing supervision and peer consultation
- Evidence-based practices
- Ethical issues in the supervision of evidence-based practices
- Purpose of supervision

DOI: 10.4324/9781003490067-5

- Managing multiple relationships and interpersonal dynamics
- Format of supervision
- Supervisor qualifications and competence
- Evaluation
- Ethics in action: Developing and maintaining written supervision contracts

Chapter 5, **When Psychotherapy Becomes a Matter of Life and Death: Supervision for Suicide Prevention**, by Helen M. Stallman, addresses the roles of support, knowledge, modelling, and reviewing session notes in supervision to support coping and thus prevent client suicidal actions. Role-play information is also provided.

Chapter themes

In this chapter you will explore the following themes:

- Support
- Knowledge
- Modelling
- Reviewing Session Notes

Chapter 6, **Addressing Supervisee Fears and Interest Areas in Supervision**, by Nadine Pelling, is a short chapter but one the reader will readily relate to and benefit from. All clinicians have some fear as they conduct their professional role, especially at the start of their career. Here the worst-case scenario idea is explored with the most frequently raised issues by counselling trainees, and thankfully some ways of responding are also included, as the reader is simultaneously reassured and validated. Recent areas of applied interest are also noted.

Chapter themes

In this chapter you will explore the following themes:

- Tell me your fears and interests
- Worst client case scenario categories
- Harm to client/client in great pain
- Difficult clients
- Danger to therapist
- Ethical responsibilities
- Questioning therapist competence
- Main interest areas
- General activities for increasing knowledge, self/other awareness, and skill

Chapter 7, **Supervision and Vicarious Trauma**, by Fran Lane, explores the real occupational hazard of vicarious traumatization. Vicarious traumatization is explored conceptually, and the chapter outlines how supervisors can be prepared to experience and support supervisees experiencing vicarious traumatization in a hopeful and forward-facing manner.

Chapter themes

In this chapter you will explore the following themes:

- Supervising counsellors for vicarious trauma
- Understanding vicarious trauma
- Constructive self-development theory
- VT Informed supervision
- Anticipate and Prepare
- Address the Signs of VT
- Transform the Pain of VT

Chapter 8, **Demonstrating hope, compassion, and justice: Supervision of family violence counsellors in Australia,** by Stephen O'Kane, addresses basic principles in family violence counselling and the importance of assessment and being aware of one's focus and avoiding bias when engaging in family violence work.

Chapter themes

In this chapter you will explore the following themes:

- Family Violence in Australia
- Principles of Family Violence Counselling practice
- Comprehensive Assessment in Family Violence Counselling Practice
- Criminogenic focus versus health focus
- Family violence counselling and stereotyping
- Avoidance of bias in reporting – community standards
- Family violence and the law
- Self-violence and threats
- Family violence and culturally and linguistically diverse (CALD) communities
- Effects on children
- Effects on mothers
- Effects on fathers
- Situational couple violence and family violence
- Compassion fatigue, burnout, and vicarious trauma

4 Ethical Issues in the Clinical Supervision of Evidence-Based Practices

Cynthia J. Osborn and Thomas E. Davis

Introduction

For as long as some form of psychotherapy has been taught, the supervision of the implementation of that psychotherapy has been practised. The earliest model of supervision, originating from the teaching and learning of psychoanalysis, resembled a master-apprentice interaction between supervisor ("master therapist") and supervisee ("novice therapist" or "apprentice"; see Binder & Strupp, 1997). As the practice of counselling and other forms of psychotherapy has expanded and evolved, so has supervision. This is particularly true with the emergence of innovative therapeutic practices, including evidence-based practices (EBPs). No longer can clinical supervision be considered a well-defined practice, one typically confined to a counselling student's formal academic training (e.g., during counselling practicum and internship), or representing the guidance or shepherding of a counsellor in the early phase of his or her career. As Milne (2007) contended, Bernard and Goodyear's (2014) long-standing definition of clinical supervision may no longer capture the varied types of counselling and the concomitant functions of supervision, nor satisfy the need for empirical support that "the evidence-based movement" has ushered in.

Although clinical supervision is now considered a discipline separate from psychotherapy or counselling, the two retain a symbiotic relationship: one cannot exist without the other. This entanglement – as with any type of professional relationship, particularly, in the intimate business of counselling – has always brought with it ethical and legal issues. However, as the type, function, and setting of counselling has changed, so has the supervision of that counselling and, in the process, new ethical considerations have arisen.

This chapter focuses on ethical issues in clinical supervision (rather than administrative supervision), particularly in the era of EBPs. Although certain ethical issues remain "standard" in clinical supervision (e.g., evaluation, power, multiple relationships) regardless of the type, function, and setting of counselling that is supervised, counselling and supervision practiced in an EBP milieu raise further ethical considerations.

The following case involves Leah, Laurie, and Dr. Bennett – all of whom are connected in the training and implementation of one EBP, multisystemic therapy (MST). After reading through the case, review the questions that follow, questions that are intended to stimulate ethical considerations that are discussed throughout the chapter.

Case study

Leah earned her master's degree in counselling three years ago and has worked in a juvenile correctional facility since graduation. Tired with what she considered to be a more punitive

DOI: 10.4324/9781003490067-6

and less remedial treatment philosophy, she pursued employment elsewhere. She was recently hired as a counsellor at a community based mental health facility, Horizons, that serves adolescents and their families. Funding sources have required the facility to render treatment services that have empirical evidence to support their efficacy and effectiveness, so-called evidence-based practices (EBPs). One of these, multisystemic therapy (MST; Henggeler & Borduin, 1990), has been adopted by the facility, requiring all front-line clinicians to obtain intensive training and ongoing supervision. The facility has contracted with a small, private training and research group, Ignite, comprised of clinicians and university faculty with expertise in MST and other EBPs (e.g., cognitive-behavioural therapy, motivational interviewing).

MST is a comprehensive treatment approach for adolescents and their families, conducted by a team of professionals that includes home-based counselling. This treatment approach is pragmatic and goal-oriented and was initially designed for serious juvenile offenders. Today, MST is appropriate for adolescents who struggle with both mental health and substance use concerns and, in the process, have become involved in the legal system (see Henggeler, Schoenwald, Borduin, Rowland, & Cunningham, 2009). Service providers receive ongoing group supervision for six months after completing an initial and intensive five-day MST training.

As a new hire at Horizons, Leah has been assigned an internal supervisor, Laurie, a social worker with 15 years of experience who oversees clinicians working with youth who have co-occurring (mental health and substance use) disorders. Laurie is new to MST whereas Leah had learned some about MST while a graduate counselling student. Both Leah and Laurie just completed the 5-day MST training, conducted by Dr. Bennett, one of Ignite's trainers and a lecturer at the local university where Leah earned her counselling degree. He taught several counselling courses in which Leah was a student.

Due to the severe, chronic, and complex nature of problems that families appropriate for MST present to treatment, a multidisciplinary treatment team approach is indicated and is the norm for direct care in MST. Each team is typically comprised of two to four practitioners, and Laurie and Leah are on the same MST team. Although each is responsible for four to six client cases (i.e., four to six adolescents and their families), MST practitioners meet regularly as a team to coordinate services to all families served at Horizons. Team members provide coverage when the primary therapist for a family is on vacation or otherwise not on-call and all team members have met all the families served by their colleagues.

MST supervision is intended to mirror that of MST direct care and thus supervision is provided to a team. Group supervision – rather than individual supervision – is therefore the standard format of MST supervision. The group format for MST supervision allows therapists to learn from one another, to work collaboratively and as a cohesive unit (as the therapists are teaching families to do), and to practise a new skill set with colleagues. To remain consistent with MST training guidelines, both Laurie and Leah will participate in ongoing MST group supervision for at least six months, and Dr. Bennett will be serving as their MST team supervisor. The purpose of supervision is to ensure therapist fidelity with or adherence to MST practice principles.

The introduction of an EBP to a mental health facility like Horizons can "shake up the system" and therefore it can have the effect of clinicians re-evaluating their priorities and practices. "Treatment as usual" may no longer be an option. "Standard supervision practice" also may no longer exist or be unrecognizable. As a result, clinicians may feel out of their comfort zone or even lost, uncertain as to how to address the new configurations and possible dilemmas that an EBP – a new and perhaps unfamiliar "standard of practice" – has ushered in.

In the preceding case, the administration at Horizons has adopted MST as the new standard of practice. How does this affect the practice of supervision? What ethical and possibly legal issues does it raise? Specifically:

- Should Leah and Laurie participate in and be members of the same MST supervision group?
- Should Dr. Bennett serve as Leah's individual MST supervisor?
- Who should (or can be) ultimately be responsible for welfare of Leah's clients – Laurie or Dr. Bennett?
- How can and should Leah's clinical skills be assessed? Would someone (Laurie or Dr. Bennett?) need to accompany her to client homes to observe her interactions with clients and their families?
- Who is responsible for Leah's clinical evaluation?
- What happens if Leah's MST skills do not meet minimum requirements at the end of the six-month training/supervision period?

Types of supervision

The case of Leah, Laura, and Dr. Bennett illustrates some of the complexities of clinical supervision, particularly in the current era of evidence-based practices (EBPs). What is the purpose of supervision of an EBP such as multisystemic therapy (MST)? How is supervision conducted? Who gets to decide? Who is ultimately responsible for the professional development of supervised counsellors and for the welfare of their clients? There is clearly not one way to conduct supervision and supervision fulfils various functions. We briefly discuss four types of supervision, each of which may raise unique ethical considerations given the purpose or intent of supervision.

Training supervision

Supervision is regarded primarily as the required teaching and clinical oversight or monitoring of persons (e.g., counsellor trainees) preparing to enter a helping profession during their formal/academic training. When counselling students are enrolled in a practicum or an internship and are delivering counselling services to clients, they are required to be supervised by a faculty member or a practitioner in the field. This is the predominant understanding of supervision and is exemplified in Bernard and Goodyear's (2014) definition of clinical supervision as:

> an intervention provided by a more senior member of a profession to a more junior member or members of that same profession. This relationship is evaluative, extends over time, and has the simultaneous purposes of (1) enhancing the professional functioning of a more junior person(s), (2) monitoring the quality of professional services offered to the client(s) she, he, or they see(s), and (3) serving as a gatekeeper of those who are to enter the particular profession.

(p. 9)

In this definition of supervision, the power differential between supervisor and supervisee is made explicit and a master-apprentice model is implied. Although this type of supervision "extends over time," its purpose is to ensure client welfare and at the same time determine whether a counsellor-in-training is prepared to practice and be recognised by a credentialing body as a professional counsellor. In this sense, supervision is time-limited and corresponds to a period of apprenticeship or probation. The supervisee must be able to demonstrate that he or she is ready to function as a professional independent of close monitoring or supervision. And the supervisor must be able to assess the supervisee's preparedness, fulfilling the role of "gatekeeper," the one who may hold the key to the counsellor trainee's induction into the profession.

Given the purpose of training supervision, evaluation is understandably an integral function of supervision and the source of much anxiety for supervisees and supervisors alike. Gould and Bradley (2001) offered some explanation for what Nelson, Barnes, Evans, and Triggiano (2008) later described as *supervisor gatekeeping anxiety*, including discomfort with what some supervisors may construe as the authoritarian and dictatorial role of evaluator. Supervisors may also be uncertain as to how to evaluate and may therefore shirk this important responsibility. This is suggested in Ladany, Ellis, and Friedlander's (1999) survey of 151 psychologists-in-training. The most frequent ethical violation of their supervisors reported by these supervisees (by 33.1% of respondents) was that of "*performance evaluation and monitoring of supervisee activities.*" Specific supervisor evaluation practices supervisees deemed unethical included giving little feedback, failing to observe recorded sessions, and proving no feedback on performance until a final assessment of performance.

Remedial supervision

Not only is evaluation integral to training supervision; it is an essential function of remedial supervision. By remedial supervision we refer to supervision that a credentialing body or professional association may require to restore to "good standing" an independently licensed/registered counsellor who has been found to be in violation of an ethical code or standard. Cobia and Pipes (2002) described mandated supervision as a mechanism "to rehabilitate impaired professionals" (p. 143). As with training supervision, remedial supervision may also be time-limited and encompass a probationary period. Unlike training supervision, however, remedial supervision is intended to be restorative, whereas training supervision is designed to be foundational and generative (i.e., launching a new counsellor into professional practice).

Although it appears that remedial supervision is not an uncommon practice (see Rapisarda & Britton, 2007), it is rather surprising that very little has been discussed in the literature about its purpose and how it should be conducted. In terms of research, Rapisarda and Britton attempted to interview supervisors in one state of the United States who provided what they referred to as sanctioned supervision, but were not successful. They conducted a focus group instead with eight clinical supervisors who had *not* conducted sanctioned supervision about sanctioned supervision. Several of the participants indicated this particular intervention resembled "clinical monitoring" rather than supervision.

Kress, O'Neill, Protivnak, Stargell, and Herman (2015) interviewed four supervisors from one midwestern state in the United States who had provided sanctioned supervision to at least one counsellor in the past year. Two themes captured these supervisors' experiences: (1) sanctioned supervision is a *different process* than traditional supervision, and (2) providing sanctioned supervision generates *supervisor ambivalence*. The first theme described sanctioned supervision as "a more active, directive supervisory stance" (p. 46) than is typical of routine supervision. The second theme reflected the ambivalence experienced by these supervisors, such as feeling good about serving the profession while at the same time being concerned about liability.

Ongoing supervision and peer consultation

Compared to training supervision and remedial supervision, ongoing supervision and peer consultation are typically voluntary (i.e., not required) and initiated by an independently licensed/registered counsellor for the purpose of his or her own continuous professional enhancement. The British Association for Counselling and Psychotherapy (BACP, 2013), however, requires that all accredited therapists (i.e., counsellors, psychotherapists, trainers, and supervisors) receive "regular and on-going formal supervision/consultative support for their work" (p. 05). Sometimes referred to as peer supervision and conducted in a group setting (see Bernard & Goodyear, 2014; Borders, 1991), ongoing supervision may be characterised as a form of clinical consultation for seasoned clinicians to offer one another support and guidance. This is particularly true for clinicians in private practice as an antidote to professional isolation. It is also true for clinicians in a group practice or a community-based agency who desire additional support and assistance with ethical dilemmas.

From interviews with 30 social workers in Australia who were willing to discuss an ethical dilemma they had experienced, McAuliffe and Sudbery (2005) found that 21 were provided with supervision (primarily administrative) by their employing organisation (often referred to as the "immediate line manager" and not necessarily social workers). Four of the 21 elected to obtain additional, external, private, and ongoing supervision to focus more on professional development and emotional support. Of the nine social workers without access to internal supervision, all had accessed external supervision from social workers, an indication that clinicians may pursue continuous supervision from members of their own profession.

Peer consultation has been proposed recently as a means of fostering supervisor development, specifically enhancing critical thinking skills when working with challenging client cases. Granello, Kindsvatter, Granello, Underfer-Babalis, and Hartwig Moorhead (2008) described their supervisory peer consultation group that met on a periodic basis to generate multiple perspectives on specific supervisory experiences of group members. One member served as the ethics consultant and offered guidance in ethical decision making. The purpose was to generate multiple perspectives about specific clinical (including supervisory) issues. In so doing, Granello et al. reported that they each learned to think more complexly about supervision and realised the importance of investing in their own development as supervisors, "with more than lip service to the idea that development must be lifelong" (p. 42).

Targeted and skill-specific supervision

A fourth type of supervision is practised for reasons similar to ongoing supervision and peer consultation (i.e., professional support and development) but is associated with specific skill sets and therapeutic approaches, namely evidence-based practices (EBPs). The adoption of any EBP and other forms of innovative practices requires initial, periodic, and often ongoing supervision to ensure fidelity to the treatment protocol. Heaven, Clegg, and Maguire (2006) referred to supervision of an EBP as the "bridge between the classroom and workplace following...training" (p. 314). With respect to cognitive-behavioural therapy (CBT), Pretorius (2006) described supervision as "quality control...during initial training and throughout therapists' careers" (p. 413).

Dialectical behaviour therapy (DBT; Linehan, 2015) has become an EBP in the treatment of borderline personality disorder (see Linehan et al., 2006). One of the five functions of a standard DBT "package" is therapist skill enhancement and motivation. Regular (i.e., weekly) counsellor training/consultation team sessions are held specifically to reduce therapist burnout, provide therapy for therapists, improve therapist empathy for clients, and offer skills training to therapists regarding specific client difficulties (Lynch, Trost, Salsman, & Linehan, 2007). Supervision in DBT is therefore not only for the purpose of ensuring that therapists deliver DBT-consistent services to clients and that clients are receiving quality care. It is also intended to "treat" the therapists at the same time that clients are being treated by DBT therapists. The focus of these DBT team meetings and ongoing supervision is on counsellor fitness and wellbeing and less on client difficulties (Lynch et al., 2007). Fruzzetti, Waltz, and Linehan (1997) asserted that supervision in DBT is designed to anticipate, minimise, or even prevent therapist burnout by enhancing "therapist training, effectiveness, and competence, and also satisfaction and enjoyment with [their] work" (p. 85). Supervision is also continuous when practising DBT. This means that as long as a clinician is practising DBT, he or she is receiving and participating in regular supervision.

As mentioned earlier in this chapter, supervision of multisystemic therapy (MST) is intended to "facilitate therapists' acquisition and implementation of the conceptual and behavioural skills required to achieve adherence to the MST treatment model" (Henggeler & Schoenwald, 1998, p. 1). As with CBT, therefore, MST supervision serves as a "quality assurance" measure, designed to ensure treatment fidelity; in other words, the purpose of MST supervision is to ensure that services clinicians have been trained to deliver to clients are actually being implemented. This function of supervision is also true for the supervision of non-clinical staff trained in a standard practice adopted by a treatment or correctional facility. For example, the supervision of probation officers is a required element in New Zealand's Department of Corrections (see Norrie, Eggleston, & Ringer, 2003) to ensure implementation of the Department's "best practices" (interpreted as providing the best services to offenders, Departmental Services, and the community).

Supervision of an EBP often has a specific purpose: to provide further and extended training in an EBP so as to facilitate the application of a specific skill set to clinicians. In this way, supervision targets a specific counselling approach or style and is intended to help clinicians transfer or apply new counselling behaviours to their work with clients. If the clinician fails to meet minimum criteria for treatment adherence or fidelity, additional and perhaps intensive supervision may be required. Although some EBPs may require supervision only until the supervisee has achieved a certain level of proficiency (i.e., time-limited supervision), other EBPs (e.g., DBT) consider supervision an essential component of the therapeutic approach and is therefore ongoing. It seems that EBP supervision contains features of the first three types of supervision discussed in this chapter: training supervision, remedial supervision, and ongoing supervision.

Evidence-based practices

The American Psychological Association (APA) has defined evidence-based practice (EBP) as "the integration of the best available research with clinical expertise in the context of patient characteristics, culture, and preferences" (APA Presidential Task Force on Evidence-Based Practice, 2006, p. 273). The purpose of EBPs has been to "raise the bar" by providing clients with services that have research support, services that have "passed the test" and can be trusted to yield beneficial therapeutic outcomes. Despite its laudatory purpose to prioritise only those therapies that have been proven to be effective, the EBP "movement" has been critisised for several reasons. These include (a) what appears to be an exclusive focus on treatment interventions rather than client or therapist factors, (b) a seeming lack of consensus as to what constitutes "evidence" (i.e., results of randomised clinical/control trials only?), and (c) the mandatory manner in which EBPs are marketed (see Cormier, Nurius, & Osborn, 2017, pp. 20–21, for further discussion).

Negative views of EBPs are therefore understandable, particularly when clinicians are required by their superiors (who may also represent sources of funding) to adopt a new skill set and to be monitored over a period of time to ensure fidelity or treatment compliance. Bohart (2005) accused advocates of EBPs as dictatorial because they restrict alternative practices. Indeed, he referred to the "hegemonic tendencies" of EBPs (p. 51) and has implied that this strong-arm approach is unethical. Depending on how EBPs are introduced to clinicians and how training and supervision are presented, clinicians may feel "manualized." It may be that Laurie, an experienced clinician introduced at the beginning of this chapter, may feel this way about her "assignment" of having to learn and practice MST under Dr. Bennett's supervision. This may be particularly true because she is expected to participate in MST training along with Leah, Laurie's new supervisee who is also new to the profession.

Although highly controversial, the focus on EBPs appears to have opened up lines of communication between practitioners and researchers, has prioritised care that is "in the best interest of the client," and has ushered in a more integrative perspective about client care. In addition, EBP has challenged clinicians to be more accountable in their practice. That is, simply following "intuition" when making practice decisions is no longer acceptable. Indeed, Reamer (2006) defined as "non-traditional and unorthodox" those interventions that are "not based on sound theory and research-based evidence" (p. 192) and argued that social workers who practise these interventions make themselves vulnerable to ethics complaints, lawsuits, and criminal charges. Falender and Shafranske's (2007) delineation of competency-based supervision is consistent with what we suspect is the increasing expectation for supervisor accountability.

Gambrill and Gibbs (2002) found that of a sample of social workers ($n=83$) and social work students (undergraduate and master's degree; $n=124$), the majority reported relying on intuition in making practice decisions (e.g., treatment planning with clients) rather than evidence- or science-based information, even after receiving training on integrating research into practice. Furthermore, the majority of this same sample acknowledged wanting their physician to make decisions about their medical care based on research findings rather than their (the physicians') intuition. Gambrill and Gibbs interpreted their findings to mean that "Social workers want their physicians to rely on scientific criteria when they make recommendations for treatment, but rely on weak evidentiary grounds such as tradition when working with clients...[or, in other words,] what's good for the goose is not viewed as good for the gander" (p. 39). This suggests that clinicians in the behavioural sciences (e.g., counselling, psychology) may have conflicting views of EBPs, believing that EBP may apply to the work of other professionals but not to their own work.

The emphasis on EBPs has at least two implications for the practice of clinical supervision. First, many if not the majority of EBPs seem to require some form of supervision to facilitate or ensure clinician proficiency in the EBP. This implies that supervisors are competent themselves in the EBP. It is unclear whether the supervisor of an EBP is required to receive training specifically in clinical supervision, and whether such training is separate from the EBP itself (i.e., training supervisors to provide training supervision). In multisystemic therapy (MST), it appears that supervisor training is specific to MST and that such training is provided by "MST consultants" (see Henggeler, Schoenwald, Liao, Letourneau, & Edwards, 2002).

A second implication of EBP in the practice of clinical supervision pertains to what may be the fracturing of clinical supervision due to the possible splintering of clinical practice itself. To explain what we mean by this we refer back to the case of Leah, Laurie, and Dr. Bennett presented at the beginning of this chapter. If Leah will be supervised by both Laurie and Dr. Bennett, how will the supervision she has received from both of them differ? If one will focus on her MST skills, what will the other supervision focus on – her overall professional skills, including clinical documentation, openness to supervision, collaboration and cooperation with colleagues? We wonder if Leah will be confused, not knowing who her "actual" or "ultimate" supervisor is and what she is expected to do. In addition, Laurie is an experienced clinician and is new to MST. By focusing specifically (and perhaps exclusively) on MST interventions, we wonder what effect this might have on her foundational skills, such as empathy. A concern might be that Laurie will be so focused on adhering to a specific skill set and protocol that certain pre-existing counsellor qualities (e.g., patience, positive regard) may suffer. This splintering may not be noticed or be of concern to Dr. Bennett if his primary focus is on ensuring that Laurie demonstrates proficiency in MST skills. Laurie's ongoing and holistic professional development – including working through ethical dilemmas that may not be specific to MST – and personal growth may therefore get overlooked.

Yet a third implication of EBP supervision is that just as EBPs have demonstrated effectiveness or even efficacy in research trials, so too may the supervision of EBPs need to demonstrate effectiveness beyond supervisee satisfaction or even supervisee competence. Although client improvement has long been proposed as the intended and defining outcome of clinical supervision, linking client improvement to supervision has proven difficult if not impossible. Supervisors of EBPs, however, may increasingly need to supply evidence that their work with clinicians yields beneficial results for clients. This is apparent in Henggeler et al.'s (2002) investigation of MST supervision in which families (i.e., clients) measured therapist effectiveness, therapists who were supervised by MST supervisors according to the MST supervision manual.

The entrée of EBP into the lexicon of counselling and psychotherapy practice will have additional implications for the practice of clinical supervision. Not only will supervisors need to be conversant – and perhaps proficient – in evidence-based *therapeutic* practices, they will need to demonstrate competence in supervision and practice according to certain evidence-based *supervisory* practices – practices that have not yet been established. Falender and Shafranske's (2007) discussion of competency-based supervision, however, may represent one effort toward determining such supervisory practices. One of their 12 recommendations for implementing competency-based supervision is that supervisors commit to practising supervision according to certain values, one of which is EBP (see p. 238). Furthermore, Milne (2007) offered a definition of supervision that he contends fulfils four criteria of empiricism (i.e., precise, specific, operational, and supported by research or corroboration): "The formal provision by senior/qualified health practitioners of an intensive relationship-based education and training that is case-focused and which supports, directs and guides the work of colleagues (supervisees)" (p. 438). These discussions in the supervision literature, coupled with increased emphasis on EBP in counselling and psychotherapy, will continue to influence how supervision is practised, and ethical issues are an integral part of this evolution.

Ethical issues in the supervision of evidence-based practices

Our discussion thus far of supervision of evidence-based practices (EBPs) has only hinted at specific ethical issues. In this section we briefly discuss five ethical issues related to the supervision of EBP: (a) purpose of supervision, (b) managing multiple relationships and interpersonal dynamics, (c) format of supervision, (d) supervisor qualifications and competence, and (e) evaluation. These do not exhaust the list of potential ethical issues but do serve to concentrate our discussion.

Purpose of supervision

Treatment fidelity is an essential aspect of any EBP. In ongoing research investigations, ensuring treatment fidelity (or construct validity) allows researchers to state with a certain degree of confidence that what was tested was indeed the actual treatment. Studies conducted on the supervision of certain EBPs have demonstrated that supervision does increase a clinician's proficiency with the specific skill set associated with an EBP. For example, Smith et al. (2007) reported that following a two-day training in the EBP of motivational interviewing (MI; Hettema, Steele, & Miller, 2005; Miller & Rollnick, 2013), clinicians who received individual supervision of five counselling sessions they conducted demonstrated an increase in MI-adherent behaviours (e.g., empathic reflections). Supervision in this study was conducted using a live and interactive teleconference format: MI supervisors wore a modified headset to allow them to hear the live counselling session and speak directly into an earpiece worn by the supervisee. During a mid-session break and at the conclusion of each counselling session, the supervisee and supervisor spoke directly to one another. Each clinician received a total of 7.5 hours of individual supervision and skill level was assessed at 20 weeks post-training and then three months later.

As already stated, it appears that a primary purpose of supervision of certain EBPs is to ensure clinician adherence to a specific EBP skill set. This focus could be viewed as *coercive* and also *exclusive*. By coercive we mean the practice of supervision that restricts supervisee and also supervisor innovation and creativity. Following a supervision manual may have this effect. Indeed, it seems somewhat ironic that EBPs could be accused of discouraging or even outright squelching innovation when most if not all EBPs began as innovative practices themselves, approaches that challenged or at least offered alternatives to the accepted standards of care at the time.

The focus of supervision of EBPs also appears to be exclusively on supervisee skill performance, which resembles the practice of "clinical monitoring" that participants in Rapisarda and Britton's (2007) study associated with sanctioned or remedial supervision.

In their review of the supervision literature, Morgan and Sprenkle (2007) identified several dimensions of or common factors in supervision, one being emphasis. They determined that the emphasis of supervision (primarily training supervision) appears to be on clinical competence (i.e., knowledge of and demonstrated skill in applying specific interventions, strategies) or professional competence (e.g., emotional management, personal growth, understanding and practice of ethical standards) or a combination of the two. They describe these emphases on a continuum, with clinical competence on one end and professional competence on the other. The purpose of supervision of EBPs is more than likely closer to the clinical competence endpoint than the professional competence endpoint. A concern with this exclusive focus is, as mentioned earlier, the potential oversight of a supervisee's professional development, such as his or her ability to work respectfully and constructively with other professionals. We believe that any type of supervision should not only be concerned with how well the supervisee is able to apply techniques that are consistent with an EBP; supervision should also attend to and encourage supervisee personal growth.

Such a "happy medium" may be the purpose of at least one EBP – dialectical behaviour therapy (DBT). As mentioned earlier in the chapter, supervision or consultation in DBT is not only intended to ensure that clients are receiving quality care but that counsellors are also being cared for (see Lynch et al., 2007). Weekly DBT consultation meetings often include practising self-care strategies (e.g., deep breathing, mindfulness exercises) and communication strategies (e.g., striving to be "radically genuine" with other members of the consultation team), the same strategies taught to and practised with clients in DBT. It could be said, therefore, that the purpose of DBT supervision is to achieve and maintain a balance of both clinical competence and professional competence. This balance itself seems to be consistent with dialectical philosophy and practice wherein a synthesis of acceptance and change is achieved. An ethical issue arises, however, when DBT supervision is more like therapy than consultation.

Managing multiple relationships and interpersonal dynamics

Managing multiple relationships is an ethical issue in any type of supervision and refers to the interactions between supervisor and supervisee, as well as relationships both parties have with others in the execution of counselling and supervision (e.g., clients, clinical director, other supervisees who are members of the same consultation team or supervision group). These professional relationships can be compromised, and ethical concerns raised when personal interests become primary. An extreme example of this is when supervisors and supervisees engage in a sexual relationship with each other. Due to the inherently hierarchical nature of most types of supervision (specifically training, sanctioned, and targeted/skill-specific supervision), the ethical issue may be how the supervisor uses or exerts his or her power in interactions with the supervisee and reciprocally, how the supervisee responds to or operates within this power dynamic. Moreover, these interactions are influenced by the predominant or preferred power base from which the supervisor operates.

Power can be thought of as the potential and actual influence that a supervisor has on a supervisee. Robyak, Goodyear, and Prange (1987) applied three types of power to supervision that Strong and Matross (1973) had originally applied to the therapeutic relationship. *Legitimate power* refers to the supervisor's sanctioned or designated position and the supervisee's perceived trustworthiness of the person in this role. Dr. Bennett, the assigned multisystemic therapy (MST) supervisor mentioned earlier in the chapter, may be thought to have legitimate power by virtue of his contract with Horizons, the facility that hired him for his expertise in MST. *Referent power* derives from the supervisor's interpersonal style and the supervisee's attraction to, resonance with, or agreement with the supervisor's values, opinions, experiences, or practices. Dr. Bennett's referent power will depend on his personal qualities and how he facilitates his interactions with Laura and Leah, particularly in group MST supervision. The third type of power, *expert power*, would be based on Dr. Bennett's advanced or specialized knowledge and skills in MST. Although Dr. Bennett may be knowledgeable in MST, his success as an MST supervisor may be evaluated by Laura and Leah according to how well he is able to assist them in learning and applying MST to their clients; that is, his supervisory knowledge and skills.

Gottlieb, Robinson, and Younggren (2007) reinforced the notion that multiple relationships are to be expected in supervision and should not be avoided unequivocally. This is true for Dr. Bennett, Laura, and Leah. Dr. Bennett is a former professor of Leah's and is now her assigned MST supervisor. Because Leah is a new counsellor at Horizons, Laura has been assigned as her internal supervisor and has 12 years more experience in mental health than Leah. Laura and Leah, however, attended the five-day MST training together and are now members of the same MST treatment team and supervision group at Horizons. In this sense, they may be considered equals. Laura is new to MST and therefore is not able to supervise Leah's MST application. For these three to be able to work together effectively, and for client care not to be compromised, Dr. Bennett and Laura may need to agree and collaborate on a distribution of power or, more precisely, how each will use his or her power as a supervisor. It may be that Dr. Bennett's power will be restricted to or prioritised as his MST expertise, whereas Laura's power will derive from her clinical mental health experience and her familiarity with Horizons and the clients and families served at the agency. It appears that Dr. Bennett's power will be time-limited (at least six months), whereas Laura's power as Leah's supervisor will extend beyond that time.

Format of supervision

Henggeler et al. (2002) suggested that "The effective transport of evidence-based models might require a major shift in current mental health supervisory and quality-assurance practices" (p. 165). This shift may include ongoing rather than time-limited supervision (consistent with DBT supervision), conducting group supervision as standard practice rather than individual supervision (consistent with MST and DBT supervision), and incorporating other means of interactions to typical face-to-face supervisory communication (e.g., live teleconference supervision; Smith et al., 2007).

The importance of ongoing supervision in learning a new skill set associated with an EBP has been suggested in studies of motivational interviewing (MI). Miller, Yahne, Moyers, Martinez, and Pirritano (2004) found an increase in MI skill proficiency among clinicians who participated in up to six 30-minute individual telephone "coaching sessions" following a two-day MI training. Schoener, Madeja, Henderson, Ondersma, and Janisse (2006) reported similar findings in their study of therapists who received approximately eight bi-weekly small group supervision sessions following a two-day MI training. The results from these and other MI supervision studies (e.g., Mastroleo, Magill, Barnett, & Borsari, 2014; Smith et al., 2007) indicate that post-training supervision in an EBP is a critical component for skill retention. Indeed, in Miller et al.'s study, clinicians who attended the two-day workshop but did not receive supervision actually demonstrated *diminished* MI skill levels at four, eight, and 12 months after the two-day training, essentially erasing skills learned at the workshop.

The need for ongoing supervision of an EBP beyond initial training may be explained by Heaven et al.'s (2006) study of clinical nurse specialists in the United Kingdom. Although the nurses received training in communication skills and not an EBP, the results are consistent with those of MI supervision research. Specifically, nurses who received 12 hours of supervision over four weeks after a three-day training improved their use of specific communication skills (i.e., open questions, negotiation, psychological exploration, and response to cues) from baseline (pre-workshop) to one month after supervision had concluded. When compared to nurses who did not receive supervision, however, there was no evidence of transfer of skills. Heaven et al. (2006) explained that some of the nurses were "deeply embedded in a philosophy of care that was diametrically opposed to the model being taught" (pp. 322–323) and supervisors lacked time to challenge in a supportive fashion these "entrenched defences" (p. 323). They speculated that "a longer period of supervision "would have [provided] an opportunity to challenge more entrenched longstanding beliefs" (p. 323).

Although ongoing supervision – and specifically group supervision – may be essential to attain proficiency in an EBP, ethical issues arise in coordinating services. For example, if MST supervision would continue beyond the first six months, would Dr. Bennett remain the MST supervisor? How would the ongoing supervision he provided, then, differ from the supervision Laura would be providing to Leah? In addition, group supervision may offer counsellors additional support from fellow counsellors, but may not provide the individualised training necessary, particularly when certain counsellors struggle with mastering specific skills. Furthermore, confidentiality in group supervision requires more careful attention than in individual supervision, although the use of additional means of communication (e.g., telephone consultation, live teleconferencing) also extends the parameters of confidentiality.

Carter (2005) described the use of a technology-mediated managed learning environment for the supervision of student teachers enrolled in practicum in Australia. Digital cameras allowed the university-based supervisor to view and collect "visual data of classroom events" (p. 487) but it is not clear how supervisory feedback was provided to the student teachers. Varied forms of technology clearly have the capacity to expand the nature of supervisory practice, particularly for the purpose of disseminating or transferring EBP from training room to counselling room. Clinicians with expertise in certain EBPs are able to provide supervision from a distance, thus augmenting or even replacing on-site supervision. Although technology affords innumerable possibilities for the supervision of EBP, ethical issues (e.g., confidentiality) must always be considered and evidence supporting technology-mediated distance supervision for supervisee skills enhancement and client wellbeing is still lacking.

Supervisor qualifications and competence

A fourth ethical issue in the supervision of EBPs pertains to supervisor competence. As discussed earlier, supervisors of EBPs such as MST, DBT, and MI need to have attained a certain level of proficiency as MST, DBT, or MI counsellors. However, skill level as a *supervisor* of an EBP remains unclear. What skills are necessary for a supervisor beyond those of counsellor proficiency in an EBP? Henggeler et al. (2002) described the MST *Supervisor Adherence Measure* (*SAM*), a means for therapists to assess MST supervisor skills on three factors: (a) the extent to which supervision emphasised the primary underpinnings of MST, (b) the extent to which the supervisor attempted to build the MST-related competencies of therapists, and (c) the supervisor's knowledge and skill in MST and EBP intervention modalities. Their investigation of 12 MST supervisors who provided supervision to 74 MST therapists working with 285 youth and their families determined that only MST supervisors' knowledge of MST principles (one of the three factors of the *SAM*) predicted only two of three MST therapist skills: ability to collaborate with families and assess family progress. These findings raise questions about MST supervisor skills *as a supervisor*, and that simply being knowledgeable in MST principles does not make one an effective MST supervisor. It may be that supervision training and practice in only one model of supervision – and a model developed solely from a specific model of therapy – may actually restrict supervisory competencies and stifle further supervisor development.

Falender and Shafranske (2012) included the practice of self-assessment and a commitment to scientific knowledge and methods evidence-based practice among their seven foundational competencies of supervision. Determining supervisor competence, however, will continue to remain problematic in the absence of empirical support.

Evaluation

Evaluation has been referred to as "one of the key definitional features of clinical supervision" (Watkins, 1997, p. 611). Bernard and Goodyear (2014) consider evaluation central to clinical supervision and listed "evaluative" as the first of three characteristics of the supervisory relationship. Holloway (1995) listed "monitoring/evaluating" as the first of five functions of the supervisor. Evaluation is therefore considered an inherent feature of supervision and a function of the counsellor supervisor that cannot be avoided.

In the supervision of EBP, however, what is being evaluated and who gets to evaluate? Henggeler et al. (2002) described the *Therapist Adherence Measure (TAM)* specific to MST and designed to be completed by clients (i.e., family members with whom the MST counsellor is working). It assesses three MST therapist skill areas: (a) ability to establish agreement with families on problems to address and collaborate with families to address these problems, (b) ability to change family interactions, and (c) ability to follow-through on treatment progress. Supervisors could assess supervisee technical performance (i.e., ability to implement MST interventions) with each family unit the supervisee is responsible for, but such an evaluation is limited to clinical competence rather than professional competence, a distinction that Morgan and Sprenkle (2007) discussed. It also limited to client perspectives of therapist proficiency and thus does not include supervisor assessment. The exclusive reliance on the TAM may therefore not provide a complete picture of an MST therapist's competence as a mental health professional.

In the supervision of EBPs, we recommend that counsellors be evaluated clinically as well as professionally. By this we mean that a supervisee's ability to adhere to a specific treatment protocol (i.e., perform specified technical skills) should only be part of the evaluation. A more comprehensive evaluation should also be considered, such as Fall and Sutton's (2004) 102-item *Supervisee Performance Assessment Instrument*. In addition to assessing supervisee intervention skills, this instrument evaluates supervisees on their conceptualisation skills, personalisation skills, professional behaviour, and supervision skills. Supervisees would thereby benefit from more extensive feedback.

Ethics in action: Developing and maintaining written supervision contracts

There are clearly ethical issues in any type of supervision conducted. The supervision of evidence-based practices (EBPs) has introduced new ethical issues to the practice of supervision or, more accurately, has generated additional and alternative perspectives about ethical practice not encountered in training supervision.

To maintain ethical practice in the supervision of EBPs, we recommend the use of a written supervision contract. Hewson (1999) described contracting in supervision as possibly "the most important task engaged in by supervisor and supervisee" (p. 81) and Storm (1997) referred to the contract as the "blueprint" for the supervision relationship. Falender and Shafranske (2007) proposed that the development of a supervisory agreement or contract signifies competency-based supervision. Contracting for supervision also appears consistent with Gonsalvez, Oades, and Freestone's (2002) objectives approach to supervision (i.e., formulating supervisor and supervisee objectives) and parallels the ethical standards (Codes 3.4.b. and 3.8.c.) of the Australian Counselling Association (2015) that counsellors contract with clients for counselling.

We believe that establishing a written supervision contract is critical in any supervisory arrangement but is particularly necessary in the culture of accountability that EBPs represent. Specifically, a written supervision contract clarifies the services to be provided, the roles and responsibilities of all parties involved, the purpose and length of supervision, and the supervisory procedures (e.g., frequency, format), including evaluation. Documenting in writing at the beginning of a supervisory arrangement these and other elements of supervision and then reviewing adherence to the contract at certain periods of time could be one measure of supervision effectiveness. Contracting for supervision can also be viewed as a quality assurance measure, thereby applying a value of EBPs to the practice of supervision. One way that the use of a contract may exemplify quality is in its function of opening up lines of communication. Nelson and Friedlander (2001) reported that most conflict occurs due to opposing expectations between supervisor and supervisee about what should take place in the supervision relationship (e.g., confusion over who was in charge, who would be evaluating). In light of this, Thomas (2007) suggested that the use of a written supervision contract could serve to curtail misunderstandings or at least lessen the extent or intensity of conflict between the supervisor and supervisee.

Although several examples of written supervision agreements exist (e.g., Haynes, Corey, & Mouton, 2003; Sutter, McPherson, & Geeseman, 2002), we are most familiar with and have routinely used the format we designed several years ago (Osborn & Davis, 1996). A current example is included in Bernard and Goodyear's (2014) book, on pages 305–307.

There are six sections of the supervision contract. The first section outlines the purpose, goals, and objectives of supervision. The second section describes the context of supervision services and includes when and how often supervision will take place, as well as the method the supervisor will use to monitor the supervisee's performance (e.g., live supervision).

The third section clarifies how the supervisee will be evaluated and refers to both formative and summative evaluations. We recommend that when the supervisor reviews the initial contract with supervisees in the first supervision session, each supervisee receive a copy of the actual evaluation form that the supervisor will use when conducting summative evaluations. In MST supervision, this may be the *Therapist Adherence Measure*. In motivational interviewing, this may include the *Motivational Interviewing Treatment*

Integrity (*MITI* 4.2) coding manual (Moyers, Manuel, & Ernst, 2014) or the *Motivational Interviewing Skill Code* (*MISC* 2.1; Miller, Moyers, Ernst, & Amrhein, 2008). The remaining three sections of the written supervision contract are separate listings of the supervisor's and supervisee's duties and responsibilities (including three or four supervisee learning objectives), procedural considerations (e.g., emergency procedures and contact, record keeping, process for addressing supervisor–supervisee disagreement), and the supervisor's competencies or scope of practice.

In the supervision of EBPs, a written supervision contract can serve to clarify the exact purpose and nature of supervision, the length and frequency of supervisory contact, the duties and responsibilities of the assigned supervisor, and what is expected of the supervisee. In the case of Dr. Bennett, Laura, and Leah, a written supervision contract could delineate Dr. Bennett's supervisory responsibilities and Laura's supervisory responsibilities. It could also explain when individual supervision would be indicated, what protocol to follow in crisis and other emergency situations, who at Horizons or Ignite would be consulted in the event of differences of opinion or outright conflict, and any expectations of professional competence in addition to skill or technical proficiency. The method of determining supervisee skills and competence should be included in the contract (e.g., live observation, supervisee self-report, client report), as well as a description of the format of supervision (e.g., group, telephone contact). In the case of Dr. Bennett, Laura, and Leah, we would recommend that one written supervision contract be drafted that all three persons would contribute to and eventually sign off on. Rather than having separate contracts for each supervisory dyad, one contract for all three would help to foster cohesion and collaboration and would also be consistent with the standard group supervision format of MST.

We believe the development and incorporation of a written contract in clinical supervision promotes ethical practice. It can be considered a tangible example of ethical principles in action. From our own use of a contract with supervisees, we believe its intent is to embody the six ethical principles outlined in the Preamble of the American Counseling Association's (ACA, 2014) *ACA Code of Ethics*: autonomy, nonmaleficence, beneficence, justice (treating individuals equitably and fostering fairness), fidelity (honouring commitments and keeping promises), and veracity (dealing truthfully with individuals). The use of a contract may also signify the supervisor's commitment to competency-based supervision, as defined by Falender and Shafranske (2007).

Conclusion

Targeted and skill-specific supervision is a type of supervision rendered when counsellors are delivering an evidence-based practice (EBP). It is a relatively new type of supervision that has been a required component of clinical trials testing EBPs. Although its primary purpose is to ensure counsellor adherence or fidelity to the therapeutic approach, we believe this type of supervision must also consider the professional competence of supervisees, especially if supervision is ongoing, as in dialectical behaviour therapy.

Ethical issues common in other types of supervision (e.g., training supervision) are also present in the supervision of EBPs. However, the nature, purpose, and format of EBP supervision highlight certain ethical issues not encountered in other types of supervision. To promote ethical practice, we recommend the use of a written supervision contract, which can serve as a quality assurance measure consistent with the culture of accountability associated with EBPs.

Educational questions & activities

1. What is the standard form of Supervision for MST?
2. In Bernard and Goodyear's definition of clinical supervision what is made explicit?
3. Two themes were captured by supervisors from one midwestern state in the United States who had provided sanctioned supervision to at least one counsellor in the past year. What were they?
4. What are the five ethical issues related to the supervision of EBP that are briefly discussed in this Chapter?
5. In EBP supervisors need skills beyond those of being a counsellor. The MST Supervisor Adherence Measure (SAM) measures three factors, what are these?

References

American Counseling Association (2014). *ACA code of ethics*. Alexandria, VA: Author.

APA Presidential Task Force on Evidence-Based Practice. (2006). Evidence-based practice in psychology. *American Psychologist, 61*, 271–285.

Australian Counselling Association (2015). *Code of conduct*. Grange Qld, Australia: Author. Retrieved July 3, 2016, from www.theaca.net.au/documents

Bernard, J. M., & Goodyear, R. K. (2014). *Fundamentals of clinical supervision* (5th ed.). Upper Saddle River, NJ: Pearson Education.

Binder, J. L., & Strupp, H. H. (1997). Supervision of psychodynamic psychotherapies. In C. E. Watkins (Ed.), *Handbook of psychotherapy supervision* (pp. 44–62). New York: John Wiley.

Bohart, A. C. (2005). Evidence-based psychotherapy means evidence-informed, not evidence-driven. *Journal of Contemporary Psychotherapy, 35*, 39–53.

Borders, L. D. (1991). A systematic approach to peer group supervision. *Journal of Counseling & Development, 69*, 248–252.

British Association for Counselling and Psychotherapy (2013). *Ethical framework for good practice in counselling and psychotherapy*. Leicestershire, United Kingdom: Author. Retrieved July 3, 2016, from www.bacp.co.uk

Carter, D. (2005). Distributed practicum supervision in a managed learning environment (MLE). *Teachers and Teaching: Theory and Practice, 11*, 481–497.

Cobia, D. C., & Pipes, R. B. (2002). Mandated supervision: An intervention for disciplined professionals. *Journal of Counseling & Development, 80*, 140–144.

Cormier, S., Nurius, P. S., & Osborn, C. J. (2017). *Interviewing and change strategies for helpers* (8th ed.). Boston, MA: Cengage Learning.

Falender, C. A., & Shafranske, E. P. (2007). Competence in competency-based supervision practice: Construct and application. *Professional Psychology: Research and Practice, 38*, 232–240.

Falender, C. A., & Shafrnaske, E. P. (2012). *Getting the most out of clinical training and supervision: A guide for practicum students and interns*. Washington, DC: American Psychological Association.

Fall, M., & Sutton, Jr., J. M. (2004). *Clinical supervision: A handbook for practitioners*. Boston: Pearson Education.

Fruzzetti, A. E., Waltz, J. A., & Linehan, M. M. (1997). Supervision in dialectical behavior therapy. In C. E. Watkins, Jr. (Ed.), *Handbook of psychotherapy supervision* (pp. 84–100). New York: Wiley.

Gambrill, E., & Gibbs, L. (2002). Making practice decisions: Is what's good for the goose good for the gander? *Ethical Human Sciences and Services, 4*, 31–46.

Gonsalvez, C. J., Oades, L. G., & Freestone, J. (2002). The objectives approach to clinical supervision: Towards integration and empirical evaluation. *Australian Psychologist, 37,* 68–77.

Gottlieb, M. C., Robinson, K., & Younggren, J. N. (2007). Multiple relations in supervision: Guidance for administrators, supervisors, and students. *Professional Psychology: Research and Practice, 38,* 241–247.

Gould, L. J., & Bradley, L. J. (2001). Evaluation in supervision. In L. J. Bradley & N. Ladany (Eds.), *Counselor supervision: Principles, process, and practice* (3rd ed., pp. 271–303). Philadelphia: Brunner-Routledge.

Granello, D. H., Kindsvatter, A., Granello, P. F., Underfer-Babalis, J., & Hartwig Moorhead, H. J. (2008). Multiple perspectives in supervision: Using a peer consultation model to enhance supervisor development. *Counselor Education and Supervision, 48,* 32–47.

Haynes, R., Corey, G., & Moulton, P. (2003). *Clinical supervision in the helping professions: A practical guide.* Pacific Grove, CA: Brooks/Cole-Thomson Learning.

Heaven, C., Clegg, J., & Maguire, P. (2006). Transfer of communication skills training from workshop to workplace: The impact of clinical supervision. *Patient Education and Counseling, 60,* 313–325.

Henggeler, S. W., & Borduin, C. M. (1990). *Family therapy and beyond: A multisystemic approach to treating the behavior problems of children and adolescents.* Pacific Grove, CA: Brooks/Cole.

Henggeler, S. W., & Schoenwald, S. K. (1998). *Multisystemic therapy supervisory manual: Promoting quality assurance at the clinical level.* Charleston, SC: MST Institute.

Henggeler, S. W., Schoenwald, S. K., Borduin, C. M., Rowland, M. D., & Cunningham, P. B. (2009). *Multisystemic therapy for antisocial behavior in children and adolescents* (2nd ed.). New York: Guilford Press.

Henggeler, S. W., Schoenwald, S. K., Liao, J. G., Letourneau, E. J., & Edwards, D. L. (2002). Transporting efficacious treatments to field settings: The link between supervisory practices and therapist fidelity in MST programs. *Journal of Clinical Child Psychology, 31,* 155–167.

Hettema, J., Steele, J., & Miller, W. R. (2005). Motivational interviewing. *Annual Review of Clinical Psychology, 1,* 91–111.

Hewson, J. (1999). Training supervisors to contract in supervision. In E. Holloway & M. Carroll (Eds.), *Training counselling supervisors: Strategies, methods and techniques* (pp. 67–91). London: Sage.

Holloway, E. (1995). *Clinical supervision: A systems approach.* Thousand Oaks, CA: Sage.

Kress, V. E., O'Neill, R. M., Protivnak, J. J., Stargell, N. A., & Herman, E. R. (2015). A qualitative study of supervisors' reflections on providing sanctioned supervision. *The Clinical Supervisor, 34,* 38–56.

Ladany, N., Ellis, M. V., & Friedlander, M. L. (1999). The supervisory working alliance, trainee self-efficacy, and satisfaction. *Journal of Counseling & Development, 77,* 447–455.

Linehan, M. M. (2015). *DBT skills training manual* (2nd ed.). New York: Guilford Press.

Linehan, M. M., Comtois, K. A., Murray, A. M., Brown, M. Z., Gallop, R. J., Heard, H. L., et al. (2006). Two-year randomized controlled trial and follow-up of dialectical behavior therapy vs. therapy by experts for suicidal behaviors and borderline personality disorder. *Archives of General Psychiatry, 63,* 757–766.

Lynch, T. R., Trost, W. T., Salsman, N., & Linehan, M. M. (2007). Dialectical behavior therapy for borderline personality disorder. *Annual Review of Clinical Psychology, 3,* 181–205.

Mastroleo, N. R., Magill, M., Barnett, N. P., & Borsari, B. (2014). A pilot study of two supervision approaches for peer-led alcohol interventions with mandated college students. *Journal of Studies of Alcohol and Drugs, 75,* 458–466.

McAuliffe, D., & Sudbery, J. (2005). Who do I tell? Support and consultation in cases of ethical conflict. *Journal of Social Work, 5,* 21–43.

Miller, W. R., Moyers, T. B., Ernst, D., & Amrhein, P. (2008). *Manual for the motivational interviewing skill code (MISC, Version 2.1).* Retrieved September 5, 2008, from https://motivationalinterviewing.org/sites/default/files/MISC2.pdf

Miller, W. R., & Rollnick, S. (2013). *Motivational interviewing: Helping people change* (3rd ed.). New York: Guilford Press.

Miller, W. R., Yahne, C. E., Moyers, T. B., Martinez, J., & Pirritano, M. (2004). A randomized trial of methods to help clinicians learn motivational interviewing. *Journal of Consulting and Clinical Psychology, 72,* 1050–1062.

Milne, D. (2007). An empirical definition of clinical supervision. *British Journal of Clinical Psychology, 46,* 437–447.

Morgan, M. M., & Sprenkle, D. H. (2007). Toward a common-factors approach to supervision. *Journal of Marital and Family Therapy, 33,* 1–17.

Moyers, T. B., Manuel, J. K., & Ernst, D. (2014). *Motivational interviewing treatment integrity coding manual 4.1.* Retrieved July 3, 2016 from http://casaa.unm.edu/download/MITI4_2.pdf

Nelson, M. L., Barnes, K. L., Evans, A. L., & Triggiano, P. J. (2008). Working with conflict in clinical supervision: Wise supervisors' perspectives. *Journal of Counseling Psychology, 55,* 172–184.

Nelson, M. L., & Friedlander, M. L. (2001). A close look at conflictual supervisory relationships: The trainee's perspectives. *Journal of Counseling Psychology, 48,* 384–395.

Norrie, J., Eggleston, E., & Ringer, M. (2003). Quality parameters of supervision in a correctional context. *New Zealand Journal of Psychology, 32,* 76–83.

Osborn, C. J., & Davis, T. E. (1996). The supervision contract: Making it perfectly clear. *The Clinical Supervisor, 14*(2), 121–134.

Pretorius, W. M. (2006). Cognitive behavioural therapy supervision: Recommended practice. *Behavioural and Cognitive Psychotherapy, 34,* 413–420.

Rapisarda, C. A., & Britton, P. J. (2007). Sanctioned supervision: Voices from the experts. *Journal of Mental Health Counseling, 29,* 81–92.

Reamer, F. G. (2006). Nontraditional and unorthodox interventions in social work: Ethical and legal implications. *Families in Society, 87,* 191–197.

Robyak, J. E., Goodyear, R. K., & Prange, M. (1987). Effects of supervisors' sex, focus, and experience on preferences for interpersonal power bases. *Counselor Education and Supervision, 26,* 299–309.

Schoener, E. P., Madeja, C. L., Henderson, M. J., Ondersma, S. J., & Janisse, J. J. (2006). Effects of motivational interviewing training on mental health therapist behavior. *Drug and Alcohol Dependence, 82,* 269–275.

Smith, J. L., Amrhein, P. C., Brooks, A. C., Carpenter, K. M., Levin, D., Schreiber, E. A., et al. (2007). Providing live supervision via teleconferencing improves acquisition of motivational interviewing skills after workshop attendance. *American Journal of Drug and Alcohol Abuse, 33,* 163–168.

Storm, C. L. (1997). The blueprint for supervision relationships: Contracts. In T. C. Todd & C. L. Storm (Eds.), *The complete systemic supervisor: Context, philosophy, and pragmatics* (pp. 272–282). Boston: Allyn and Bacon.

Strong, S. R., & Matross, R. P. (1973). Change processes in counseling and psychotherapy. *Journal of Counseling Psychology, 20,* 25–37.

Sutter, E., McPherson, R. H., & Geeseman, R. (2002). Contracting for supervision. *Professional Psychology: Research and Practice, 33,* 495–498.

Thomas, J. T. (2007). Informed consent through contracting for supervision: Minimizing risks, enhancing benefits. *Professional Psychology: Research and Practice, 38,* 221–231.

Watkins, C. E. (1997). Some concluding thoughts about psychotherapy supervision. In C. E. Watkins (Ed.), *Handbook of psychotherapy supervision* (pp. 603–616). New York: John Wiley.

5   When Psychotherapy Becomes a Matter of Life and Death

Supervision for Suicide Prevention

Helen Stallman

Background

Psychotherapists who work with people with suicidality often have two main fears. Firstly, the healthcare consumer may die, and, secondly, if the person dies, the therapist will be held responsible for the death by themself, the organisation, the family of the person who died, or the coroner (Farberow, 2005). The first of these, fear for the consumer's life, may inadvertently harm the consumer when the therapist tries to manage risk and try to make the consumer safe rather than using the interaction with the consumer to meet their needs for support, interpersonal connectedness, and care that can prevent suicide (Stallman, 2018). The fear of blame is based on suicide-related stigma—the deeply embedded cultural judgements about suicide (Keller, McNeill, Honea, & Paulson Miller, 2019). These fears can make suicide prevention therapy stressful and affect outcomes.

The Health Theory of Coping conceptualises coping strategies as either healthy or unhealthy (Stallman, 2020a). Both healthy and unhealthy coping strategies are likely to reduce acute distress; but unhealthy coping strategies may also have unwanted adverse consequences. Categories of coping strategies can be conceptualised on a Coping Continuum (Figure 5.1) from low-intensity to high-intensity and low harm to high harm. Unhealthy coping strategies are used when healthy coping strategies are overwhelmed, not in the absence of healthy coping strategies (Stallman, Beaudequin, Hermens, & Eisenberg, 2021). Asking for professional support is a strength and healthy coping strategy, irrespective of the use of unhealthy coping strategies, including suicidality. The therapist's role is to meet the need for additional social support to reduce distress and be a buffer against death.

Care Collaborate Connect is a consumer-centred approach to suicide prevention that attends to the needs of the person asking for help (Stallman, 2018; Stallman & Allen, 2021). It differs from traditional approaches that rely on calculating the probability of a future event (risk) that has poor validity (Franklin et al., 2017). Care Collaborate Connect is the only strengths- and needs-based acute suicide prevention counselling approach (Stallman & Allen, 2021), that is, it attends to the needs for additional support by the person sharing suicidal ideation, rather than the needs or desires of the helper. It recognises sharing thoughts and feelings as a healthy coping strategy. Care Collaborate Connect is the first step in suicide prevention—attending to acute distress—followed later by an assessment of the drivers of overwhelming distress and evidence-based interventions for the drivers of distress (Stallman, 2020c). These may be environmental (physical, social, cultural, economic), developmental deficits (healthy identity, emotional and behavioural regulation, interpersonal skills, problem-solving skills), sense of belonging, health behaviours (sleep,

DOI: 10.4324/9781003490067-7

Coping continuum

Unpleasant emotions		Distress		Overwhelming distress				
COPING								
Healthy				Unhealthy				
Self-soothing	Relaxation/ distraction	Social support	Professional support	Negative self-talk	Harmful activities	Social withdrawal	Suicidality	
Coping self-talk paced breathing mindful awareness crying	Activities that are personally relaxing or briefly distracting	Friends, family, community	Trusted healthcare professionals	Negative thoughts about self, others, future, suppression, rumination	Eating sleeping aggression (verbal or physical) alcohol drugs self-harm	Cease doing regular work, recreation or social activities	Thoughts actions	Death
Low-intensity			High-intensity	Low harm				High harm

Figure 5.1 Coping continuum (Stallman, 2019)

nutrition, exercise, pleasurable and mastery activities), perception of innate resilience or effective treatment of illnesses (Stallman, 2018, 2020c).

Two primary supervision foci—restorative and formative (Milne, 2009)—can improve consumer outcomes and therapist experience in suicide prevention. Restorative supervision encourages emotional processing and reflection. Formative supervision involves facilitating counsellor competence, capability, and effectiveness. Supervision can include each at different times or both in the same supervision session. Restorative supervision always comes before formative supervision, when needed, as emotion impairs cognitive functioning and, therefore, needs to be addressed before reflection and learning. This chapter will review supervision strategies to improve the content and process of psychotherapy suicide prevention.

Supervision

Support

When a therapist is upset about suicidality or death by suicide—or indeed any issue—the supervisor's immediate tasks are Care, Collaborate, and Connect. The first step is to make time and Care. Allow the therapist time to explore and express emotions they are feeling (e.g., sad, anger, shame, guilt, worry) and the thoughts driving those emotions. Provide empathy and validation.

When the therapist feels calmer, help them reflect on their thoughts and emotions. Use Socratic questioning to help them challenge unhelpful or stigma-based thoughts. Notice the responsiveness of the therapist to thought-challenging. This may be an opportunity for the therapist to reflect on any cognitive dissonance of using a coping framework with consumers but a stigma-based framework themselves.

Collaborate with the therapist to explore how they have been coping with their distress and their plans to cope after the supervision session. Assess their needs for additional professional support and explore the therapist's thoughts about accessing professional support, if needed. Make them aware that you will follow up with them and when you will do that, for example, later the same day, the next day, or in a few days, as appropriate.

Follow up with the therapist to monitor their thoughts, emotions, and coping and provide appropriate support as needed. Be aware of unhealthy coping behaviours that may indicate overwhelming distress, including negative self-talk (doubts about skills and competence, blame), harmful activities (e.g., irritability with others, emotional eating, alcohol, drugs, self-harm), social withdrawal, or suicidality or mention of reduced health behaviours (sleep, nutrition, exercise). These indicate the need for professional support to help them cope with their distress in addition to supervision.

In the case of a death by suicide, take steps to ensure that a coping narrative is used in documentation and discussions with others, including the organisation and family of the deceased. Destigmatising suicide potentially reduces secondary stressors on the therapist from criticism and blame from other staff or academic faculty criticism.

Knowledge

Active skills training in Care Collaborate Connect (Stallman, 2019) is needed to provide consumer-centred care for distress and suicidality. Training helps the therapist learn a) a biopsychosocial model of health and wellbeing, b) the differences between consumer-centred care and risk and safety frameworks, c) how overwhelming distress fits within the continuum of coping strategies, and d) how to use Care Collaborate Connect skills in psychotherapy.

Further training in bereavement resilience (Stallman, 2021) provides psychotherapists with knowledge about how language affects distress and coping after a death by suicide and why some people may be more vulnerable to suicidality when someone they know dies by suicide (Stallman, 2023). Bereavement resilience helps prevent adverse outcomes for the therapist after a death by suicide (Farberow, 2005) and the knowledge to support consumers to prevent overwhelming distress and suicidality in those bereaved.

Suggestions for further reading are provided at the end of this chapter for therapists to cement their understanding of underlying theory and practice (Stallman, 2020a, 2020c; Stallman et al., 2021).

Modelling

Modelling is an important teaching tool, particularly when changing a deeply entrenched social stigma about suicide that is perpetuated through language. Modelling can include routinely and consistently using a) Care Collaborate Connect when the therapist is upset, b) non-stigmatising language, and c) consumer-centred conceptualisations.

The word *consumer* is used throughout this chapter to focus attention on the needs of the person seeking a service rather than on the service provider. The terms *client* and *patient* are therapist-centred. The word *my* implicitly precedes each of these words—*my consumer, my patient*—denoting ownership. Table 5.1 gives some examples of consumer-centred language supervisors can use routinely to develop a consumer-centred supervision space. The greater exposure to consumer-centred language and thinking, the more likely therapists will adopt the language and translate it into therapeutic practice.

Discussions

Supervision discussions can help clarify, reinforce, and challenge therapists to enhance their understanding of the Health Theory of Coping, needs-based support, suicide prevention

Table 5.1 Unhelpful and helpful suicide prevention language

Unhelpful	Helpful
mental health problems	overwhelmed, upset, distressed or the actual name of a psychiatric disorder e.g., Major Depressive Disorder
anxious, depressed	worried, sad, frustrated, annoyed, disappointed
suicidal, not coping, at-risk	distressed, upset, coping
failed suicide attempt	suicide attempt
committed suicide, killed himself	died by suicide

strategies, and stigma. The use of analogy can be helpful at times. Comparing a death by suicide to death by a heart attack, for example, is a useful strategy to identify stigma. If thoughts or language would differ between the two causes of death, they are likely to be stigmatising. For example, someone was to blame, or the person was selfish for causing their death.

Role-plays

Role-plays can help therapists practise applying the knowledge gained in training to enhance their therapeutic and communication skills (Rønning & Bjørkly, 2019). Role-playing in supervised groups can promote reflection and insight for those in the consumer and therapist roles and peers observing role-plays. Role-plays facilitate helper–consumer equality (needed for consumer-centred care) and increase involvement, self-efficacy, and empathy(Rønning & Bjørkly, 2019).

Videotaping can increase the precision of evaluating competencies and refining actual practice rather than perceived practice. Videotaped sessions provide a space to reflect on one's own experience and the consumer's experience. By watching one's practice as an observer, the therapist can reflect on specific therapy moments to consider their thoughts, their practice, the needs of the consumer at that moment, and the consumer's experience of the therapist's verbal and non-verbal behaviour. The supervisor can identify and highlight moments that the therapist might have overlooked.

Key role-plays to practise to develop and refine Care Collaborate Connect competencies are:

1. Care. The competency to practise here is to listen with the sole purpose of understanding the cause of distress and validate and normalise experiences until their distress is reduced or resolved.
2. Collaborate. The two essential skills to practise are 1) making a smooth transition between Care and Collaborate, for example, "How do you cope when you feel so worried?" and 2) conducting a coping assessment and coping planning comprehensively and without repeating content.
3. Connect. The two skills to practise for this competency are 1) collaboratively identifying the consumer's needs for additional professional support and 2) working collaboratively with consumers with moderate or high needs for additional professional support who are reluctant to use adequate professional support.

4. Discussing a death by suicide. This competency involves 1) providing a coping-based cause of death; 2) using Socratic questioning to challenge stigma-based narratives of a cause of death by suicide; and 3) supporting healthy coping.
5. Mood and coping review. This competency involves assessing mood, coping, needs, and the effectiveness of the consumer's coping plan without becoming derailed by the presenting problem.

Reviewing session notes

Session notes tend to reflect the level of competence of practice. Errors may include stigmatising language, omissions or commissions, or incorrect needs assessment.
   Common errors include:

- imprecise or unconcise language
- insufficient detail to understand the presenting problem and impact (triggers, thoughts, emotions, behaviour, impact)
- not assessing/recording the consumer's reaction to coping psychoeducation
- insufficient detail of social or professional supports (i.e., names of supports)
- not assessing/recording previous history of suicidality
- not recording details of suicidality (thoughts, plans, intent)
- incorrect needs assessment
- moderate or high needs for additional professional support without noting discussions or decisions to meet those needs
- no record of the plan with the consumer for further contact after hospitalisation in the case of a consumer connected for immediate high needs for professional support
- listing coping strategies randomly in mood and coping review rather than in sequential order according to the coping continuum and under the relevant coping category necessary to understand how overwhelmed the consumer is.

The process of editing session notes and discussing edits with the therapist provides further opportunities for the therapist to reflect on each session and their practice, identify assumptions or misunderstandings, and set goals for change.

Concluding statement

Historically, suicide has been shrouded in stigma—a negative communal moral judgment. While professional help-seeking is a healthy coping strategy when people feel overwhelmed—including experiencing suicidality—the usefulness of professional help-seeking depends on the quality of care provided. The consumer's need for additional support must be met to prevent adverse experiences and ensure consumer outcomes. Care Collaborate Connect is a consumer-centred model of social and professional support. It attends to the needs of the person asking for help. After Care Collaborate Connect training, supervision helps refine knowledge and skills to ensure skill refinement and treatment integrity. In addition to improving consumer outcomes, this consumer-centred care model of support improves therapist wellbeing and coping self-efficacy (Stallman, 2020b).

Educational questions & activities

1. What are your thoughts about suicide and people who have suicidal thoughts or die by suicide? Do you notice any thoughts that reinforce suicide-related stigma?
2. Find a media story about a death by suicide and reframe the narrative of the cause of death using the biopsychosocial domains that caused overwhelming distress and the coping continuum.
3. Think of recent stressful events in your life. Using the coping continuum, identify all the healthy and unhealthy coping strategies you used to feel better.
4. Download the *My Coping Plan* app and enter your healthy coping strategies. Notice if having an explicit coping plan changes how you think about or what you do to feel better when you have unpleasant emotions.

References

Farberow, N. L. (2005). The mental health professional as suicide survivor. *Clinical Neuropsychiatry: Journal of Treatment Evaluation, 2*(1), 13–20.

Franklin, J. C., Ribeiro, J. D., Fox, K. R., Bentley, K. H., Kleiman, E. M., Huang, X., . . . Nock, M. K. (2017). Risk factors for suicidal thoughts and behaviors: A meta-analysis of 50 years of research. *Psychological Bulletin, 143*(2), 187–232. doi:10.1037/bul0000084

Keller, S., McNeill, V., Honea, J., & Paulson Miller, L. (2019). A look at culture and stigma of suicide: Textual analysis of community theatre performances. *International Journal of Environmental Research and Public Health, 16*(3), 352. doi:10.3390/ijerph16030352

Milne, D. (2009). *Evidence-based clinical supervision. Principles and practice.* Chichester, UK: BPS Blackwell.

Rønning, S. B., & Bjørkly, S. (2019). The use of clinical role-play and reflection in learning therapeutic communication skills in mental health education: an integrative review. *Advances in Medical Education and Practice, 10*, 415–425. doi:10.2147/AMEP.S202115

Stallman, H. M. (2018). Coping planning: A patient-centred and strengths-focused approach to suicide prevention training. *Australasian Psychiatry, 26*(2), 141–144. doi:10.1177/1039856217732471

Stallman, H. M. (2019). *Care · collaborate · connect: Suicide prevention training.* Adelaide: Care Collaborate Connect Pty Ltd.

Stallman, H. M. (2020a). Health theory of coping. *Australian Psychologist, 55*(4), 295–306. doi:10.1111/ap.12465

Stallman, H. M. (2020b). Online needs-based and strengths-focused suicide prevention training: Evaluation of care · collaborate · connect. *Australian Psychologist, 55*(3), 220–229. doi:10.1111/ap.12419

Stallman, H. M. (2020c). Suicide following hospitalisation: Systemic treatment failure needs to be the focus rather than risk factors. *The Lancet Psychiatry, 7*(4), 303. doi:10.1016/S2215-0366(19)30528-0

Stallman, H. M. (2021). *Bereavement resilience program.* Adelaide: Care Collaborate Connect Pty Ltd.

Stallman, H. M. (2023). Intergenerational transmission of suicidality or shared stressors? *Psychological Medicine, 53* (3). doi:10.1017/S0033291721001884

Stallman, H. M., & Allen, A. (2021). Acute suicide prevention: A systematic review of the evidence and implications for clinical practice. *Journal of Affective Disorders Reports*, 5, 100148. doi:10.1016/j.jadr.2021.100148

Stallman, H. M., Beaudequin, D., Hermens, D. F., & Eisenberg, D. (2021). Modelling the relationship between healthy and unhealthy coping strategies to understand overwhelming distress: A Bayesian network approach. *Journal of Affective Disorders Reports*, 3, 100054. doi:10.1016/j.jadr.2020.100054

6 Addressing Supervisee Fears and Interest Areas in Supervision

Nadine Pelling

Tell me your fears and interests

I begin almost all my counselling and clinical skills classes in the same manner. Specifically, I ask participants to take some time and list their worst imagined client case scenarios, anonymously, on poster paper during class. I also ask students to list their main areas of interest broadly. This includes populations, settings, and issues and diagnoses. In other words, I ask participants to share their fears regarding their approaching work with clients and what areas they would like to know more about. After I gain a listing of participant worst client case scenarios and interest areas, I take them home and organise them into groupings which are clearly related. I type up the results for dissemination to the entire class. As a result, a rough qualitative analysis of student fears is conducted and reflected back to the group. Further, a list of general interest areas are also identified along with resources for students to find additional information. The following is a summary of my experiences in asking supervisees about fears and interest areas (Pelling, personal communication, October 20, 2022).

Over the next few classes participants' concerns and interests are directly addressed through discussion of the issues raised, exercises, and related role plays. In this manner some of the content of our supervisory work is determined by those in training. This focus honours supervisee needs. Moreover, participants can experience the fact that others have fears too when it comes to their upcoming work with clients, which has a normalising and anxiety reducing effect. They can also be made aware of the diversity and commonality of various applied work interest areas presented.

I am often amazed by the level of detail some have woven into their most concerning imagined client interactions. However, the general content presented by participants tends to be somewhat stable. I am also impressed by the variety of interest areas presented by students. What follows are the five main areas into which the worst client case scenarios of many therapists in training can be placed. This presentation includes brief suggestions relating to the therapist knowledge, self/other awareness, and skills that are need addressing relating to each scenario category presented. Some recent counselling and clinical skills classes' interest area groupings are then presented. This chapter ends with a short overview of some general activities that aid in therapist knowledge, self/other awareness, and skill development.

DOI: 10.4324/9781003490067-8

Worst client case scenario categories

I have come across five general worst client case scenario categories: harm to client/client in great pain, difficult clients, danger to therapist, ethical responsibilities, and therapist competence. Of course, these categories can overlap and specific examples in each category can vary but I have included for illustrative purposes some general examples of each that I have come across in my supervision work.

Harm to client/client in great pain

It should be no surprise that having a client demonstrate any level of suicidality or overwhelming emotional pain can be anxiety provoking for beginning level therapists. The most common fear listed regarding this category in my classes has been having a client overtly state an intention to kill oneself. Such an issue needs to be addressed regarding therapist knowledge, self/other awareness, and skill. Specifically, therapists need to know ethically what the limits to confidentiality entail as well as the basic risk factors relating to self-harm and suicide. Regarding self/other awareness, therapists need to know the content areas that trigger their own emotions and the difference between empathy and identification. Finally, all therapists need to be taught the basic skills needed to assess lethality and follow through actions needed to protect client wellbeing and help identify, with clients, how to assist clients in coping through such challenging times. Extensive role play activities can be very helpful in reducing supervisee anxiety and increasing confidence when working with clients in great pain. Entire supervision sessions can be spent on these and related harm to client/client in great pain factors.

Difficult clients

What is a difficult client? According to many of my past students difficult clients include those that confront the therapist verbally, have difficulty expressing themselves verbally, those who are resistant and mandated to treatment, anyone who is sarcastic, and, my personal favourite, malevolent clients who simply enjoy being difficult. Once again, the issue of difficult clients needs to be addressed regarding therapist knowledge, self/other awareness, and skill. Specifically, therapists need to know the roots of resistance and understand that therapy is a joint venture; not one in which a therapist can metaphorically drag a client along to experience. Through experience and support therapists can learn that basic counselling skills, such as listening and reflecting feeling, can help address the issues that difficult clients might raise. Regarding self/other awareness, I encourage therapists to remember that 'salt only hurts when it is rubbed in an open wound' and thus once again therapists need to know the content areas that trigger their own emotions and the difference between empathy and identification. The supervisor can demonstrate through empathetic listening that the best way to address difficult clients is to work with, not against, client resistance. Understanding that ambivalence and self-protection are common in humans can help one not overact to such occurrences. This type of work turns theory into practice in a manner that can directly be beneficial for clients.

Danger to therapist

I must have been somewhat naive as a therapist in training as I do not personally remember fearing for my safety when beginning work with clients. Nevertheless, many students have indicated that they fear clients being physically confronting to or specifically threatening the therapist if they do/do not do something that the client is against/requests. For instance, many students have indicated a concern over a client threatening them if they rightly engage in their mandatory reporting obligations regarding suspected child abuse and/or neglect. Once again, therapists need to know ethically what the limits to confidentiality entail and follow through with their mandatory reporting requirements. Basic safety and security measures also need to be in place when and where clients are to be seen. Regarding self/other awareness, therapists need to understand that clients may become upset in session and that we might be able to help them express their concerns in a socially appropriate manner. Therapists need to be skilled in remaining calm when working with clients, how to excuse themselves from a dangerous situation or how to make an appropriate referral to another professional if needed. Numerous role-play scenarios, self-exploration exercises, and literature searches regarding such topic areas could be conducted as part of supervision.

Ethical responsibilities

Ethics are taught differently in different training programmes. Some integrate ethical training across all their classes while others have a specific class regarding professional and ethical behaviour. Each method of ethical training has its benefits and drawbacks, and experienced professionals know that ethics are not static but ever evolving to fit our current culture and knowledge base. The most common fears regarding one's ethical responsibilities I have encountered as an instructor and supervisor involve mandatory reporting requirements and romantic or personal, not professional, connections with clients. A lack of therapist knowledge of ethics is fairly easy to address via the reading of one's relevant ethical codes and ethical case books which include not just a list of 'dos and do not dos' but principals which highlight the why behind such ethical codes. Also, knowing one's own self and vulnerabilities as well as the need to respect clients can be key to ethical behaviour. Role playing scenarios in which a therapist must clearly define the professional nature of their relationship with a client or in which a mandatory reporting situation has occurred can help build one's skill in these areas. Similarly, keeping in regular collegial contact with other therapists, possibly in a supervision group, can help therapists determine what is considered standard practice and thus generally on safe ethical footing in their own geographical/specialty area. Of course, when in doubt regarding practice one can contact their relevant professional organisation for advice or referral to a supervisor or colleague for discussion (please see Part 7 of this book for various country-based counselling/psychology associations that generally provide a code of ethics/conduct for their members).

Questioning therapist competence

When I first started my psychological practice, a very mature female client (50+ years older than I) that I had just finished seeing told my supervisor that she did not want to "see that little blonde chickie again." in retrospect I understand her concern since I might not like to see a 23-year-old psychologist if I was in my 70s either. At the time I was at a loss for words and was not certain what to do. One needs to know referral sources in their area so that if needed an appropriate referral can be made. Regarding self/other awareness my supervisor challenged me to acknowledge that not every therapist can see every client and that the only way to move forward when someone questions your competence is to empathically listen to them, discuss the matter, and if needed make an appropriate referral. This tends to be the case if you are considerably younger/older than a client, you are/are not a parent and thus may have difficulty understanding where a client is coming from regarding parenting, or if you have just been told that therapy with you, or in general, is useless as an activity. Being skilled in listening and exploring expectations and views is a way forward. Therapist defensiveness needs to be explored personally by the therapist and supervisor, but therapy needs to remain focused on the client. Therapists need to be aware that client ambivalence and resistance can occur and that such things need to be worked with not against. By discussing such things in supervision the supervisor can model how to be supportive, understanding, and encouraging.

Main interest areas

Regarding interest areas, over the last two decades my students have shown great variety in what they are interested in related to their applied work. The populations students state they are interested in working with include teens, young adults, and the elderly. More counselling than clinical students note an interest in children.

Most in training with me report being interested in working in a private practice setting. Private practice is where most practicing psychologists work. Students believe that they will require additional experience after their training and initial registration before engaging in private practice. Thus, students note they will seek employment in various group, not-for-profit, and government-based settings focusing upon teens and adults prior to eventually moving into private practice. Over the last few years, however, there has been a trend in the clinical psychology students I have taught. Namely, many of them indicate little interest in practice with clients in an ongoing fashion. Instead, many of these clinical psychology students already have their doctoral research-based degrees and are seeking applied credentials so as to focus their academic careers on clinical research. Many of these clinical students indicate little interest in seeing clients past the experience needed to gain registration, endorsement, and approved psychology supervisor status. This may be, however, an artifact of how a university selects students for the clinical psychology programme (possibly preferencing those who already have a PhD for interview) and manages various applied staff (no longer universally allowing/counting applied client work in academic workloads). For counselling students, providing support that is covered thought the National Disability Insurance Scheme (NDIS) is often noted. Most students do not mention work support/return to work agencies nor family/couple therapy and mediation focused agencies such as Relationships Australia. The issues and diagnoses students indicate they are interested in are varied and include domestic and family violence, substance abuse, and gender dysphoria. Most indicate an interest in anxiety, depression, and trauma.

When one has a list of student related interest areas, materials can be provided to students that encourage them to further explore related populations, settings for work, and issues and diagnoses. This may include the provision of speciality interest area groups that provide specialist training in such things as EMDR (Eye Movement Desensitisation and Reprocessing) therapy. For students who will eventually conduct research as part of their training, interest area identification can aid in their finding and developing an area of investigation.

General activities for increasing knowledge, self/other awareness, and skill

Models, methods, and modes used in supervision abound. Indeed, much of this book outlines various interventions used in supervision. What follows here are simply an outlining of a few of my more favoured activities for expanding therapist knowledge, self/other awareness, and skill (Kocarek & Pelling, 2003).

Knowledge

Read, research, and collegial discussion are my favourite methods for increasing knowledge. Specific topic areas such as mania or addiction can be researched, one's local ethical code can be obtained and read, one can attend regular research or journal meetings at which topics are discussed.

Self/Other awareness

Generally one can increase self/other awareness through many of the techniques used with clients but with a focus on how such an increase in awareness is likely to impact one's therapeutic work. For instance, timelines, genograms, an examination of personal views, counselling, keeping a journal, attending to self-care, and examining multicultural issues can all be beneficial. Specifically, if working with a client with an addiction problem, a therapist could examine via a timeline how their views of or experiences with substances that are commonly the focus of addiction have shaped their thinking and emotional reactions to addiction and how this can impact their client work.

Skill

Knowledge and awareness are wonderful but eventually one needs to develop client skill if one is to have a successful client practice. How can one build skill? Role play activities, self-examination of one's work via video review and requesting specific feedback from colleagues, supervisors, and clients can be helpful. There is also volunteer work, training placements, practice, and supervised practice. Specifically, in order to increase therapeutic skill, one needs to work in a reflective manner. This takes targeted time and effort as well as personal fortitude.

Concluding statement

Therapists in training have some common fears regarding their impending work with clients. Some common interest areas also can be identified. As supervisors we can address these and thus show an acceptance of our supervisees and encourage their growth as therapists through aiding an increase in their knowledge, self/other awareness, and clinical skill. Addressing common client fears can be accomplished in numerous ways but often requires therapist courage and the support of a knowledgeable, understanding, and supportive supervisor. What do your trainees fear/find interesting and how are their fears/interest areas being addressed?

Educational questions & activities

1. What are the five general worst client case scenario categories outlined by Dr Pelling?
2. Create a possible client scenario to go with each category and do either a literature search on the topic (knowledge), write your thoughts and feelings down about the topic (self/other awareness), or engage in an extended role place as client and then counsellor regarding the topic.
3. What is your favourite way of enhancing your knowledge on a topic?
4. What is your favourite way of developing your self/other awareness?
5. What is your favourite ways of developing your counselling skills?
6. What are your interest areas relevant to populations, settings, and issues/diagnoses?

References

Australian Institute of Health and Welfare (2022). Mental health services in Australia. www.aihw.gov.au/reports/mental-health-services/mental-health-services-in-australia

Pelling, N., & Kocarek, C. (2003). Beyond knowledge and awareness: Enhancing counsellor skills for work with gay, lesbian, and bisexual clients. *Journal of Multicultural Counseling and Development, 31*(2), 99–112.

Pelling, N., & Proeve, M. (2006). Australian and New Zealand university clinical and counselling psychology staff: Maintaining practice in academe. *Australian Psychologist, 41*(2), 112–119.

Pelling, N., & Renard, D. E. (1999). The use of videotaping within developmentally-based supervision. *Journal of Technology in Counselling, 1*(1). http://techcounseling.net/Archive/vol1_1/index.htm

Stallman, H. M. (2019). An ethical response to disclosures of suicidal ideation or behaviour. In N. Pelling & L. Burton (Eds.), *The elements of ethical practice: Applied psychology ethics in Australia* (pp. 155–166). Abingdon, Oxon: Routledge.

7 Supervision and Vicarious Trauma

Fran Lane

Counsellors often find themselves working with clients who have experienced trauma. When that trauma impacts counsellors professionals tend to talk about burnout or counter-transference, compassion fatigue, and vicarious trauma. In the following pages, vicarious traumatisation is defined and explored as it exists in counselling contexts.

Supervising counsellors for vicarious trauma

All counsellors regardless of their work setting will find themselves working with clients who have experienced trauma. From the time that trauma effects were recognised the impact of working with those who had experienced traumatic events was noted. Historically the adverse reactions of counsellors to client trauma were viewed as burnout or counter-transference (Figley, 1995). In many cases burnout, compassion fatigue, and vicarious trauma were conflated as secondary traumatic stress (Figley, 1995; McCann & Pearlman, 1990). However, studies have since identified differences between these concepts, and vicarious traumatisation (VT) is now seen as a separate theory based construct with observable symptoms (Pearlman & Mac Ian, 1995; Pearlman & Saakvitne, 1995a, 1995b).

Understanding vicarious trauma

Vicarious traumatisation is defined 'as the transformation that occurs within the therapist (or other trauma worker) as a result of **empathic engagement** with clients' trauma experiences and their sequelae' (Pearlman & Mac Ian, 1995, p. 558 emphasis added). We know from research on the therapeutic alliance that the bond or connection between therapist and client is integral to a successful therapeutic outcome (Bordin, 1979; Duff & Bedi, 2010).

Difficulty has surrounded the formulation of a universal definition of empathy. Goleman defined empathy as 'the ability to know how another feels' (1996, p. 98). Looking at a scaffolded development of empathy from infancy, the concept of empathy was proposed as being composed of two forms, an affective and a cognitive form of empathy (van der Graaff et al., 2014). Goleman also proposed a third type that he called 'empathic concern' (2007). In neuro-scientific study Decety and Meyer (2008) distinguish between empathic mimicry and true empathy, noting that true empathy allows for an understanding that the emotions are external to the self, and derived from the other's experience of their environment and the meaning they make of that interaction. Decety and Yoder have framed empathy as 'a multifaceted construct used to account for the capacity to share and understand the

DOI: 10.4324/9781003490067-9

thoughts and feelings of others' (2016). The neuroscience of empathic functioning derives from a number of mechanisms within the brain such as mirror neurons.

Mirror neurons are a mechanism involved in observational learning with Ramachandran referring to them as a 'subset of motor neurons' that perform a 'virtual reality' (2011). Further discussions have raised the perspective of two differing systems; one system is involved in the sharing of experience (empathy), and the other system involves cognitively understanding what it might be like to have that experience (Bloom, 2016). Bloom argues that these two systems represent the concepts of communion and agency, and speaks of 'unmitigated communion' (2016, p. 140) in connection to individuals who experienced a form of chronic empathic distress.

Although much of the writing on VT revolves around mental processes, thoughts and awareness, it must be emphasised that individuals also experience the world through their bodies (Herman, 2015; Rothschild, 2003, 2006, 2014; Van der Kolk, 2014). Studies in neurodevelopment (Decety, 2010) demonstrate that empathy connects and interacts with various neural regions, as well as the autonomic nervous system and the neuroendocrine processes that are involved in emotional states and social behaviours (Decety, 2010). Walker (2009) described how working with clients who have experienced abuse can physically effect the counsellor, while Rothschild (2006) referred to these experiences as 'somatic countertransference' where the action of mirror neurons together with body mimicry can result in a 'contagion' of affect that manifests itself physically, emotionally, and cognitively. A study of 35 counsellors over a six-month period showed that 70% experienced sleepiness, muscle tension, unexpected shift in the body, yawning, and tearfulness. Among some of the other effects experienced were headaches (54%), stomach disturbance (41%) loss of voice (32%), nausea (23%), and numbness (29%).

Pearlman and Mac Ian (1995) noted 'just as PTSD is viewed as a normal reaction to an abnormal event, we view vicarious traumatisation as a normal reaction to the stressful and sometimes traumatizing work with victims' (p. 146). With what seems to be a therapeutic imperative to establish a therapeutic alliance through empathic engagement (Bordin, 1979; Safran & Muran, 2000; Safran, Muran, & Proskurov, 2009) coupled with the difficulty to anticipate the level of empathic distress that may be experienced by therapists, it seems therapists are caught in a paradoxical dilemma.

The key distinguishing characteristic of VT is its transformative nature (Pearlman & Mac Ian, 1995). Exposure to the trauma stories of clients can alter the perceptions of therapists, changing the way they view themselves, other people, and the world (Figley, 1995; Pearlman, 2012; Pearlman & Saakvitne, 1995b). These cognitive distortions (McCann & Pearlman, 1990) can impact on the psychological functioning of the therapist. VT has been conceptualised as being worsened by, possibly even based in, the therapeutic connection or empathic engagement with the client that is inherent in all counselling (Pearlman & Saakvitne, 1995b; Saakvitne, Gamble, Pearlman, & Tabor, 2000).

Constructive self-development theory

Since VT is described as a progressive and adaptive process Constructive Self Development Theory (CSDT) (McCann & Pearlman, 1992) is useful in understanding this progression. CSDT frames the changes in counsellor's cognitive schemas as being pervasive, across all spheres of the counsellor's life, and cumulative, with each traumatised client contact providing reinforcement to these changes. Saakvitne and Pearlman (1996) proposed that distorted beliefs and VT reactions arose out of five areas. These areas are outlined as

i) frame of reference, ii) self-capacities, iii) ego resources, iv) psychological needs, and v) cognitive schemas (Saakvitne & Pearlman, 1996). The individual's sense of self and their perception of reality are developed out of these five areas (Saakvitne & Pearlman, 1996). The combination of perceived self and perceived reality provides the individual's context or framework for viewing the world. It is within these five areas that the vulnerability to adaptation, as a result of clients' stories, can result in disruptions and disorientation, and an emergence of VT in counsellors.

The CSDT model is also helpful in the development of strategies to deal with VT (Saakvitne et al., 2000). As VT is framed as an adaptive process it can be viewed as being on a continuum, based not on the accumulation of client trauma stories, but on the shifts that occur in the adaptive process. Saakvitne et al.'s suggested approach (2000) is to antici-pate and prepare, address signs as they arise, and to transform the pain of VT.

It becomes the responsibility of counselling supervisors to provide a VT-informed ser-vice to counsellors that is knowledgeable, supportive, and VT-preventative.

VT-informed supervision

Using the CSDT model Saakvitne et al. (2000) suggested taking the following approach to working in an VT informed manner: Anticipate and prepare, address signs of VT, and transform the pain of VT.

Anticipate and prepare

Each individual therapist needs to be cognisant of their own unique protective factors and their risk factors. Understanding of the interplay of these factors allows for an informed construction of a self-care plan that is specific and unique to the individual. Supervisors can facilitate these understandings by having conversations that allow the counsellor to iden-tify their own unique personal risk, and protective factors, such as:

- Personality and coping style
- Current life circumstances
- Personal history
- Social supports
- Work style
- Spiritual connection and resources

Some studies have found that engaging in any coping strategy recommended for redu-cing distress did not have an impact on immediate trauma symptoms, and cautioned that focusing on the use of individual coping strategies might imply that those who feel traumatised may not be balancing life and work adequately by not be making effective use of leisure, self-care, or supervision, thus in effect blaming the victim (Bober, 2005; Bober, Regehr, & Zhou, 2006). Rather than constructing a generic work/life balance self-care plan the informed counselling supervisor can facilitate an understanding of the specific risk factors for an individual counsellor, and assist in the identification, reinforcement and employment of the counsellor's unique protective factors.

Working with protective factors includes examining the meaning-making of the coun-sellor around their work and clients and the usual personal intersecting issues that may arise. Working with CSDT the counselling supervisor can explore:

- Frameworks utilised by the counsellor to interpret experience
- Abilities that enable the individual to maintain a sense of self as consistent and coherent across time and situations; intrapersonal
- Abilities that enable the individual to meet psychological needs and to relate to others; interpersonal

Meaning-making is particularly affected by long term, continuous exposure to trauma stories. With empathic engagement the counsellor has a narrowed focus on a single, identified individual. Work in the cognitive sciences has acknowledged that such a singular focus can skew moral judgements and ethical decision-making (Bloom, 2016; Zaki, 2017). Checking in with the counsellor on the meaning they place on the work that they do; the stories that they hear; the therapeutic interventions they choose; will assist the supervisor to detect the subtle changes to the counsellor's point of view or frame of reference. Encouraging the counsellor to be cognitively aware of their frame of reference, and any movements or changes promotes the management of vicarious trauma symptoms. The facilitation of choice in ways of working with changes involves activating coping and managing strategies and the utilisation of resources.

The domains that CSDT note of particular importance to meeting psychological needs and supporting existing cognitive schemas are:

- Safety
- Esteem
- Trust/dependency
- Control
- Intimacy

Regular self-reflection and the development of a capacity for personal insight are protective factors for VT. Awareness around cognition and meaning-making coupled with a preparedness to work openly with vulnerability is necessary for the counsellor and supervisor to work in this area.

Promoting counsellor awareness of body sensations arising during counselling sessions will assist the supervisor to address body state countertransference. A number of mindful interventions are now incorporated into therapeutic modalities for trauma symptoms. The awareness of body sensations arising can be developed and supported through a variety of mindful meditation/awareness techniques. Counsellors should be encouraged to develop sufficient skill in conducting a body-scan on themselves, to the point of being able to easily check-in on themselves intermittently through their working day.

Rothschild strongly recommends a sense of calm detachment when working with clients trauma stories (2014) and a strong recommendation for therapists to be aware of motion within the therapeutic space. The body mimicry that results in postural mirroring links to how the action of mirror neurons may result in unconscious automatic somatic countertransference.

In Egan and Carr's study of trauma counsellors (2008) they noted a correlation between the 'degree to which a therapist reports experiencing countertransference at the somatic level in response to their clients and the amount of sick leave they need to take' (p. 5).

Supervisors may also find themselves hearing about organisational issues, and how the environment impacts the counsellors' capacity to delivery therapeutic services. Conversations regarding the environmental/organisational contexts are also a source to identify the risk and protective factors that are inherent within the counsellors work context. The three work areas of concern for vicarious trauma risk factors are:

- The organisational environment
- Working with clients
- Counsellor experience

The organisational environment expresses the policies and procedures applied by the organisation. The organisation may have a mission statement that aligns with the counsellor's however it is in the application that values conflicts may arise. Some organisations have a required number of client sessions per day. Other organisations may not have any such requirement, however the workload balances maybe a problem. When an organisation is funded to deliver services to a particular client demographic the counsellor may find they only ever see clients who have been severely traumatised. Community attitudes to the client demographic as well as the availability of community resources can place added stress on the counsellor. Supervisors of clients not in general counselling need to be particularly aware of the inherent risks in the delivery of therapeutic services within single demographic funded projects.

Inadequate training may also be viewed as a VT risk factor for counsellors. Again, counsellors trained for general practice may find themselves working within a specific field of counselling for which they feel ill equipped. It is important not only for the ongoing learning process of counsellors to be offered appropriate training, but also to the meaning-making the counsellor makes regarding the value and meaning in their work as well as their beliefs around their own competency.

Address the Signs of VT

In 1996 Saakvitne and Pearlman developed a Self-Assessment Scale to aid workers in addressing their self-care needs (Saakvitne & Pearlman, 1996). Other scales and assessment tools have been developed for use: the Traumatic Stress Institute Belief Scale (Pearlman, 1996), the Trauma and Attachment Belief Scale (Pearlman, 2003), and the Secondary Traumatic Stress Symptoms (Bride, Robinson, Yegidis, & Figley, 2004). It has been suggested that using the self-assessment tool periodically might assist in tracking changes (Quitangon & Evces, 2015) in counsellors exposed to trauma stories.

Counsellors working with trauma may find themselves caught in a state of preoccupation with the trauma stories their clients bring to them. They may find themselves caught in a state of constant arousal as a result of repeatedly being triggered by these trauma stories, or they may become numbed. When a counsellor is caught in the cognitive and physical tension of their responses to the traumatic experiences of others it can impact not only their professional life, but also their physical and emotional health, and their relationships with friends and family.

In such instances counsellors will question their frame of reference, world-view or spirituality. The domains of safety, esteem, trust/dependency, control, and intimacy will all be disrupted. Belief in self-capacity will be diminished; challenging the counsellors ability to have view of a positive self, their ability to self-modulate, and to maintain a strong sense of connection to self.

Counsellors may present with doubts regarding their work, low motivation, avoidance of trauma clients, over involved in details, lack of flexibility, critical attitude towards colleagues, and withdrawing from community and training activities. They may feel undervalued, or believe that their work makes no difference. Such changes to professional performance and functionality may lead to errors in judgement. A reluctance to work collaboratively can also lead to isolation and withdrawal from colleagues and may result in job changes or poor-quality work.

On a personal level the same feelings of hopelessness, anger, apathy, negative perception, and low self-image may lead the counsellor to reject any personal or emotional support available from friends and family. This detachment comes in the form of isolation, poor communication and conflictual relationships.

All of the above and more are signs and symptoms of vicarious traumatisation. They may manifest in varying degrees of seriousness. Since we understand VT to be a cumulative and transformative phenomenon then it is possible to view it as being on a continuum.

Taking a continuum viewpoint fits with the approach of anticipate/prepare, manage, and transform. Along the continuum are a number of decision or action points that can provide the braking and/or reversing of an identified progression of vicarious trauma that without action will lead to a full effect experience of vicarious trauma.

Within the therapeutic environment strategies to employ include:

- Balance the level of empathic engagement. Make empathy conscious and disconnect from traumatic experiencing.
- Employ somatic and mindful awareness interventions. Break the mirroring process, moderate arousal, and work on grounding, centering and boundaries.
- Strengthen resilience working through the five domains detailed in CSDT.

With an increased awareness of bodily sensations, the counsellor has an opportunity to recognise when they enter into a state of empathic distress. Empathy activates in the insular and anterior cingulate cortex. It is a 'self'-related emotion producing negative feelings (stress) that over time leads to poor health, withdrawal and non-social behaviours (Singer & Klimecki, 2014). Utilising empathy to springboard to compassion may assist the counsellor to bypass empathic distress. Compassion activates in the medial orbitofrontal cortex and ventral striatum. Compassion is 'other' related, promotes positive feelings, good health and allows for prosocial motivation (Singer & Klimecki, 2014). While future research is required, studies show that the plasticity around these emotions is encouraging and training in compassion would prove beneficial to those exposed to empathic distress.

Outside of the therapeutic environment it may also be necessary to consider the contribution of the workplace. For the health and wellbeing of the counsellor, framing vicarious trauma as an occupation health and safety issue may assist in identifying workplace practices that are increasing counsellor risk factors. Organisational change may not be possible, however the supervisor may facilitate a discussion with the counsellor regarding what they may be prepared to raise with their coordinator/manager, such as reduced client hours, or changing one to one counselling with some psycho-educational group work.

A review of the existing self-care plan of the counsellor may also be due, to further assess which needs are being met and those that need more support. Personal replenishment activities will vary, and it may be necessary for the counsellor and supervisor to consider personal therapy as a safe option for facilitated self-examination of the counsellor's thoughts and feelings.

The informed counselling supervisor who has worked with the counsellor on anticipation and preparation for VT need only identify the signs/symptoms, to implement the coping and managing strategies that will address that particular manifestation for that particular individual. There is no magic one size fits all solution to something as complex as vicarious trauma, experienced by someone as unique as any human being. The response needs to be crafted to suit the signs/symptoms and the individual and their context.

Transform the Pain of VT

The full range of the effects of vicarious traumatisation is spread across five categories: emotional, behavioural, physiological, cognitive, and spiritual.

- Emotional – feeling unsafe, experiencing anxiety or grief, feeling angry or irritable. Distraction and changes in mood and/or sense of humour can also be felt.
- Behavioural – isolation, changes in eating or sleeping habits, increase in alcohol or substance use. Difficulty separating work and personal life, increased workloads, and sometimes engagement in risky behaviours may also be present.
- Physiological – depletion of physical wellbeing may be evidenced in headaches, rashes, ulcers or heartburn as well as more serious physical complaints.
- Cognitive – difficulty concentrating, changes to negativity or cynicism in points of view, and difficulty separating from the trauma experienced by clients.
- Spiritual – disconnect from others and the world, loss of hope, decreased sense of purpose and feelings of unworthiness.

Untreated this constellation of symptoms can become very debilitating, and a need for a combined mental and physical health approach may be required. As the revised criteria for PTSD in the Diagnostic and Statistical Manual of Mental Disorders (American Psychiatric Association, 2013) has been expanded to include 'repeated exposure to aversive details' of a traumatic event some of those suffering from vicarious trauma may be diagnosed with PTSD. Therapy is definitely recommended in such cases.

Summary

All counsellors will be exposed to the risks of vicarious trauma in their working life. For some those risks will be balanced by protective factors that are intrinsic to them or structurally available through their work organisation (such as supervision) or safety plans. For others, though a more fraught journey on the vicarious trauma continuum is experienced. The message is that vicarious trauma is not some random phenomenon that may or may not occur. Through the intervention of aware supervision counsellors can be empowered to construct a practice that acknowledges the possibility of being effected by symptoms of vicarious traumatisation, and goes on to structure strategies to cope with risk factors, strengthen protective factors and monitor movement on the continuum initiating braking strategies where necessary.

There is a need to recognise that the transformative effect of vicarious traumatisation is not only cognitive but also somatically expressed. The development of mindful awareness of self – bodily sensations, emotions and thoughts is a strong protective factor for all in the field. Training in compassion may also provide the counsellor with a strong protective approach to the presence of distress within the empathic engagement.

Educational questions & activities

1. In a neuro-scientific study, Decety and Meyer (2008) distinguish between empathic mimicry and true empathy. How do they explain true empathy?
2. What did a study of symptoms of somatic transference of 35 counsellors over a six-month period show?
3. What does Rothschild strongly recommend when working with client's trauma stories?
4. What is the key distinguishing characteristic of VT, what is its transformative nature?
5. It has been suggested that using self-assessment tools periodically might assist in tracking changes in counsellors exposed to trauma stories. In 1996 Saakvitne and Pearlman developed a Self-Assessment Scale to aid workers in addressing their self-care needs. Name three other assessment tools used for this purpose?
6. Empathy activates in the insular and anterior cingulate cortex. It is a 'self'-related emotion producing negative feelings (stress) that over time leads to what?

References

American Psychiatric Association (2013). *Diagnostic and statistical manual of mental disorders* (5th ed.). American Psychiatric Publishing. https://doi.org/10.1176/appi.books.9780890425596

Bloom, P. (2016). *Against empathy*. The Bodley Head/Vintage.

Bober, T. (2005). Strategies for reducing secondary or vicarious trauma: Do they work? *Brief Treatment and Crisis Intervention*, 6(1), 1–9. https://doi.org/10.1093/brief-treatment/mhj001

Bober, T., Regehr, C., & Zhou, Y. (2006). Development of the coping strategies inventory for trauma counselors. *Journal of Loss and Trauma*, 11(1), 71–83.

Bordin, E. S. (1979). The generalizability of the psychoanalytic concept of the working alliance. *Psychotherapy: Theory, Research & Practice*, 16(3), 252–260. https://doi.org/10.1037/h0085885

Bride, B., Robinson, M. R., Yegidis, B., & Figley, C. R. (2004). Development and validation of the Secondary Traumatic Stress Scale. *Research on Social Work Practice*, 14, 27–35.

Decety, J. (2010). The neurodevelopment of empathy in humans. *Developmental Neuroscience*, 32(4), 257–267. https://doi.org/10.1159/000317771

Decety, J., & Meyer, M. (2008). From emotion resonance to empathic understanding: A social developmental neuroscience account. *Development and Psychopathology*, 20, 1053–1080.

Decety, J., & Yoder, K. J. (2016). Empathy and motivation for justice: Cognitive empathy and concern, but not emotional empathy, predict sensitivity to injustice for others. *Social Neuroscience*, 11(1), 1–14. https://doi.org/10.1080/17470919.2015.1029593

Duff, C. T., & Bedi, R. P. (2010). Counsellor behaviours that predict therapeutic alliance: From the client's perspective. *Counselling Psychology Quarterly*, 23(1), 91–110. https://doi.org/10.1080/09515070003688165

Egan, J., & Carr, A. (2008). Body-centred countertransference in female trauma therapists. *Éisteacht/Irish Association for Counselling and Psychotherapy*, 8(1), 24–27.

Figley, C. R. (1995). Compassion fatigue: Toward a new understanding of the costs of caring. In B. H. Stamm (Ed.), *Secondary traumatic stress: Self-care issues for clinicians, researchers, and educators* (pp. 3–28). The Sidran Press.

Goleman, D. (1996). *Emotional intelligence: Why it can matter more than IQ*. Bloomsbury Publishing.

Goleman, D. (2007). *Social intelligence*. Bantam Dell.

Herman, J. L. (2015). *Trauma and recovery: The aftermath of violence, from domestic abuse to political terror*. Basic Books.

McCann, I. L., & Pearlman, L. A. (1990). Vicarious traumatization: A framework for understanding the psychological effects of working with victims. *Journal of Traumatic Stress*, 3(1), 131–149. https://doi.org/10.1007/BF00975140

McCann, I. L., & Pearlman, L. A. (1992). Constructivist self-development theory: A theoretical framework for assessing and treating traumatized college students. *Journal of American College Health*, 40(4), 189–196. https://doi.org/10.1080/07448481.1992.9936281

Pearlman, L. A. (1996). Psychometric review of TSI Belief Scale. In B. H. Stamm (Ed.), *Measurement of stress, trauma, and adaptation* (pp. 415–417). The Sidran Press.

Pearlman, L. A. (2003). *Trauma and attachment belief scale*. Western Psychological Services.

Pearlman, L. A. (2012). Vicarious trauma. In C. R. Figley (Ed.), *Encyclopedia of trauma*. Sage Publications.

Pearlman, L. A., & Mac Ian, P. S. (1995). Vicarious traumatization: An empirical study of the effects of trauma work on trauma therapists. *Professional Psychology: Research and Practice*, 26(6), 558–565. https://doi.org/10.1037/0735-7028.26.6.558

Pearlman, L. A., & Saakvitne, K. W. (1995a). *Trauma and the therapist: Countertransference and vicarious traumatization in psychotherapy with incest survivors*. W. W. Norton.

Pearlman, L. A., & Saakvitne, K. W. (1995b). Treating therapists with vicarious traumatization and secondary traumatic stress disorders. In C. R. Figley (Ed.), *Compassion fatigue: Coping with secondary traumatic stress disorder in those who treat the traumatized* (pp. 150–177). Brunner/Mazel.

Quitangon, G., & Evces, M. (2015). *Vicarious trauma and disaster mental health: Understanding risks and promoting resilience*. Routledge.

Ramachandran, V. S. (2011). *The tell-tale brain: A neuroscientist's quest for what makes us human*. W. W. Norton & Co.

Rothschild, B. (2003). *The body remembers*. W. W. Norton & Co.

Rothschild, B. (2006). *Help for the helper*. W. W. Norton & Co.

Rothschild, B. (2014). Motion in the consulting room is more contagious than we thought. *Psychotherapy Networker*. Retrieved from www.psychotherapynetworker.org/blog/ details/387/ mirror-mirror

Saakvitne, K. W., Gamble, S., Pearlman, L., & Tabor, B. (2000). *Risking connections: A training curriculum for working with survivors of childhood abuse*. The Sidran Press.

Saakvitne, K. W., & Pearlman, L. A. (1996). *Transforming the pain: A workbook on vicarious traumatization*. W. W. Norton & Co.

Safran, J. D., & Muran, J. C. (2000). The therapeutic alliance. Introduction. *Journal of Clinical Psychology*, 56(2), 159–161. https://doi.org/10.1002/(sici)1097-4679(200 002)56:2<159::aid-jclp2>3.0.co;2-d

Safran, J. D., Muran, J. C., & Proskurov, B. (2009). Alliance, negotiation, and rupture resolution. In R. R. Levy & S. J. Ablon (Eds.), *Handbook of evidence based psychodynamic psychotherapy* (pp. 201–205). Humana Press.

Singer, T., & Klimecki, O. M. (2014). Empathy and compassion. *Current Biology*, 24, 875–878.

van der Graaff, J., Branje, S. T. J., de Wied, M., Hawk, S. T., van Lier, P. A. C., & Meeus, W. H. J. (2014). Perspective taking and empathic concern in adolescence: Gender differences in developmental changes. *Developmental Psychology*, 50(3), 881–888. https://doi.org/10.1037/a0034325

Van der Kolk, B. (2014). *The body keeps the score*. Penguin Group.

Walker, L. E. (2009). *The battered woman syndrome* (3rd ed.). Springer Publishing Company.

Zaki, J. (2017). Moving beyond stereotypes of empathy. *Trends in Cognitive Sciences*, 21(2), 59–60. https://doi.org/10.1016/j.tics.2016.12.004

8 Demonstrating Hope, Compassion, and Justice

Supervision of Family Violence Counsellors in Australia

Stephen O'kane

Supervision of family violence counsellors is a nuanced and complex process involving agreed practice principles, adherence to ethical standards, monitoring and managing complex client presentations. Family violence counselling supervisors have a challenging and difficult task to ensure that the family violence counsellor works within their scope of practice, maintains effective client engagement, meets rapidly changing legislative requirements and maintains a demonstrated commitment to professional development. Delivery of responsive and effective Family Violence counselling requires the supervisor to ensure the promotion of safety for both the client and the counsellor, the avoidance of bias, and ensuring that all clients receive a professional service based on hope, compassion, and justice.

Family violence in Australia

The true incidence of family violence and sexual assault in Australia is unknown. Incidence can only be estimated because of under reporting and the observed differences between personal safety and crime victim surveys, with official crime statistics. Nevertheless, owing to many factors relating to societal changes – tougher legislation in a number of Australian jurisdictions, greater community awareness and public reporting, and Royal Commissions in a number of states – more than ever counsellors are being exposed to clients with family violence presentations.

Family violence can affect anyone in the community regardless of age, location, gender, socio-economic or health status, culture, ethnicity, ability, sexual identity, or religion (Isacco & Wade, 2019; Murdolo & Quiazon, 2016; O'Brien, 2016). Violence can be perpetrated by any member of a family or society against any other, however the available data show it is more likely to be perpetrated by men against women and children.

With this emphasis being placed on family violence, counsellors are not immune. Counselling supervisors need to develop a set of family violence principles and practices to assist counsellors to effectively respond to such matters. Counselling supervisors need to adopt a caring and nurturing response to family violence counsellors, but at the same time challenge and help define (and refine) the emerging family violence counselling practice of counsellors.

DOI: 10.4324/9781003490067-10

Principles of family violence counselling practice

The principles that counselling supervisors need to encourage in all counsellors engaged in family violence practice are:

- All clients involved in any family violence system who present to a counsellor deserve a professional service delivered without judgement.
- All clients who present for family violence counselling deserve and are entitled to be treated with hope, compassion, and justice.
- In a civil society, the rule of law is pre-eminent, and the role of the family violence counselling supervisor is to challenge the practise of counsellors to ensure that they are not involved in questions of guilt or innocence (which is a matter for the courts) or engaging in moralising behaviour towards clients.
- Counsellors must meet all statutory obligations (which will vary between jurisdictions), including mandatory reporting obligations, adherence to child safe practices and the sharing of appropriate information to meet statutory reporting obligations.
- Client and counsellor safety are paramount.
- In areas of uncertainty, practitioners must adhere to ethical codes and the codes of practice presented by the appropriate practitioner registration bodies.
- Counselling supervisors must ensure that counsellors have and maintain a comprehensive understanding of family violence practice and do not engage in any conduct which may involve collusion in condoning behaviours which involve violence, threats, coercive conduct, or control of one person over another.
- Counselling supervisors must ensure that counsellors understand current approaches and contemporary practices relating to Family Violence Risk Assessment.
- Family violence counsellors have a strong understanding of the factors leading to psychological distress in their clients and engage in trauma informed practice in the conduct of their work.
- Family violence counselling supervisors must regularly challenge any underlying stereotypes used by counsellors in their family violence counselling practice (e.g., that all men are violent; that all women are nurturers).
- Family violence counselling supervisors ensure that family violence counsellors are aware of the effects of vicarious trauma and have an adequate and effective regime in place to practice self-care.
- Family violence counsellors have access to established and up to date resources that relates to their local geographical area, to enable secondary referrals to take place where required (e.g., mental health services, homelessness services, alcohol & drug detoxification, and rehabilitation services).
- Any public advocacy on behalf of clients must be consistent with the ethical codes and the codes of practice presented by the appropriate practitioner registration bodies.

Comprehensive assessment in family violence counselling practice

It is important in our counselling work, particularly in the context of family violence presentations, that counsellors treat all clients or potential clients in a non-judgemental way. This presents counselling supervisors with an obligation to ensure that family violence counsellors practice their craft in a way which is effective, knowledgeable, respectful, and without harm. It is also important to relieve the psychological distress of clients by acknowledging their lived experience and, further, to encourage them to maintain some ongoing contact with established health and welfare systems. Whilst an understanding of gender is an important component of family violence practice it is not the only component. Practitioners have a duty of care to all clients to ensure that they are safe and are left with a sense of hope. To adopt a lesser standard of practice would only lead to a greater propensity for the client to engage in harmful behaviours.

Traditionally, because of paradigms that are in some cases rigidly gender based, some counselling clients of family violence systems feel disenfranchised, and may become less engaged and less visible as a result. In court systems currently, those groups who tend to receive less services and less available public resources include:

- Female perpetrators of family violence
- Male victims of family violence
- Elderly members of the community who are abused by younger family members
- Members of the Lesbian, Gay, Bisexual, Transgender, Intersex, & Queer Communities who are subjected to threats of outing

All family violence counsellors have an obligation in their practice to ensure that clients are provided with a professional service which provides hope, compassion, and justice for that particular client. This can provide a considerable challenge for many family violence counsellors. Counselling supervisors have a particular obligation to note instances of transference and countertransference in their practice. This should be openly discussed in supervision.

In order for family violence clients to be effectively engaged and listened to by counsellors, supervisors must have explicit conversations with family violence counsellors about the differences between sympathy and empathy (Jenkins, 2001). Sympathy involves revealing to the client that you are aware of their distress and that you have compassion for them. Empathy, however, involves not only the expression of compassion but demonstrating a deeper understanding by entering into the other person's lived experience. In many family violence client presentations, the expression of sympathy alone may leave the client feeling that people have taken pity on them, or feel sorry for them, which can create a sense of inferiority and disempowerment. The nuanced response required in family violence cases, however, is that this deeper level of engagement be done without colluding with any violent or controlling behaviours exhibited by the client. If such counselling approaches are practised effectively, it provides the opportunity to get to the circumstances leading to the violence.

In employing such counselling approaches, the following issues have typically been revealed:

- Behaviours that resulted in family violence were intergenerational and were modelled on that provided by one or both parents, or the absence of parents
- There were poor communication practices and fractured relationships in the person's family of origin
- Basic life skills are often missing (e.g., basic literacy where the client has no reading or writing abilities or comprehension)
- The tone or language of the sessions can be focussed on the past incidences of violence exclusively, or oriented towards resilience and hope for the future, acknowledging the

client's inner strengths. Indeed, it may be appropriate to do elements of both within sessions, when openly discussed with the client

Counselling supervisors must make sure that counsellors expand the narrative and develop a deep understanding of the client's circumstances at the early stages of client engagement. In undertaking initial assessments of the family violence client, whether the client has committed family violence or has been subjected to it, a comprehensive assessment of the client is needed. This would typically include:

- Client income sources (e.g., employed/unemployed or Centrelink recipient)
- Family structure (e.g., birth order, only child, adopted, step-family, orphan)
- Current Accommodation or Homelessness status (e.g., couch surfing)
- Mental health issues (current or past)
- Use of drugs and/or alcohol (current or past)
- Circles of support (e.g., family/friends)
- Language and communication skills
- Nationality or visa status
- Legal issues (e.g., current fines, criminal & civil matters, litigation)
- Physical health status (e.g., attends GP or psychiatrist, current medication, history of injury)
- Education levels (literacy, capacity to understand directions/ documentation)
- Any intervention Orders (current or past)
- Prior counselling history (if any)
- Any other community service agency or service providers (e.g., community transport; National Disability Support)
- Current suicide ideation, previous actions, psychiatric admission)

Criminogenic focus versus health focus

Counsellors practising in family violence should discuss with their supervisor how they are able to maintain a client focus offering hope, compassion, and justice in the context of their current working environment. In some jurisdictions family violence counselling may be associated with understanding how intervention orders or other criminal proceedings work and may immediately affect the client. This may mean that a client may not be able to see his or her children for an extended period of time as determined by a court. It is particularly important that the client feels supported by the family violence counsellor regardless of decisions made by courts or child protection agencies. It is important that some ongoing level of engagement is maintained, as if the client doesn't access counselling or secondary referrals then they can't be assisted.

It may be that the client is unable to fully access counselling at the time of initial presentation. They may be experiencing the immediate effects of family violence (e.g., anxiety, hypervigilance) and require a more immediate crisis response from the family violence counsellor. In other cases, they may have recently experienced a relationship breakdown but have the desire to have longer-term counselling support to engage in Family Dispute Resolution procedures (e.g., developing a parenting plan for their children).

It is important that by engaging in supervision the family violence counsellor is able to develop understanding of the differences between a crisis response to family violence presentations and practising a series of more structured responses. Over time, the impact of immediate legal proceedings, the current feelings that the client has about current safety and security, and their most immediate needs (e.g., homelessness, food, medical issues). This well-developed and nuanced understanding of the client is what is needed to increase effectiveness in family violence counselling.

Family violence counselling and stereotyping

Counsellors need to be aware of where there is a social context to support stereotyping. Family violence counsellors in particular, need to be aware of factors such as gender-based discrimination and age discrimination to ensure that they make a conscious effort to deactivate such bias and ensure they are fully present for all clients (Stangor, 2009).

In the Queensland Royal Commission into Family Violence (trends are mirrored in all Australian jurisdictions) they outline that:

> Domestic and family violence awareness and prevention messages have been a prom-inent theme in our national discourse ... The majority of people who experience domestic and family violence in Queensland are women. This is not to say that women cannot be the perpetrators of fear and violence upon male victims. Men can be and are victims of violence and coercive control and are victims of domestic and family violence homicides. Any domestic and family violence, regardless of who the victim and per-petrator are, is unacceptable... . The Taskforce also recognises that there are particular groups more vulnerable and at risk of being abused in a domestic or family situation, than others in the community. These vulnerable groups face challenges unique to them. Aboriginal and Torres Strait Island Australians, people from culturally and linguistically diverse backgrounds, the elderly, people with a disability, people in rural and remote communities, people who identify as lesbian, gay, bisexual, transgender and intersex, and children, are all at significantly higher risk from the incidences and impacts of domestic and family violence
>
> (Special Taskforce on Domestic and Family Violence in Queensland, 2017)

Avoidance of bias in reporting – community standards

The mainstream media significantly influences the perceptions of all those affected by or involved with family violence practice, including clinicians. Whilst family violence is a ser-ious cause of public concern, there is now much more public reporting than has been in the past. Society viewing family violence as an essentially private matter is no longer compatible with mainstream reporting. The Australian Press Council has now issued an advisory framework to assist editors and journalists to carefully exercise judgement in reporting. In part the Guidelines advise:

> The relationship between the alleged offender and the victim is the key. Violence inflicted by a stranger would rarely be conceptualised as family violence. The coverage of a breaking story may need to respond adeptly to subsequent information from police or other sources when what first appeared to be an ordinary crime or a tragic accident might now be viewed through the lens of family violence
>
> Victoria Police, 2004

Reporting of family violence is currently impacted by more than 40 often-inconsistent Commonwealth as well as State and Territory laws to ensure that reporting does not interfere with court proceedings or pre-empt the findings (Australian Press Council, 2018).

Family violence and the law

Family violence counselling supervisors need to ensure that they are able to provide support to family violence counsellors. Counsellors may need assistance in:

- Understanding how legal protections for those subjected to family violence work in the jurisdiction within which their counselling takes place
- Providing broad guidance about accessing legal and court processes (as opposed to legal advice)
- Understanding legal and protection orders and variations, and also orders made under the Commonwealth Family Law Act 1975
- Organising a pre-court visit or orientation session or participate in one organised by various courts in their local jurisdiction
- Understanding what Safety Planning means in a Family Violence context
- Consider accessing targeted training in giving evidence, referral, advocacy, and applicable documentation/case note writing relevant to their jurisdictions

In Victoria, since August 2004 there has been a Code of Practice for the Investigation of Family Violence. Whilst this is not counselling information per se, it does help in the understanding of, and provide some context for what some presenting clients may have experienced prior to attending counselling. It includes processes such as:

- Police will respond to the needs of children individually
- Police will treat every report of family violence as genuine and respond and act on all reports, regardless of where the reports have originated
- Police will assess the immediate risks and threats to victims and manage each incident
- Police will assess the level of future protection required for victims
- Stronger emphasis will be placed on police recognition that diverse communities and some incidents may require a different approach
- All reported incidents of family violence must be recorded to allow identification of recidivist offenders, monitoring of trends and identification of persons at risk
- Referral will be a mandatory component of any police response (Victoria Police, 2004)

Given the background in which the Law and Family Violence interact, counsellors need to provide their family violence clients with a psychologically safe place and prioritise what they say and believe. This does not mean that they act on everything a client says, as often perpetrators of family violence can play the role of victim or deflect or minimise their role in the violence. This is part of the skill counsellors need in being able to provide a nuanced response, including being skilled in the application of their clinical intuition.

Self-violence and threats

Professionals are responsible for the care and safety of consumers at elevated risk for suicidal behaviours in all settings and across the age span. This applies to family violence
counsellors also.

As part of the counselling supervision process it is an important competency requirement that family violence counsellors possess the necessary skills to reduce mental health
consumer morbidity and mortality by standardising the detection, assessment, and management of all clients at elevated risk for self-directed violence, in all settings and across the
age span. Many counsellors have undertaken Applied Suicide Intervention Skills Training
(ASIST)or similar and should be able to clearly identify those participants in the family violence process who are at elevated risk of suicide. The family violence counselling supervisor
needs to ensure that the counsellor has the core competencies required of professionals
responsible for the care and safety of consumers detected to be at elevated risk for suicidal
self-directed violence. Their micro-counselling skills need to reflect the ability to be comfortable conducting an interview designed to elicit perceived burdensomeness, suicidal
ideation, intent, capability, and buffers against suicide. Based on the quality of the therapeutic relationship, the difficulty of the interview, and the reliability of any data collected,
family violence counsellors learn to make informed risk stratification decisions to determine the level of care recommended or required and implement risk mitigation strategies.
This typically involves making sure that the family violence counsellor has left the client
with collaborative crisis safety planning, and input to managing/monitoring risk over time
and documentation.

In some family violence cases, threats of ongoing violence can be used as a form of coercion in relation to the other party, and should always be taken seriously by the counsellor
until determined otherwise.

As part of their regular practice, family violence counsellors are likely to encounter
presentations with clients before, during, and after violence is identified, and may receive
client referrals in a variety of contexts. Therefore, the cycle of violence needs to be well
understood in order for effective counselling interventions to occur. The supervision of
family violence counsellors must therefore be designed in ways that support practitioners to
work (depending on the participants) in both a child focussed and a relationally reparative
context with individuals, parents, and children following experiences of family violence.

Family violence and culturally and linguistically diverse (CALD) communities

Family violence counsellors who work with CALD, migrant, and refugee communities
require significant support by supervisors. Intimate partner violence takes place in Australia
across all cultures and faith groups. In addition to sexual and physical violence, women
from refugee backgrounds are particularly vulnerable to reproductive coercion, financial
abuse, and immigration related violence (Australian Human Rights Commission, 2017).
They are often subjected to pre-arrival traumatic experiences, as well as social isolation, and
the stresses associated with adapting to a new culture and way of life. In recent years there
has been a greater emphasis on involving men in violence prevention, the rationale being
that whilst the majority of men are not physically violent, gendered violence is perpetuated
overwhelmingly by men against women. What is not well understood is the ways in which

gender and culture intersect and the potential role of men from immigrant and refugee communities might have in family violence prevention (El-Murr, 2019).

A study of community attitudes demonstrated that people from countries in which the main language is not English were more likely to have low levels of understanding of what constitutes violence against women, to have a low level of support for gender equality, and were least likely to reject attitudes explicitly supportive of violence (VicHealth, 2014). What is still being developed is knowledge about the diversity of views regarding men and women's lived experiences, culturally bound experience, place of birth migration experiences, and religious beliefs.

Effects on children

Children experience loss as a result of family violence. It often disconnects them from their place in the world, their family, and their community. They sometimes have to leave their home, their room, their neighbourhood, their school, or their childcare. They miss their teachers and their friends. Part of the family violence supervision process of counsellors is to ensure that they have the necessary skills and experience to bring the voice of the child into the room. It may be that formal training in child inclusive practice and trauma informed practice forms a necessary discussion with the counsellor about practical considerations in their ongoing professional development.

An important supervision question that needs to be discussed with family violence counsellors for their work with children and young people, is their understanding and construction of the question: What does the idea of home mean for the child? Family violence can affect issues such as the young person's sense of self. Home may be associated with family, ease, relaxation, sense of belonging, security, oppression, marginalisation, kinship/culture, fear, or indeed feeling connected or not to the world (VicHealth, 2014).

Effects on mothers

Finding the courage to leave a violent relationship and rebuild the life of their family requires a mother to meet many complex challenges. It may impact the ways in which the mother and child interact in an ongoing way. It may be that the child did not feel protected or safe. It can affect the confidence of mothers to understand and meet the developmental needs of their children. As a part of this there will also be a need to understand whether and how to involve the parent who has acted violently. This is nuanced work through which the family violence counsellor needs to be supported by their supervisor and also not be afraid about raising such complexities in an ongoing way as part of supervision. Family violence counsellors need to be aware that violence against women in Australia is disturbingly high and can take many forms (VicHealth, 2014). These forms include domestic violence, sexual assault, online violence and harassment (including social media), and intimate partner violence. Other forms include violence against women experiencing social inequality, disability, or refugee and migrant status, or who are of Aboriginal or Torres Strait descent.

Effects on fathers

Men who present to counsellors for family violence may present as lost, not in control, remorseful, angry, disrespected, sad, lacking skills in parenting, and grieving. Family violence counsellors need to be in a position to respond effectively to any or all of such presentations (Ashfield, 2011).

There has been and continues to be considerable debate in the counselling and psychotherapy profession about whether there has been a feminisation of psychotherapy and whether counsellors have adopted standard approaches to family violence that only involve the consideration of Gender to the exclusion of developing a deeper understanding of men and their needs. Indeed, as far back as 2011 it was highlighted that men had been abandoning the field of psychotherapy for decades and that, for example, women outnumbered men enrolled in United States doctoral psychology programmes by a ratio of at least 3 to 1 (Carey, 2011).

This is not to say that females or males make better family violence counsellors or psychotherapists, but that a male counsellor may be more effective for some clients than others, as female counsellors may have more success with certain clients than their male counterparts.

Supervisors of family violence counsellors should not shy away from discussion of these important nuanced issues. Personality style, extraversion, introversion, and self-confidence are inevitably linked to gender and may impact how the client's story is heard. This forms part of the discussions of countertransference and biases about which we all need to be aware in counselling work (Diamond, 2012).

Situational couple violence and family violence

Counselling supervisors need to educate family violence counsellors in the differences between situational couple violence and family violence. Not only are they different in a practical sense, but the counselling treatment offered by the counsellor needs to take into account the nuances associated with these differences.

To be clear, no violent or abusive relationship is acceptable. Having said that, the distinguishing feature of what is commonly understood, regardless of jurisdiction, as family violence is that it is a pattern of behaviour. This abusive behaviour has been ongoing in some way for a consistent period of time and may present in the form of psychological abuse, financial abuse, physical abuse, sexual abuse, or emotional abuse.

By contrast, situational violence does not necessarily form a pattern of behaviour. It differs from family violence in that it is generally minor in nature and specific to the situation. It does not escalate over time and whilst one partner or the other (or both) may use violence to gain control during a fight, there is generally not an ongoing effort to exert power and control over the other between fights.

Both men and women engage in situational couple violence (Kelly & Johnson, 2008). Often those who engage in this type of violence do so because they are poor communicators who do not know how to argue without resorting to verbal or physical aggression. This does not excuse the behaviours described above, nor does it suggest that assaulting someone isn't a crime, because it is. Any use of violence to solve a problem is wrong. There are many examples that family violence counsellors regularly see that involve verbal aggression and insults that turn physical.

Part of effective family violence counselling involves understanding the client, the type of problem-solving models they adopt, where they learned this model from, and how they might change this model in order to be better or more effective communicators into the future. For example, one model adopted by perpetrators of violence is the EITHER/OR model. The basis of this model is a win/lose posture. It is either my way or your way and one is determined to win and make it their way. An alternative that the client can be introduced to is the BOTH/AND model. The basis of this model is a shared modality. How can "we" ensure that it is both my way AND your way. This facilitates forward joint decision making. during family violence counselling it is useful to explore the decision-making model that existed in the client's family of origin and how they learned their current behaviours.

It is also a useful counselling strategy to explore the differences in communication between men and women and the tools and techniques used by each party to get their messages across to the other. This includes issues such as the number of ideas to be communicated, the length of the message, the frequency of communication, the timing of communications to maximise effectiveness, effective listening, communication spoilers and the history of communication between the parties.

Taking the time to understand and explore interactions are critical in understanding situational couple violence and family violence. This assists with determining what interventions are appropriate and at what times (McCarthy & McCarthy, 2015).

Often presentations resulting from childhood trauma influence how effective communications and escalation between parties occur into adulthood. A significantly under explored variable in men, and to a lesser extent in women, is literacy. Often poor communication, disrespect, hurt, and embarrassment occur in the first instance as one or both of the parties lack the basic skills to read and write, and even speak with one another respectfully (Golden, 2000). It's sad to think this is the case in a modern society like Australia, however this is a reality. It doesn't excuse the use of violence, but it is helpful in understanding what contributing factors have led to this occurring.

The family violence counsellor and the family violence counselling supervisor need to discuss the significant contribution that psychoeducation can make to the client. It would be most appropriate in sessions that the use of specific psychoeducation materials is discussed and retained in an ongoing resource kit developed for this purpose.

Compassion fatigue, burnout, and vicarious trauma

One of the most difficult issues to deal with in counselling supervision in general, but with family violence counsellors in particular, is the acknowledgement and ongoing monitoring of counsellor fatigue and vicarious trauma and burnout. This is difficult and challenging work. There needs to be a regular system put in place to protect family violence counsellors. In cases where family violence counsellors are sole practitioners, they need to seek external supervision and to regularly practice self-care.

Some strategies that should be discussed in supervision regularly include:

- Decreasing the frequency and duration of caregiving
- Arranging work cycles to allow for brief breaks between sessions to allow time to refocus, recharge, and to stop patterns of compassion fatigue
- Monitor and reduce feelings of pressure and encourage informal conversations with colleagues which support and allow the spread of emotionally demanding or time- consuming tasks
- Encouraging professional development activities or group work to vary counselling routines
- Promote the autonomy of Family Violence Counsellor self -care strategies such as walking, mindfulness and meditation
- Encouraging the regular taking of annual leave and leisure time

Fortunately, the counselling profession is starting to provide more focus on family violence counsellors having their personal needs and mental health attended to on a more regular basis (Australian Childhood Foundation, 2019). This in turn promotes recovery, practitioners becoming less stressed, and having more confidence in their own ability to cope. It is essential that family violence counsellor wellbeing is the primary focus of every supervision session, because if the family violence counsellor is not functioning well then their ability to help their clients effectively is also diminished (Centre for Excellence in Therapeutic Care, 2019; Denborough, 2008).

Concluding Remarks

The underlying philosophy of family violence counselling practice is that all clients must be treated with hope, compassion, and justice. There is an obligation for counselling supervisors to ensure that all family violence counsellors operate within their current scope of practice, conform to relevant standards and codes of ethics, and meet all legislative requirements applicable to the jurisdictions in which they practice. There is often uncertainty about what issues (see Appendix C) need to be brought by family violence counsellors to their clinical counselling supervision sessions.

Counselling supervisors must ensure that all family violence counsellors do no harm. By the very nature of being involved in the family violence process clients have already been harmed in some way. Counsellors have an obligation to ensure that processes are in place to ensure the safety of both the family violence counsellor and the family violence client and that these aspects are regularly reviewed in supervision sessions with their supervisor.

Because of the nature of all family violence counselling presentations, there is a requirement to engage in trauma informed practice. Consideration should be given to increasing the frequency of counselling supervision sessions to provide more regular family violence counsellor support as a result. It is essential in the family violence domain that family violence counsellors actively seek out supervision as they are particularly and frequently exposed to people who are in or who have witnessed family and personal crises.

This is challenging, difficult professional work. In this context family violence supervisors are a major resource which needs to be utilised by the counsellor. The family violence domain in Australia and in the entire western world is rapidly changing as societal norms shift. In various jurisdictions mandatory reporting regimes are being created and implemented by governments. New accountability guidelines are being implemented and gender roles are becoming less certain than in the past.

It is of concern that in this rapidly changing environment that family violence counsellors may forget that they are not there to judge clients, to usurp the role of courts and magistrates, or to impose their own values or beliefs on clients. They for example should not assume that all men are violent, or all women are nurturers, or that all children are not affected by family violence. Whether the client is a sex offender or a victim of a violent crime, everyone deserves to receive a professional service.

Family violence counsellors need to demonstrate hope, compassion, and justice for all clients. Anyone who works in this difficult area of professional counselling practice can experience ethical conflict, transference, trauma, and doubt. It is tough work. And that is the reason why family violence supervision is so essential. Effective counselling supervision is a mandatory professional requirement. Family violence supervisors are there to ensure that family violence counsellors are mindful of their own competence and standards of ethical practice.

Educational questions & activities

1. When legal questions arise, what two behaviours does the FV Counselling Supervisor need to challenge in FV Counselling practice?
2. If there are "grey" areas of FV Practice, how are these issues resolved?
3. What protective mechanisms need to be in place to ensure the welfare of FV Counsellors?
4. To effectively understand the reasons for FV presentations, what three issues are often present?

References

Ashfield, J. (2011). *Doing psychotherapy with men: Practising ethical psychotherapy and counselling with men*. Peacock Publications.

Australian Childhood Foundation (2019). *Practice guide: Creating positive social climates and home-like environments in therapeutic care*.

Australian Human Rights Commission (2017). *Violence against women in Australia: Submission to the UN Special Rapporteur on violence against women*.

Australian Press Council (2018). *Advisory guideline on family and domestic violence reporting*.

Carey, B. (2011, May 21). Need therapy? A good man is hard to find. *New York Times*. www.nytimes.com/2011/05/22/health/22therapists.html

Centre for Excellence in Therapeutic Care (2019). *Practice guide: Secondary traumatic stress and staff well-being: Understanding compassion fatigue, vicarious trauma and burnout in therapeutic care*.

Denborough, D. (2008). *Collective narrative practice: Responding to individuals, groups and communities who have experienced trauma*. Dulwich Centre Publications.

Diamond, S. A. (2012, October 5). End of men: The "feminization" of psychotherapy. *Psychology Today*. www.psychologytoday.com/intl/blog/evil-deeds/201210/end-men-the-feminization-psychotherapy

El-Murr, A. (2019). *Intimate partner violence in Australian refugee communities* (CFCA Paper No. 50). Australian Institute of Family Studies.

Golden, T. (2000). *Swallowed by a snake: The gift of the masculine side of healing* (2nd ed.). GH Publishing.

Isacco, A., & Wade, J. C. (2019). *Religion, spirituality and masculinity: New insights for counsellors*. Routledge.

Jenkins, A. (2001). *Invitations to responsibility: The therapeutic engagement of men who are violent and abusive*. Dulwich Centre Publications.

Kelly, J. B., & Johnson, M. P. (2008). Differentiation among types of intimate partner violence: Research update and implications for interventions. *Family Court Review*, 46(3), 476–499. https://doi.org/10.1111/j.1744-1617.2008.00215.x

McCarthy, B., & McCarthy, E. (2015). *Therapy with men after sixty: A challenging life phase*. Routledge.

Murdolo, A., & Quiazon, R. (2016). *Key issues in working with men from immigrant and refugee communities in preventing violence against women*. White Ribbon Australia.

O'Brien, C. (2016). *Blame changer: Understanding domestic violence*. Threekookaburras.

Special Taskforce on Domestic and Family Violence in Queensland (2017). *Not now, not ever: Putting an end to domestic and family violence in Queensland*. Queensland Government. https://www.justice.qld.gov.au/initiatives/end-domestic-family-violence/about/special-taskforce

Stangor, C. (2009). The study of stereotyping, prejudice, and discrimination within social psychology: A quick history of theory and research. In T. D. Nelson (Ed.), *Handbook of prejudice, stereotyping, and discrimination* (pp. 1–22). Psychology Press.

VicHealth (2014). *Australians' attitudes to violence against women.* Victorian Health Promotion Foundation.

Victoria Police (2004). *Code of practice for the investigation of family violence.*

Part 3

The Approaches

Part 3, The **Approaches** section, comprising six chapters, will enable both trainees and supervisors to re-examine the important role of the working alliance in facilitating change through supervisory encounters, while furthermore exploring the major models and processes used to enhance learning. Chapter 9 explores the main models of supervision and moving from theory to practice. Chapter 10 focuses upon the alliance in supervision to enhance client outcomes. Chapter 11 outlines a solution-focused approach to supervision. Chapter 12 explores various processes and interventions that can be used in supervision. Chapters 13 and 14 explore Christian counselling and social work counselling, respectively.

Chapter overview

Chapter 9, **Models of Supervision: From Theory to Practice**, by Bert Biggs, Matt Bambling, and Zoë Hazelwood, clearly and methodically presents each of the major models of supervision, and associated components, and then follows up each with interesting practical examples that elucidate the concepts. The reader will review the chapter several times, because of the concentration of terms and notions, but will be thankful to do so as it will significantly enhance both clinical interventions and the process of supervision. The enumerated *secrets that supervisors and trainees keep from each other* is a list that will easily stimulate quality dialogue in supervision, and aid enormously in the development of ultimately collegial relationships with supervisees.

Chapter themes

In this chapter you will explore the following themes:

- The psychodynamic model of supervision
- The behavioural and cognitive models of supervision
- The developmental model of supervision

Chapter 10, **Alliance Supervision to Enhance Client Outcomes**, by Matt Bambling, provides a very interesting and timely model for supervision that addresses brief therapy, clinical outcomes, empirically research, and non-approach bound concepts – all themes that have received popular backing in recent decades. Bambling's innovative model, which is explained in some detail, has a significant orientation towards examining and developing the interpersonal and alliance-related factors in supervision. This is one of the few research

DOI: 10.4324/9781003490067-11

focused chapters in the text, and is thus not only a welcome addition but an opportune reminder of the scientist-practitioner model clinicians adopt as they work. As with other chapters, the case examples are additive to the reader's understanding of concepts and processes, which are also well explicated.

Chapter themes

In this chapter you will explore the following themes:

- Why focus on alliance?
- Three-stage alliance supervision
- Case examples of TSAS
- TSAS supervision insights

Chapter 11, **Solution-Focused Supervision,** by Ann Moir-Bussy, explores the supervisory relationship and techniques in supervision that focus on the present as well as goals versus problems.

Chapter themes

In this chapter you will explore the following themes:

- Present focus
- Goal focus
- Wu-Wei and Cross-Cultural Utility

Chapter 12, **Processes and Interventions to Facilitate Supervisees' Learning,** by Keithia Wilson and Alf Lizzio, comprehensively addresses one of the most basic yet significant questions asked of supervision: 'How does it impact learning?' This chapter identifies that if we are clear about what we ultimately want from the process, and we know how best we learn, as well being cognisant of the power of reflective practice, there is a greater likelihood of the supervisory experience being powerful and positive for all involved. Central to the development of this chapter is the focus on the supervisory relationship as a critical variable that impacts supervisee growth and development. Wilson and Lizzio's chapter is replete with many challenging questions and numerous helpful suggestions that will enable the reader to systematically grasp, in due course, the more effective ways of facilitating learning in meaningful ways.

Chapter themes

In this chapter you will explore the following themes:

- Establishing an effective working alliance
- What learning goals shall we pursue?
- What approach to learning suits our circumstances?
- What type of relationship do we wish to have?
- What management processes do we wish to establish?
- Supervisor reflection

- Supervisee reflection
- Initial contracting
- Ongoing review
- Supervisory meta-competencies
- Processes for constructive feedback
- Forms of participation and voice
- Facilitating reflective practice
- Specific supervisory methodologies
- Case studies
- Observation
- Role play
- A contextual model for role play

Chapter 13, **Chrisitan Counselling Supervision,** by Shannon Hood and Tracey Milson, explores the unique character of Christian counselling supervision and the types of Christian counselling provided to clients, including professional and pastoral.

Chapter themes

In this chapter you will explore the following themes:

- Christian counselling supervision
- Christian counselling
- In partnership with the Holy Spirit
- To accompany … on the journey of life
- Types of Christian counselling
- Professional Christian counselling
- Professional counselling by a Christian
- Pastoral counselling
- Lay Christian counselling
- Professional Christian supervised supervision

Chapter 14, **Supervision of Social Workers,** by Rebecca Braid, examines the unique components of supervision that are relevant to social workers.

Chapter themes

In this chapter you will explore the following themes:

- Supervision of social workers
- Components of social work supervision
- Changes to social work standards for supervision
- Case Example: The changing face of supervision

9 Models of Supervision

From Theory to Practice

Herbert Biggs, Matthew Bambling, and Zoë Hazelwood

Introduction

This chapter will address psychodynamic, cognitive-behavioural, and developmental models in supervision by initially considering the historical underpinnings of each and then examining in turn some of the key processes that are evident in the supervisory relationships. Case studies are included where appropriate to highlight the application of theory to practice and several processes are fully elaborated over all models to enable a contemporary view of style and substance in the supervision context.

The psychodynamic model of supervision

Psychodynamic supervision is grounded in Freud's psychoanalytic theory,[1] and many of the processes and relationships that are addressed in psychoanalytic psychotherapy are also present in the psychodynamic supervisory relationship. This section will first consider the historical underpinnings of psychodynamic supervision and some of the key processes that are prevalent in the psychodynamic supervisory relationship. The extent to which the supervisory relationship can be considered similar to the therapeutic relationship has been the focus of substantial debate and will therefore also be briefly discussed.

Historical background

Historically, psychodynamic supervision owes its beginnings to Freud's psychoanalytic model of psychotherapy. Indeed, Freud is often labelled as the first psychotherapeutic supervisor (Bernard & Goodyear, 2004), with informal supervision sessions designed to educate analysts and discuss each other's work. Riess and Herman (2008) describe this as the 'master–apprentice' model of supervision, and one can imagine Freud firmly positioned as the master, holding court to a gathering of inspired apprentices.

By the 1920s, formal training standards were introduced by the International Psychoanalytic Society. The standard was set requiring analysts to participate in their own personal analysis and to participate in supervision, referred to as 'control analysis' (Ekstein & Wallerstein, 1976). In this approach, the supervising analyst was responsible for performing both the role of supervisor and personal analyst for the trainee psychoanalyst. Not surprisingly, it was not long before some psychoanalysts began to question the wisdom of having these dual roles in place. By the 1930s the substantial debate that surrounded this issue resulted in a professional division. The Budapest School continued with the practice of using supervision as both an instructional tool and a means for personal

DOI: 10.4324/9781003490067-12

analysis, whereas the Institute in Vienna argued that both roles could not be fulfilled by the one person and mandated psychoanalysts seek personal analysis as separate from the supervisory relationship (Bernard & Goodyear, 2004). The Hungarian argument promoted supervision as an extension or continuation of personal analysis, where supervision would address both transference from therapy and countertransference from supervision. On the other hand, the Austrian approach argued the two should remain separate because supervision was designed to teach and the analyst's personal problems and issues needed to be raised in a different forum, during personal analysis. Therefore, psychodynamic supervision can be thought of as providing the historical foundation for the classic controversy that is still apparent today (Carroll, 2007); how do you distinguish between therapy and supervision?

Psychodynamic supervision processes

Andersson (2008) suggests the key element of psychodynamic supervision is to explore the supervisee's conscious and unconscious reactions to clients and the process of therapy. Many of the processes that are drawn upon in a psychodynamic supervision session will seem familiar to therapists from a number of orientations as they are concepts that have been adopted quite widely. Terms such as 'alliance,' 'parallel processes,' and 'transference' have all derived from early psychoanalytic theory. A few of the key psychodynamic processes often utilised and reflected upon in supervision will be discussed.

Working alliance

With early links to psychoanalytic theory (e.g., Greenson, 1967; Sterba, 1934), the supervisory working alliance closely mirrors that of the client–therapist therapeutic alliance. Now widely considered to be pantheoretical, and conceptualised best by Bordin (1983), the supervisory working alliance is 'that sector of the overall relationship between the participants in which supervisors act purposefully to influence trainees through their use of technical knowledge and skill and in which trainees act willingly to display their acquisition of that knowledge and skill' (Efstation, Patton, & Kardash, 1990, p. 323). The working alliance is a collaborative relationship where the personal and interpersonal qualities of both the supervisee and supervisor are used to formulate a relationship based around trust and security, not unlike Bowlby's (1973/1998) attachment paradigm.

Progressing towards a successful working alliance involves addressing three aspects of supervision: the supervision bond, mutually understood goals of supervision, and agreed tasks of supervision (Bordin, 1983). The supervision bond develops as the relationship grows, with trust, caring, empathy, and liking increasing over time. Goals of supervision often include the acquisition of technical skills and knowledge, improved understanding of self and others, developing comfort with process issues in therapy, and overcoming obstacles that may impact on a therapist's progress with a client. The tasks of supervision will be the actions agreed upon by supervisor and supervisee that assist with achieving the supervision goals. When these three components are strong and mutually satisfying, an effective working alliance is in place.

Substantial research has investigated the predictors and outcomes of a successful working alliance (see Bernard & Goodyear, 2004 for a comprehensive review). Self-disclosure in supervisees is greater in supervisory relationships where the quality of the alliance is rated as strong compared to when quality is considered poor (Webb & Wheeler, 1998). The working alliance also impacts elements of the therapist's work, with greater rapport and a stronger alliance related to greater job satisfaction compared to less rapport and poorer alliance (Mena & Bailey, 2007). Recent research tends to suggest that a strong working alliance between supervisor and supervisee is important for buffering the impact of traumatic work environments and reducing the risk of vicarious traumatisation (Dunkley & Whelan, 2006). The working alliance has also been linked to therapist ratings of self-efficacy, although the results appear to be confusing. Ladany and colleagues (1999) suggest the strength of the working alliance does not appear to have a strong impact on therapist ratings of self-efficacy but a more recent study by Lent et al. (2006) suggests otherwise. In any event, a strong working alliance between supervisor and supervisee can contribute positively to supervisee development.

Parallel processes

Another term used frequently across models of supervision but that also developed out of psychoanalytic theory is the notion of the parallel process. Friedlander, Siegel, and Brenock (1989) defined this concept as involving behaviour where supervisees will 'unconsciously present themselves to their supervisors as their clients have presented to them. The process reverses when the supervisee adopts attitudes and behaviours of the supervisor in relating to the client' (p. 149). Therefore, the supervision dyad begins to mirror the therapy dyad in a meaningful and instructional manner. If a therapist experiences a problem in supervision when discussing a particular client, this can represent an unconscious expression of a client's problem in therapy (Andersson, 2008; Ekstein & Wallerstein, 1976).

Parallel processes in psychodynamic supervision involve bringing that which is unconscious into the conscious so that it can be reflected upon, discussed, and resolved. Often the first sign that a parallel process is evolving is unusual or atypical behaviour in the therapist during supervision sessions (Deering, 1994). Once the supervisor has drawn attention to the existence of this parallel process, the therapist may appear less confused or better able to understand the feelings they were experiencing.

Case Example – Parallel Process. Isabella is a trainee psychotherapist who has been having supervision sessions with Helen, a psychodynamic supervisor, for almost a year. In her latest supervision session, Isabella began discussing a recent therapy session with a new client, Ray, a troubled and angry adolescent who presents as sullen and disengaged during sessions. He regularly tests the therapeutic boundaries and Isabella's patience. When Isabella presents this case to Helen she unconsciously re-enacts Ray's in-session behaviour during her supervision session, questioning Helen's words, and making statements that test her relationship with Helen. The 'mood' of her therapy sessions with Ray is mirrored during this supervision session with Helen. Helen is able to recognise the parallel process that Isabella is unconsciously adopting and uses her role as supervisor to illustrate how Isabella might want to proceed in her sessions with Ray and how she may best handle his behaviour. In effect, Helen models to Isabella an appropriate course of action to take in future sessions with Ray. By questioning Isabella's assumptions and feelings about Ray's behaviour, both explicitly and implicitly, Helen slowly draws out Isabella's unconscious beliefs and motivations surrounding Ray's therapy. She then openly voices her observations and she and Isabella finish the session by reflecting on the parallel process that occurred. The next time Isabella sees Ray she presents herself to Ray much as Helen did during supervision, adopting Helen's supervisory manner and approach and using it in the therapy session.

Isabella's behaviour during supervision illustrates what Deering (1994) refers to as an upward parallel process. Isabella's subsequent therapeutic approach with Ray could be classified as a downward parallel process. In this case, the downward process was therapeutic and directed towards improving client outcome. Not all downward parallel processes may be so positive. Deering (1994) provides the example of a supervisor pushing their supervisee towards the achievement of a goal too quickly and the supervisee responding by placing similar pressure on their client.

Transference and countertransference

Another essential element of psychodynamic supervision is the processing of transference and countertransference experiences. Transference refers to the client's unconscious feelings and behaviour directed towards the therapist which stem from the client's background and early experiences (Andersson, 2008). Countertransference refers to the feelings and impulses a therapist experiences as a result of interacting with a particular client (Ladany, Friedlander, & Nelson, 2005; Rosenthal, 1999) that may result either from the client's behaviour (objective countertransference), or from the therapist's background (subjective countertransference). Thus the psychodynamic supervision triangle of client, therapist, and supervisor has the potential to influence two relationships: the supervisory relationship and the clinical relationship (Beck, Sarnat, & Barenstein, 2008).

During supervision the psychodynamic supervisor will encourage their supervisee to process and reflect on the transferences and countertransferences that occur as a function of the therapeutic and supervisory relationships. 'When disturbing states of mind are transmitted from client to supervisee, they are often subsequently enacted with the supervisor rather than verbally described to him or her. By attending to the supervisee's countertransference experience and to the supervisory relationship, such states become accessible for processing' (Beck et al., 2008, p. 69).

While there is a tremendous amount of theoretical writing and many narrative case studies describing the usefulness of transference and countertransference as a supervisory process, there isn't a great deal of empirical literature on the topic. Zaslavsky, Nunes, Eizirik, and Nurse (2005) explored supervisory countertransference and concluded that countertransference became more direct and objective as the supervisory relationship continued, and the supervisors in their study (at an institution accredited by the International Psychoanalytical Association) see it as quite important to hold up the distinction between supervision and personal analysis for trainee analysts.

Case Example – Countertransference. Joan is in her mid-30s and is a trainee psychoanalyst who has been separated from her husband for almost three years. She is raising her daughter as a single parent while beginning her career as an analyst. She has been undertaking her own personal analysis since her divorce and is proud of the fact that she is commencing a new career while single-handedly raising her daughter and is financially independent of her ex-husband. One of Joan's regular clients is Sammie, who started seeing Joan following her own relationship breakdown 12 months earlier. She presents as someone who is helpless and unsure of her place in the world, who cannot see herself coping without a partner in her life, and who has repeatedly expressed a desire to reconnect with her ex-husband. She is reliant on her ex-husband for financial support and remains unmotivated to find employment or 're-enter' the world.

During supervision, Joan tells her supervisor, Robert, about Sammie's latest behaviour and she feels she has stalled in her sessions with Sammie. Joan describes Sammie as unmotivated and unwilling to change. After some careful questioning by Robert, Joan expresses a frustration with what she sees as Sammie's laziness and believes Sammie is taking the easy way out of her problems. Joan is critical of Sammie's reliance on her ex-husband for support and believes that Sammie is capable of achieving quite a lot if she puts her mind to it.

Robert must tread carefully here for he recognises that Joan's reaction to Sammie's behaviour is tied up not only in Joan's frustration with Sammie's perceived unwillingness to change (objective transference) but also in Joan's beliefs about what women can achieve and her own experience as a successful single-parent (subjective transference). Robert prompts Joan to reflect on her reactions to Sammie's motivations and defence mechanisms, and points out the obvious countertransferences that Joan appears to be expressing. He helps Joan to recognise how her own beliefs have influenced her perceptions of Sammie's behaviour and encourages Joan to discuss these beliefs and their historical development with her analyst at their next session. He and Joan then go on to discuss Sammie's behaviour and formulate a plan for how to genuinely explore with Sammie her goals for life and therapy.

This example illustrates the delicate boundaries that psychodynamic supervisors must navigate as a part of the supervisory relationship. Indeed, even very early psychoanalytic theorists (e.g., Searles, 1955) distinguish between 'disturbing experiences with the patient [that are] reframed as crucial data, diagnostic of the patient's problems, rather than as intrusions that should be relegated to the therapist's personal therapy' (Sarnat, 1992, p. 389). Thus we see the aforementioned divide occurring between those analysts who believe supervision can include personal therapy, and those who see supervision as quite distinct from the analyst's own personal therapy.

Teach or Treat?

The historical foundations of psychodynamic supervision mean that many of the practices used in this supervisory approach parallel those used in the provision of psychodynamic psychotherapy, so it's hardly surprising that therapy and supervision are often confused. It is beyond the scope of this chapter to engage in lengthy discussion of this issue, however it is important to acknowledge the distinction. Wheeler (2007) argues that 'a balance needs to be struck that enables exploration and support, but avoids supervision becoming therapy' (p.247). Freud might have seen himself as both master analyst and supervisor for his trainee analysts, but the contemporary ethical view is to encourage the supervisee to seek personal analysis outside the supervisory relationship. This is not to say that counter-transference is avoided in supervision, but that the focus of processing countertransferences is to use them as an instructional, education tool rather than a personally therapeutic process (Sarnat, 1992).

When considering the distinction between psychodynamic supervision as therapy and supervision as supervision, it is important to consider some of the key differences between the two, differences that see the analyst and supervisor performing very different roles. As Hyman (2008) discusses, unlike therapy, supervision is not confidential especially if conducted within a training course/university. In addition, the supervisor is responsible for addressing issues such as poor progress, lack of ethical behaviour, and poor record keeping which may need to be addressed with an institutional supervisor. Also the supervisor may need to address supervisee behaviour such as lateness or missed appointments in a manner that is different to how a therapist deals with the same behaviour in a client.

A final important distinction is that supervisors evaluate their supervisees, whereas psychodynamic psychotherapists rarely formally evaluate their clients in the same manner.

Seeking personal analysis appears to be beneficial to analysts on a number of levels. In addition to providing the opportunity to work through transference and countertransference processes and discussing the therapist's own defence mechanisms, it seems that analysts undertaking their own personal therapy outside the supervisory relationship make for better therapists. An interesting study Coleman (2002) surveyed a sample of community clinicians and trainees and found that analysts who undergo their own personal therapy are given higher ratings of empathy and warmth compared to those therapists not currently seeking personal therapy. Not only does the therapist benefit from therapy but it appears the therapist's clients can too.

Conclusion

Psychodynamic supervision has developed considerably since Freud's master–apprentice model of psychoanalytic supervision. Contemporary approaches argue in favour of distinguishing between supervision as an instructional tool versus supervision as a therapeutic tool. Many of the processes that occur in supervision, however, form the basic tenets of psychoanalytic psychotherapy. For example, the notion of the working alliance stems from discussions of the therapeutic alliance; downward parallel processes can impact on a client just as strongly as they impact on a therapist; reflection on transferences and countertransferences have become as much a part of supervision as they are a hallmark of discussions about psychoanalytic therapy sessions. While it is important to remember that psychodynamic supervision cannot replace individual personal therapy, quality supervision invariably involves more than just the technical presentation and teaching of skills. Psychodynamic supervision forms a type of secure base from within which the trainee analyst can explore their feelings and impulses and as such psychodynamic supervision is most effective when it embraces a therapist's experiences, feelings and reactions towards both client and supervisor, and the supervisor's similar experiences, feelings and reactions.

The behavioural and cognitive models of supervision

Historical background

Historically, therapy, and counselling texts have separated behavioural and cognitive theory and methods. In more recent times, however, there has been a therapeutic and praxis rapprochement whereby those interested in behavioural change have developed a more cognitive orientation, and cognitive theorists and practitioners have integrated behavioural techniques as part of a broader treatment suite.

Behavioural therapy's aetiology is heavily influenced by the work of Pavlov, Watson, and Skinner, and their premise that our behaviour is determined by what happens to us as a result of our behaviour. The concept of reinforcement is critical. If we are reinforced for our behaviour, then most likely we will continue to engage in that behaviour. If we are ignored or punished, the behaviour is likely to abate or cease. In this classic view of behaviourism, internal processes and cognitions are given little emphasis. The focus is on direct and observable behaviour. Behavioural therapy, as summarised by Mischel (1971) has three common features:

- Behaviour therapies attempt to modify the problematic behaviours themselves
- Like the social behaviour theories that guide them, behaviour therapies emphasise the individuals' current behaviours rather than the historical origins of the problems
- Belief in a general assumption that undesired behaviour can be understood and changed using the same learning principles that govern desired behaviour

These features underpin three other important principles which form part of the scientific basis of behaviour therapy and an empirical approach to the modification of human functioning:

- It is based on the results of empirical research using rigorous scientific methodology
- It applies behaviour change principles that have been demonstrated by basic research
- Its clinical and applied approaches must continually meet benchmark scientific standards

Bandura (1989) emphasised that the client should be deeply involved in the choice and direction of treatment and moved behaviourism towards behavioural humanism. His concept of self-efficacy emphasised individual rights and collaboration in the counselling and treatment process, by emphasising that individuals develop best when they have control of their own destiny. This view and following important work by Meichenbaum (1991), which emphasised person-environment interaction, gave focus to a view of behaviour being reciprocally influenced by thoughts, feelings, physiological processes and the consequences of behaviour. There was a de-emphasis of the centre of control being in the external environment, and a shift to a centre stage role for the client. The fusion of these approaches has produced a cognitive-behavioural therapy and counselling approach (CBT) which has become a potent dynamic in counselling and psychotherapy.

Cognitive and Behavioural fundamentals

The cognitive contribution to CBT has been heavily influenced by the work of Albert Ellis. His model of rational-emotive therapy (RET) was a pioneering method of CBT (Ellis, 1983). Fundamental principles include unconditional acceptance of all clients, encouragement to clients to think rationally and be in touch with their emotions, and a strong emphasis on follow up activity by the client after the counselling session. This 'homework' seeks to have clients apply ideas from the counselling sessions to their daily lives as important to the change process. A process result is to aim for the client to decide on an action for logical reasons that are also satisfactory emotionally. Hence the term rational-emotive. The individual must both think and feel that a decision is correct. RET endeavours to correct thought patterns and minimise irrational ideas, while simultaneously attempting to change dysfunctional feelings and behaviours. An important pneumonic coined by Ellis conveniently shapes the process:

A – the objective facts, events, behaviours that an individual encounters
B – the person's belief about A
C – the emotional consequences, or how a person acts and feels about A
D – disputing irrational beliefs and thinking
E – the effect of disputation in D on the client
F – new feelings and emotions associated with the situation

An analogous technique identifying faulty thought patterns was pioneered by Beck (1991). An eradication of harmful automatic thoughts, an examination of current thinking processes and an eventual development of new forms of cognition characterise the constructs. The following steps summarise the process:

- Recognising maladaptive thinking and ideation
- Noting repeating patterns of ideation that tend to be ineffective
- Distancing and decentring help clients remove themselves from the immediate fear, thought, or problem so that they can think about it from a distance
- Changing the rules of thinking

Both theories and therapeutic approaches place the client as a principal agent of change, who is challenged by the 'here and now' imperative and where solutions are not necessarily found by delving into past history.

The behavioural contribution to CBT has been heavily influenced by the work of Pavlov, Watson, and Skinner as previously noted. Ivey, Ivey, and Simek-Morgan (2007) describe some of the key behavioural change procedures:

- Pinpointing behaviour
  - Move from general observations of, e.g., *this hyperactive child is difficult to control* to noting precise observable behaviours such as the number of times the child interrupts the teacher or the number of times the child leaves the chair.
- Positive reinforcement
  - The provision of rewards for desired behaviour. Use of learning theory concepts such as extinction, shaping, and intermittent reinforcement to elicit and maintain desired behaviour.
- Charting
  - Charting or diary entry of the number of occurrences of important behaviours before, during, and after treatment. Assists in observing whether a behaviour is maintained after treatment and whether a new strategy should be tried.
- Relaxation training
  - Client mastery of simple relaxation techniques, allow further exploration to solve more complex issues.
- Biofeedback and self-regulation
  - Instrumentation is now readily available for biofeedback to assist in a variety of client tension patterns.
- Systematic desensitisation
  - Consists of three primary steps: (1) Training is systematic deep muscle relaxation, (2) construction of anxiety hierarchies, and (3) matching specific objects of anxiety from the hierarchy with relation training
- Modelling
  - Seeing and hearing directly, either live or via film or digital media, brings home a message more clearly and directly than advice or description.
- Social skills training
  - Skills training often involves the following cognitive-behavioural components: (a) Rapport/structuring; cognitive and emotional preparation for the instruction, (b) Cognitive presentation and cueing; explanation and rationale for acquisition of the skill, (c) Modelling; role plays, digital media, demonstrations enacted,

(d) Practice; mastery of the skill to a high level through practice, (e) Generalisation; movement of the skill from the training session to in vivo application.
- Assertiveness training
  - A balance of learning to stand up for individual rights (overt behaviour) and simultaneously consider the thoughts and feelings of others (client cognitions).
- Stress inoculation and management
  - Training for (a) A cognitive understanding of the role of stress in an individual's life, (b) specific coping skills, and (c) working with thoughts and emotions attendant to the stress situation to motivate remedial action.

Supervision

Supervision plays an essential role in the benchmarking and quality assurance of practitioners during initial training and throughout a professional career. What, then, are the elements of good supervision, and what can be expected from their adoption by the therapist? Pretorius (2006) asserts the primary goal of CBT supervision is to help the therapist adopt the philosophy of CBT as the basic approach for changing clients' cognitions, emotions, and behaviours to facilitate improvement or recovery. A secondary goal is to teach the therapist specific skills or techniques. There are striking similarities between both goals. Both are systematic, goal-directed, structured, time-limited, collaborative, person-focused, confidential and active. Both emphasise mutual trust, openness, practice, experience, change facilitation, building on existing strengths and skills, and response to feedback.

Perris (1993) argues that CBT supervision tends to follow a relatively didactic model. Leise and Beck (1997) and Liese and Alford (1998) suggest the following structure for each CBT session: checking in; setting the agenda; bridging from the previous supervision session; enquiring about previously supervised cases; reviewing homework; prioritising of agenda items; discussing an individual recorded case; using direct instruction and guided discovery; using standardised supervision instruments; assigning new relevant homework; and eliciting feedback from the supervisee. This framework has been overlaid by Armstrong, Twaddle, and Freeston (2003) who identify and describe four interacting levels for the CBT supervision framework. The first level, *primary inputs*, includes the context in which the supervision occurs, the clients' impact on supervision, and the selectivity with which the supervisee reports therapy – a subject to which we will return later in this chapter. The second level, *parameters*, outlines the nature and development of the supervisory project. The third level, *dynamic focus*, examines the changing emphasis on case conceptualisation, technique, and the therapeutic relationship. The fourth level, *learning process*, is an experiential process of learning with stages outlined for supervision to proceed to achieve new knowledge, skill and application.

Most commentators agree that the nature and quality of the relationship between supervisor and supervisee is paramount to successful supervision, but there is no universal agreement as to how this can be achieved. For example, Dobson and Shaw (1993) suggest that the three principal activities of cognitive therapists and supervisors are, in descending order, relationship activities, case conceptualisation, and learning techniques. However, in a survey of UK cognitive-behavioural psychotherapists, Townend, Iannetta, and Freeston (2002) confirm that 16 topics were discussed during supervision and were, in descending order of frequency: case formulation; cognitive analysis; cognitive interventions; behavioural interventions; three systems analysis; functional analysis; application of techniques;

emotional responsibility; goal setting; therapeutic bond; client safety; homework; ethical issues; evaluation methods; therapist safety; and exclusion criteria. In the evidence of the latter study, it has to be assumed that relationship activities are occurring in a less overt way, if at all, than in the conceptualisation of Dobson and Shaw.

An insightful and frank set of observations by Ladany (2004) helps gain some understanding of an elusive and perhaps fruitless search for a supervision template in the cognitive and behavioural therapy environment. Ladany commences by stating 'There is a theory which states that if ever anyone discovers exactly what the Universe is for and why it is here, it will instantly disappear and be replaced by something even more bizarre and inexplicable' (p. 1). He follows by noting from the beginning of his psychotherapy training how he was struck by how fabulously incompetent were those he deemed *supervisors*, that it was not until he received the title of supervisor himself that he learnt how fabulously incompetent he also could be. Ladany presents his investigations into psychotherapy supervision research by posing a series of four questions.

If nothing else what should a supervisor do? Drawing on his own experience of supervision, Ladany notes the few superb supervisors who shaped him demonstrated great skilfulness at developing a strong supervisory alliance along with providing a good mix of challenge and support that allowed him to grow as a therapist-in-training. He recommends that supervisors attend to the development of a strong supervisory alliance using and generalising their psychotherapy skills (e.g., empathy, clarification). The alliance, developing as it does most readily in the early relationship, should be considered as figure-ground in the supervisory work. That is, attend more to the alliance when the relationship is developing or when there is a rupture in the alliance, and attend to it less when supervisor technical skills are needed to focus more on the trainee's development.

What are some of the worst things a supervisor can do? First, ignore the supervisory working alliance which only creates a weak foundation on which to facilitate change in the trainee. Second, use developmental cookie-cutters to treat trainees. It seems likely there are trainee and supervisor factors that account for more of the variance in how a trainee will respond to supervision and among them are trainee tolerance for ambiguity, experience with the specific client base, general clinical experience, past effective supervision experiences, conceptualisation ability, and supervisor personality and ability factors. Third, approach supervision with the belief that supervisor ethics are for wimps. Ladany and colleagues (1999) proposed supervisor ethical guidelines and then determined how well practising supervisors adhered to them. The guidelines were an amalgam of several well-published professional body guidelines. This work yielded 18 ethical categories relevant to supervisors. Fifty-one percent of the respondents reported their supervisors violated at least one of these guidelines. Why? Many supervisors never received training to become a supervisor and in addition many supervisors may judge the 'critical feedback' role as being counterintuitive to the non-judgemental and supportive roles typically adopted in supervision.

Fail to tell trainees how they will be evaluated and then evaluate them capriciously. Ladany notes that a variety of studies point to the difficulty supervisors have in providing evaluations of trainee performance. There is little evidence that it is done well, with subjective and qualitative measures lacking rigour, and quantitative measures having poor psychometric properties (Ellis & Ladany, 1997). Ladany and Muse-Burke (2001) suggest that for any evaluation approach a series of components needs to be considered. Among them are the mode of therapy (e.g., individual, group, family or couples), the domain of supervisee behaviours (e.g., psychotherapy or supervision), the area of competence (e.g., psycho-therapy techniques, theoretical conceptualisation, assessment), methods (e.g., trainee self-report, case notes, audiotape, live supervision), proportion of caseload (e.g., all clients, subgroup of clients, one client), and evaluator (e.g., supervisor, clients, peers, objective raters). Although not all of these parameters could or should be considered in any given evaluation approach, the value of any approach can be determined based on how well each of these components are incorporated.

Demonstrate you are racist, sexist, or homophobic both overtly and subtly. Ladany notes often witnessing how supervisors can act overtly bigoted when he was a trainee but in other venues come across as champions of multiculturalism. His research findings indicated clearly that self-reported multicultural competencies are not related to demonstrated multicultural competencies. The development of the Heuristic Model of Nonoppressive Interpersonal Development codes individuals into one of two groups: a socially oppressed group (SOG), female, person of colour, gay/lesbian/bisexual, disabled, working class; or a socially privileged group (SPG), male, white, heterosexual, physically able, middle to upper class. Irrespective of group, individuals also move through similar phases of means of interpersonal functioning (MIF); e.g., thoughts and feelings about oneself as well as the behaviours based on one's identification with a given demographic variable. The phases of MIF are adaptation, incongruence, exploration, and integration. Individuals can be more advanced in terms of their MIF for one variable over another. For example, a supervisor in the adaptation phase in terms of gender identity, will likely minimise and dismiss a trainee's desire to consider gender issues in relation to client conceptualisation. To better under-stand the multiple identity interactions that occur in supervision, Ladany hypothesises four supervisor–supervisee interpersonal interaction types for each demographic variable: pro-gressive, in which the supervisor is at a more advanced stage than the trainee; parallel-advanced, in which the supervisor and trainee are at comparable advanced MIF stages; parallel-delayed, in which the supervisor and trainee are at comparable delayed MIF stages; and regressive, in which the trainee is at a more advanced stage than the supervisor. Each of these interaction types has implications for trainee and client outcome. Specifically, the facilitation of trainee outcome is predicted to occur from most to least for the following types: parallel-advanced, progressive, parallel-delayed, and regressive.

What secrets do supervisors and trainees keep from each other? Ladany reports sets of both supervisor and supervisee non-disclosures. The items listed in Table 9.1 are noted as rarely disclosed in supervision:

The overall assessment on both sets of non-disclosures probably inform us more of issues of power differential deference, impression management, fear of political suicide, and choice of client development over supervisee development. The reasons for non-disclosure will invariably be multidimensional, and closely related to the strength of the working alliance. The best that could be said is that both supervisors and supervisees should be aware of what is generally omitted in order to realistically evaluate what can be profitably and developmentally disclosed in their own relationship. It involves judgement replete with all the elements of good supervision referred to earlier, namely mutual trust, openness, practice, experience, change facilitation, building on existing strengths and skills, and response to feedback.

Table 9.1 Secrets kept in supervision

Supervisee	Supervisor
Negative reactions to their supervisors	Negative reactions to counselling and professional performance
Personal issues	Supervisor personal issues
Clinical mistakes	Negative reactions to supervisee's supervision performance
Evaluation concerns	
General client observations	Supervisee's personal issues
Negative reactions to the client	Negative supervisor self-efficacy
Countertransference	Dynamics at training site
Client–counsellor attraction issues	Supervisor's clinical and professional issues
Positive reactions to the supervisor	Supervisee appearance
Supervision setting concerns	Positive reactions to therapy and professional performance
Supervisor appearance	
Supervisee–supervisor attraction issues	Attraction to supervisee
Positive reaction to the client	Reaction to supervisee's clients
	Experience as a supervisor with other supervisees

The behavioural and cognitive approaches share much of the supervision challenge with the other contemporary approaches discussed in this chapter. At the core of the matter, supervision is a dynamic that should be aimed at the most efficient and effective process to enable an intending therapist to both inculcate the philosophy of the technique and gain knowledge and skills in the application of the therapy.

The developmental model of supervision

The developmental model is a unique approach to supervision as it is not bound to psychotherapy theory. The developmental model has its strongest conceptual links with educational theory. It has had considerable influence on the practice of supervision across all theoretical orientations, and has been subject to more empirical research than any other approach to supervision. Three areas will be addressed in this section: (1) defining the key assumptions and principles of developmental supervision, specifically the Integrated Developmental Model of Supervision (IDM); (2) demonstrating how IDM supervision is used in practice; and (3) examining the research to assess the efficacy of the developmental approach.

Developmental supervision defines good supervision as occurring when supervisors assess supervisee experience-based skill factors and use these to structure a learning environment that meets individual supervisee learning goals. In the most basic terms, the developmental model purports that experience level is the key factor that should mediate supervisory structure and supervisee learning needs.

The integrated developmental model of supervision

There are a number of developmental models of supervision that share key assumptions regarding the structuring of learning environment based on supervisee experience level. For the purposes of this discussion the focus will be on the integrated developmental model (IDM) as informed by the work of Stoltenberg, McNeill, and Delworth (1998).

Essentially IDM describes a process where the supervisor modifies the structure of supervisory activity on a continual basis to match the growing clinical experience of the supervisee. The importance of altering supervisory structure to match growing supervisee competency cannot be overemphasised as it provides the method by which more advanced skills are developed (Hansen, & Barker, 1964; Hogan, 1964; Litterell, Borden, & Lorenz, 1979; Loganbill, Hardy, & Delworth, 1982; Stoltenberg, 1981; Stoltenberg & Delworth, 1987). IDM supervisory structure is conceptualised as a series of experience related pre-defined levels through which the emerging therapist must progress to gain clinical competence with defined supervisor behaviours for each level of progression (Litterell, Borden, & Lorenz, 1979; Loganbill, Hardy, & Delworth, 1982; Stoltenberg, 1981).

Supervision that is structured and directive is hypothesised as optimal for beginning supervisees, whereas supervision that is collegial and consultative is optimal for advanced supervisees. In practical terms the supervisor makes an assessment of experience level and competency of the supervisee and prescriptively matches supervisory activity, teaching strategies in accordance with the appropriate developmental level. The model is relatively structured and prescriptive and the capacity for a supervisee to prioritise his or her own learning goals with a supervisor is limited. Development occurs across a number of overriding structures and associated specific domains (see Table 9.2 Overriding Structures and Associated Domains) and over a set number of developmental levels (Table 9.3 Levels of Supervisee Development).

Applying IDM overriding structure to competency domains

The supervisor goals are to facilitate the IDM overriding structures – motivation, autonomy, and awareness – as these are the desired internal supervisee characteristics that allow the supervisee to engage with the domain categories (Table 9.2). These domain categories may be considered competencies that will be achieved to differing degrees at each developmental level and mastered through progress to higher levels (Table 9.3). Motivation, autonomy, and awareness are mediated by the interpersonal and structural environment of supervision. Initially the supervisor develops a purposeful supervisor–supervisee relationship, which enables communication and trust and creates a shared understanding of roles, responsibilities, and boundaries of supervision. Emphasis is then placed on clarifying expectations, developing goals in clinical work and professional development, and how work will be evaluated, for example, observation of videotaped work. The supervisor

Table 9.2 Overriding structures and specific domains (Stoltenberg & Delworth, 1987)

Overriding structures	Specific domains
Self and other awareness	Intervention
	Assessment techniques
	Interpersonal assessment
Motivation	Client conceptualisation
	Individual differences
	Theoretical orientation
Autonomy	Treatment plans and goals
	Professional ethics

Table 9.3 Levels of supervisee development (Stoltenberg & Delworth, 1987)

Experience Level	Supervisee Characteristics	Supervisory Environment
Level 1 Motivation Autonomy Awareness	*Relationship building and goal setting* Focused on: • Own anxiety Dependent on external authority • Motivated to learn techniques • Imitative • Limited self-awareness and conceptual or categorical thinking In transition towards level 2: become anxious regarding new approaches and have unrealistic expectations	*Trust builder and contractor* Structure to manage anxiety Training in domain competencies is: • Prescriptive • Instruction • Supportive • Interpretative • Modelling approaches • Skills training • Feedback on strengths and weaknesses.
Level 2 Motivation Autonomy Awareness	*Affective issues and skills deficits* Focused on: • Dependency – autonomy conflict. • Fluctuating motivation. greater understanding of client, confusion, and/or defensiveness In transition towards level 3: increased desire to personalise orientation, conditional autonomy, understands limitations, beginning awareness of self in client work	*Counsellor and teacher* Training in domain competencies is: • Through providing less structure • Through modelling greater autonomy. • Encouraging higher levels of involvement • Support more so for difficult issues only. • Communication of ambivalence. • Providing difference perspectives • Pore focus on process issues
Level 3 Motivation Autonomy Awareness	*Confidence in expertise* Focused on: • Emotional impact on self. Confidence in ability. Autonomy. • Motivated to understand strengths and weaknesses. Professional identity focus. Personal responsibility. • High degree of empathy and understanding In transition to level 4: will demonstrate stability of operation across all domains (see Table 1a)	*Colleague* Training in domain competencies is: • Through mutual sharing • Involvement as peer • Exemplification • Confrontation and challenging interventions with client • Conceptualisation • Deal with affective reactions • Observation • Engage in more complex cases
Level 4 Motivation Autonomy Awareness	*Self responsibility and autonomy* Master Counsellor Focused on: • Moving conceptually and behaviourally move across domains (table 1a). Professional identity stable across domains • Personal understanding across domains • Aware of impact of personal on professional work	*Consultant* Training in domain competencies achieved by: • Being collegial • Allowing the supervisee to provide more structure • More focus on personal and professional integration • Clinical integration • Personally confronting • Change orientated to prevent stagnation • High process and experience of case focus

may at this stage assess the level of the model that suits the supervisee and structure the learning environment accordingly.

The supervisor will then observe supervisee practice in domain related areas such as interpersonal skills, clinical skills, case management skills, the client–therapist relationship, achievement of standards and use of models and theory. The supervisor then assesses these observations to evaluate the specific skill and professional development needs of the supervisee which is provided as feedback. The supervision meeting serves as the primary mode of providing feedback and skills training, communication, problem solving and the opportunity for the supervisor to model the required target skills. Importantly the supervisor follows up all agreed leaning and treatment planning tasks with the supervisee ensuring they provide the appropriate training and the agreed client plans have been implemented.

A typical developmental supervision scenario and experience – level related structure

Trevor was supervising Jennifer on her first clinical placement. Jennifer was anxious as she had not seen many clients before and was unsure she could deal with the type of problems clients might present. Trevor spent some time getting to know her and developing a positive working relationship. He talked with Jennifer about her previous therapy experience, her studies, understanding of the therapeutic process and client change as well as her personal fears and doubts. Thinking in IDM terms, Trevor realised she was a beginning level therapist and would need a high level of direction and structure in supervision (Level 1). This assessment was confirmed after Trevor viewed her first videotaped therapy session. Trevor assessed supervisory activity should focus on teaching Jennifer case conceptualisation, and formulate and implement treatment plans (domain competencies), and to manage her anxiety and fears about conducting therapy.

In negotiation with Jennifer, Trevor formulated a set of learning goals for supervision based around level 1 goals. Jennifer agreed with these goals and wanted to include her own goal to learn how to recognise and work with process issues in therapy such as defences, resistance, and transference. Trevor noted that these were more advanced skills and probably related to issues of ambivalence regarding competency and autonomy and dependence that might be played out in supervision when Jennifer progressed to level 2. Trevor said that he would provide her with instruction in recognising these issues in supervision when appropriate, but the main focus of supervision would relate to the agreed learning goals (as her learning needs related more to level 1 issues). Trevor explained that these core learning goals were foundational good therapy, and their mastery would provide a base to build more advanced skills. He assured Jennifer that there would be plenty of time to explore process issues as she became more confident with the basics of treatment. Supervision was conducted in a formal and structured way with Jennifer presenting her cases in supervision from detailed notes and occasional videotapes of therapy. The supervisory discussion focused on the agreed goals. Soon Trevor was confident that Jennifer was developing competency in foundational skills and was well on the way to achieving level 1 learning goals. As Jennifer's confidence increased Trevor decided to use a few supervision strategies based on level 2. He raised issues regarding the dynamics of therapy and interpreted client behaviour to help Jennifer understand therapeutic process. Trevor noticed Jennifer was beginning to explore her own emerging autonomy as a therapist sharing her views and ideas about therapeutic process.

Trevor also began to expect Jennifer to process her own reactions to client work in supervision. Trevor noticed that even though Jennifer was progressing well in developing skills and achieving learning goals, the focus of supervision was still educational. Jennifer easily felt unsure of herself and Trevor often had to provide support and encouragement aimed at helping her manage her anxiety about not recognising therapeutic issues or not being a perfect therapist. Trevor realised that even though Jennifer was doing some work in supervision consistent with level 2, her needs for supervision structure were still related to level 1 and she was in a transition between levels. He also realised that this experience of supervision would be formative to Jennifer's emerging professional identity as a therapist.

Trevor noted after six months of weekly supervision that Jennifer had increased in confidence in therapy and could conceptualise the important issues of a case and formulate and implement basic treatment plans. Trevor and Jennifer felt that the initial learning goals were achieved and developed new goals that focused more on treatment dynamics and process issues in therapy as well as more advanced treatment skills and interventions. Trevor reduced the level of structure of supervision and provided direct training only as needed and began to encourage Jennifer's autonomy by developing her own hypotheses and testing these out in therapy. Jennifer responded by becoming more autonomous in supervision, occasionally asserting herself regarding preferences for supervisory activity and structure and expressing more confidence in client work. At other times Jennifer appeared somewhat ambivalent about the reduction in supervision structure and her emerging autonomy. Trevor recognised that Jennifer was well established in level 2 of the developmental process and making good progress.

About the same time, the service employed a graduate therapist in a senior position. Liz was a very experienced therapist having graduated from a clinical doctoral programme. As principal staff supervisor, Trevor met with Liz and quickly assessed she was likely competent across all domains and did not need a structured learning environment and could set her own agendas in supervision to meet her goals. Trevor conducted supervision with Liz in a very collegial way giving a great deal of autonomy allowing her to structure the supervision according to her needs in accordance with level 4 of the developmental model. His assessment of her skills was confirmed when he observed her first contracted video of a client session where she demonstrated a high level of skill in all domain competencies. He noticed that in supervision Liz did not often discuss case conceptualisation and treatment planning, but rather focused on her own reactions to the case and deep insights into client dynamics and process of treatment as well as issues relating to her own ongoing professional development.

Research and the developmental model

The case examples above demonstrate the common sense appeal of IDM that supervisee experience level should determine the structure of the supervisory environment and assessment of learning needs. Does the evidence support this proposition? The answer is not as straightforward as it might seem. Research into what constitutes optimal supervisory structure has provided results that in some cases are contradictory and in others difficult to interpret. The assumption of a relationship between experience and supervision structure has been criticised by a number of researchers. Holloway (1987), Roehlke (1984), and Ellis, Ladany, Krengel, and Schult (1997) concluded there was little evidence to establish any developmental processes in supervision or that any supervisee learning needs were related to experience level and that developmental theory is prescriptive and therefore cannot accommodate other factors that might mediate supervisee learning needs. However, when the evidence is examined in detail, important conclusions can be made.

The changing needs of the supervisee

Worthington (1987) found that beginning level supervisees preferred structure and direction by their supervisor and experienced supervisees preferred less structure and direction. While providing some support for experience level being the key mediating variable in supervision an unexpected finding was that some supervisee preferred supervisory behaviour was not consistent with experience level. Experience level might mediate case conceptualisation, experienced supervisees focus on transference and countertransference, self-efficacy and self-awareness when conceptualising cases, whereas new therapists focus on the technical skills necessary to conceptualise cases. No effect was found for intermediate or transitional levels of the model in any study (Borders & Leddick, 1988; Holloway & Wompold, 1986; Holloway, 1987, 1992; Winter & Holloway, 1992; Worthington & Stern, 1985). Interestingly, any effect for developmental level was lost when situational factors were evidence such as when a supervisee engaged a new supervisor or dealing with a crisis situation. In these instances, the need for structure and support was present in supervision regardless of experience level (Krause & Allen, 1988; Miars et al., 1983; Wiley & Ray, 1986). Supervisors are also able to recognise variation in the needs of beginning and advanced level supervisees (Krause & Allen, 1988; Miars et al. 1983; Wiley & Ray, 1986; Holloway, 1987, 1992).

These studies demonstrate some support for the view that the experience level of the supervisee can influence supervisory structure, but only between novice and experienced supervisees. No effect is evident for intermediate experience levels on supervisory structure; nor do these studies demonstrate how experience level can mediate the transition of the therapist through intermediate stages of supervision. Further, these studies identify variance in the needs of supervisees for structure that cannot be explained by experience level alone.

The effect of supervisee characteristics

An alternative argument suggests that it is the characteristics of a supervisee, such as facilitative skills (Carlozzi, Campbell, & Ward, 1982), cognitive style (Holloway & Wampold, 1986; Winter & Holloway, 1992), and level of ego development as defined by attitudes and rigidity of thinking (Borders, Fong, & Cron, 1988) determines the preference for structure in supervision. These characteristics might exert an influence on supervision that is independent of experience level.

The evidence appears somewhat contradictory with support for both experience level and individual characteristics as defining supervisee preferences for structure in supervision and little relationship with supervisee skill level. These disparate positions can be reconciled by a novel study (Tracey & Sherry, 1993) that suggests experience level and individual characteristics of supervisees interact to structure the supervisory environment.

Conclusion

A number of findings regarding the IDM from the literature appear reasonably robust:

• Research only demonstrates an effect on supervisee preference for supervisory structure between lowest and highest levels of experience,

- There is no evidence, as predicted by developmental theory that supervisees progress through intermediate levels of supervisory structure based on increasing experience level,
- The relationship between experience level and skill development is not strong.

There is reasonably strong evidence that several additional factors may mediate the experience-supervisory structure of supervision. These factors are:

- That individual supervisee characteristics and situational factors in supervision strongly influence the relationship between experience level and structure in supervision,
- In some cases, individual characteristics exert more influence on the structural preference of supervisees for supervisory environment than experience level alone.

The evidence suggests IDM supervision might be a more effective model if the structure of supervision is adapted to include the needs created by supervisee characteristics, in addition to experience level. In fact, supervisors should assess and prioritise individual characteristics of supervisees and situational factors when considering the best learning structure-experience level combination for the supervisory environment.

Conclusion

From its earliest foundations in psychoanalytic psychotherapy to contemporary approaches like IDM, supervision in the helping professions remains dynamic and multifaceted. Despite the often-vast differences between these three approaches to supervision, it is worth noting all endorse a strong supervisory alliance as fundamental to the success of supervision. Psychodynamic supervision utilises processes not out of place in a cognitive-behavioural supervision session; IDM is equally as reliant on supervisee characteristics and environmental factors as is psychodynamic supervision. Another characteristic shared by all three approaches to supervision is the relative dearth of empirical evidence investigating the efficacy of each supervisory approach. While each approach has attracted research into the processes that take place during the supervision session, thus providing evidence of the mediated components of each model, there is little evidence testing the overall impact of any one complete model of supervision. Whether this reflects a reliance on an eclectic approach to supervision, whether it reflects difficulty identifying and articulating markers of efficacy in supervision, or whether if reflects a lack of agreement surrounding who supervision ultimately benefits the most (client or supervisee), the stage is set for a greater research focus in the area of psychotherapeutic supervision.

Educational questions & activities

1. In groups discuss the following:
   a. Define the key principles of psychodynamic, CBT, and IDM models of supervision.
   b. How do they differ in theoretical assumptions, processes, and techniques?
   c. What is the contribution of each approach to supervisee skill development?
   d. Which approach do you like best and why?

e. Can these approaches be integrated into your supervision practice? Provide a rationale?
2. What does a psychodynamic supervisor do in supervision?
   a. Teaches treatment planning skills and therapeutic techniques
   b. Develops a positive supervisory alliance with their supervisee
   c. Assesses supervisee skill and experience and structures the learning environment accordingly
   d. Helps the supervisee understand the interpersonal processes and intrapsychic issues that occur in therapy
   e. Both b and d.
3. Why do psychodynamic, CBT, and IDM supervision prioritise the importance of a good working relationship between supervisor and supervisee?
   a. All approaches assume that a positive working relationship will assist in achieving supervisory learning goals
   b. Supervisors want their supervisee's to have a good experience working with them
   c. It is important to feel good when in supervision
   d. A good supervisory alliance makes it possible to give honest feedback to each other.
4. If your supervisee reports they are not making progress in therapy with a client what should you do from a CBT supervision perspective?
   a. Revisit the treatment plan and provide more skilful techniques
   b. Examine the interpersonal dynamics of the case
   c. Decide how to address supervision session learning outcomes based on the developmental level of the supervisee
   d. Examine how the supervisee really feels about working with their case.
5. There is little evidence of efficacy for psychodynamic, CBT, or IDM supervision. Consider the following:
   a. What is the real value of supervision?
   b. How do you know if supervision works?
   c. How should supervision be evaluated?
   d. Who is supervision ultimately for, the supervisee or the client?

Selected references for further reading

Allen, G. J., Szollos, S. J., & Williams, B. E. (1986). Doctoral students' comparative evaluations of best and worst psychotherapy supervision. *Professional Psychology: Research and Practice, 17*, 91–99.

Bambling, M., & King, R. (2000). Supervision and the development of counsellor competency. *Psychotherapy in Australia, 6*(4), 58–63.

Note

1 For the purposes of this brief overview, the authors use the term 'psychodynamic' to encompass all related contemporary psychoanalytic theories, whereas 'psychoanalytic' is used to represent only Freudian theory.

References

Andersson, L. (2008). Psychodynamic supervision in a group setting: Benefits and limitations. *Psychotherapy in Australia, 14,* 36–41.

Armstrong, P., Twaddle, V., & Freeston, M. (2003). *Supervision: Integrating Practical Skills with a Conceptual Framework.* Unpublished manuscript. Newcastle, UK: Newcastle Centre for Cognitive and Behavioural Therapy.

Bandura, A. (1989). Human agency in social cognitive theory. *American Psychologist, 37,* 122–147.

Beck, A. (1991). Cognitive therapy: A 30 year retrospective. *American Psychologist, 46,* 368–375.

Beck, J. S., Sarnat, J. E., & Barenstein, V. (2008). Psychotherapy-based approaches to supervision. In C. A. Falender & E. P. Shafranske (Eds.), *Casebook for Clinical Supervision: A Competency-Based Approach* (pp. 57–96). Washington, DC: American Psychological Association.

Bernard, J. M., & Goodyear, R. K. (2004). *Fundamentals of Clinical Supervision* (3rd ed.). Boston: Pearson Education.

Borders, L., Fong, M., & Cron, E. (1988). In session cognitions of a counselling student: A case study. *Counselor Education and Supervision, 17,* 7–12.

Borders, L. D., & Leddick, G. R. (1988). A nationwide survey of supervision training. *Counselor Education and Supervision, 27,* 271–283.

Bordin, E. S. (1983). Supervision in counseling: II. Contemporary models of supervision: A working alliance based model of supervision. *The Counseling Psychologist, 11,* 35–42.

Bowlby, J. (1973/1998). *Attachment and Loss: Vol. 2. Separation: Anxiety and Anger.* London: Pimlico.

Carlozzi, A., Campbell, N., & Ward, G. (1982). Dogmatism and externality in locus of control as related to counsellor training skill in facilitative responding. *Counselor Education and Supervision, 21,* 227–236.

Carroll, M. (2007). *Effective Supervision for the Helping Professions.* Thousand Oaks: SAGE.

Coleman, D. (2002). Personal therapy: A catalyst to relational awareness. *Irish Journal of Psychology, 23,* 73–85.

Deering, C. G. (1994). Parallel process in the supervision of child psychotherapy. *American Journal of Psychotherapy, 48,* 102–110.

Dobson, K. S., & Shaw, B. F. (1993). The training of cognitive therapists: What have we learned from treatment manuals? *Psychotherapy, 30,* 573–577.

Dunkley, J., & Whelan, T. A. (2006). Vicarious traumatisation in telephone counsellors: Internal and external influences. *British Journal of Guidance & Counselling, 34,* 451–469.

Efstation, J. F., Patton, M. J., & Kardash, C. M. (1990). Measuring the working alliance in counselor supervision. *Journal of Counseling Psychology, 37,* 322–329.

Ekstein, R., & Wallerstein, R. S. (1976). *The Teaching and Learning of Psychotherapy.* New York: International.

Ellis, A. (1983). The origins of rational-emotive therapy (RET). *Voices, 18,* 29–33.

Ellis, M., Ladany, N., Krengel, M., & Schult, D. (1997). Clinical supervision research from 1981 to 1993: A methodological critique. *Journal of Counseling Psychology, 43,* 35–50.

Ellis, M. V., & Ladany, N. (1997). Inferences concerning supervisees and clients in clinical supervision: An integrative review. In C. E. Watkins (Ed.), *Handbook of Psychotherapy Supervision* (pp. 567–607). New York: Wiley.

Friedlander, M. L., Siegel, S. M., & Brenock, K. (1989). Parallel process in counseling and supervision: A case study. *Journal of Counseling Psychology, 36*(2), 147–157.

Greenson, R. (1967). *The Technique and Practice of Psychoanalysis.* New York: International Universities Press.

Hansen, J., & Barker, E. (1964). Experiencing and the supervisory relationship. *Journal of Counseling Psychology, 11,* 107–111.

Heppner, P. P., & Roehlke, H. J. (1984). Difference among supervisees at different levels of training: Implications for a developmental model of supervision. *Journal of Counseling Psychology, 31,* 76–90.

Hogan, R. A. (1964). Issues and approaches in supervision. *Psychotherapy: Theory, Research and Practice, 1,* 139–141.

Holloway, E. (1987). Developmental models of supervision: its development? *Professional Psychology: Research and Practice, 19,* 138–140.

Holloway, E. (1992). Supervision: a way of teaching and learning. In S. Brown & R. Lent (Eds.), *Handbook of Counselling Psychology.* New Jersey: John Wiley & Sons.

Holloway, E., & Wampold, B. (1986). Relation between conceptual level and counselling related tasks. A meta-analysis. *Journal of Counseling Psychology, 33,* 310–319.

Hyman, M. (2008). Psychoanalytic supervision. In A. K. Hess, K. D. Hess, & T. H. Hess (Eds.), *Psychotherapy Supervision: Theory, Research, and Practice* (2nd ed., pp. 97–113). New Jersey: John Wiley & Sons.

Ivey, A. E., Ivey, M. B., & Simek-Morgan, L. (2007). *Counselling and Psychotherapy: A Multicultural Perspective.* Boston: Pearson.

Krause, A., & Allen, G. (1988). Perceptions of counselor supervision: An examination of Stoltenberg's model from the perspectives of supervisor and supervisee. *Journal of Counseling Psychology, 35,* 77–80.

Ladany, N. (2004). Psychotherapy supervision: What lies underneath? *Psychotherapy Research, 14,* 1–19.

Ladany, N., Ellis, M. V., & Friedlander, M. L. (1999). The supervisory working alliance, trainee self-efficacy, and satisfaction. *Journal of Counseling & Development, 77,* 447–455.

Ladany, N., Friedlander, M. L., & Nelson, M. L. (2005). *Critical Events in Psychotherapy Supervision: An Interpersonal Approach.* Washington, DC: American Psychological Association.

Ladany, N., Lehrman-Waterman, D. E., Molinaro, M., & Wolgast, B. (1999). Psychotherapy supervisor ethical practices: Adherence to guidelines, the supervisory working alliance, ands supervisee satisfaction. *The Counselling Psychologist, 27,* 443–475.

Ladany, N., & Muse-Burke, J. L. (2001). Understanding and conducting supervision research. In L. J. Bradley & N. Ladany (Eds.), *Counselor Supervision: Principles, Process, & Practice* (3rd ed., pp. 304–329). Philadelphia: Brunner-Routledge.

Leise, B. S., & Alford, B. A. (1998). Recent advances in cognitive therapy supervision. *Journal of Cognitive Therapy: An International Quarterly, 12,* 91–94.

Leise, B. S., & Beck, J. S. (1997). Cognitive therapy supervision. In C. E. Watkins (Ed.), *Handbook of Psychotherapy Supervision* (pp. 113–133). New Jersey: John Wiley & Sons.

Lent, R. W., Hoffman, M. A., Hill, C. E., Treistman, D., Mount, M., & Singley, D. (2006). Client-specific counselor self-efficacy in novice counselors: Relation to perceptions of session quality. *Journal of Counseling Psychology, 53,* 453–463.

Littrell, J., Lee-Borden, N., & Lorenz, J. (1979). A developmental framework for counselling supervision. *Counselor Education and Supervision, 19,* 129–136.

Loganbill, C., Hardy, E., & Delworth, U. (1982). Supervision: A conceptual model. *The Counselling Psychologist, 10,* 3–42.

Meichenbaum, D. (1991). Evolution of cognitive behaviour therapy. In J. Zeig (Ed.), *The Evolution of Psychotherapy II* (pp. 95–106). New York: Brunner/Mazel.

Mena, K. C., & Bailey, J. D. (2007). The effects of the supervisory working alliance on worker outcomes. *Journal of Social Service Research, 34,* 55–65.

Miars, R., Tracey, T., Ray, P., Cornfeld, J., O'Farrell, M., & Gelson, C. (1983). Variation in supervision process across trainee experience levels. *Journal of Counseling Psychology, 30,* 403–412.

Mischel, W. (1971). *Introduction to Personality.* New York: Holt, Reinhart and Winston.

Perris, C. (1993). Stumbling blocks in the supervision of cognitive psychotherapy. *Journal of Clinical Psychology and Psychotherapy, 1,* 29–43.

Pretorius, W. M. (2006). Cognitive behavioural therapy supervision: Recommended practice. *Behavioural and Cognitive Psychotherapy, 34,* 413–420.

Riess, H., & Herman, J. B. (2008). Teaching the teachers: A model course for psychodynamic psychotherapy supervisors. *Academic Psychiatry, 32,* 259–264.

Rosenthal, L. (1999). Group supervision of groups: A modern analytic perspective. *International Journal of Psychotherapy, 49*, 197–213.

Sarnat, J. E. (1992). Supervision in relationship: Resolving the teach-treat controversy in psychoanalytic supervision. *Psychoanalytic Psychology, 9*, 387–403.

Searles, H. (1955). The informational value of the supervisor's emotional experiences. *Psychiatry, 18*, 135–146.

Sterba, R. (1934). The fate of the ego in analytic therapy. *International Journal of Psychoanalysis, 15*, 117–126.

Stoltenberg, C. (1981). Approaching supervision from a developmental perspective: The counsellor complexity model. *Journal of Counseling Psychology, 28*, 59–65.

Stoltenberg, C. D., & Delworth, U. (1987). *Supervising Counsellors and Therapists: A Developmental Approach*. San Francisco: Jossey-Bass.

Stoltenberg, C. D., McNeill, B., & Delworth, U. (1998). *IDM supervision: An integrated developmental model for supervising counselors and therapists*. San Francisco: Jossey-Bass.

Townend, M., Iannetta, L., & Freeston, M. H. (2002). Clinical supervision in practice: A survey of UK cognitive behavioural psychotherapists accredited by the BABCP. *Behavioural and Cognitive Psychotherapy, 30*, 485–500.

Tracey, T., & Sherry, P. (1993). Complementary interaction over time in successful and less successful supervision. *Professional Psychology: Research and Practice, 24*, 304–311.

Webb, A., & Wheeler, S. (1998). How honest do counsellors dare to be in the supervisory relationship? An exploratory study. *British Journal of Guidance & Counselling, 26*, 509–524.

Wheeler, S. (2007). What shall we do with the wounded healer? The supervisor's dilemma. *Psychodynamic Practice: Individuals, Groups and Organisations, 13*, 245–256.

Wiley, M., & Ray, P. (1986). Counselling supervision by developmental level. *Journal of Counseling Psychology, 33*, 439–445.

Winter, M., & Holloway, E. (1992). Relation of trainee experience, conceptual level and supervisory approach to selection of audiotaped counselling passages. *The Clinical Supervisor, 9*, 87–103.

Worthington, E. (1987). Changes in supervision as counsellors and supervisors gain experience: A review. *Professional Psychology: Research and Practice, 18*, 189–209.

Worthington, E., & Stern, A. (1985). The effects of supervisor and supervisee degree level and gender on the supervisory relationship. *Journal of Counseling Psychology, 32*, 252–262.

Zaslavsky, J., Nunes, M., Eizirik, C., & Nurse, G. (2005). Approaching countertransference in psychoanalytical supervision: A qualitative investigation. *International Journal of Psychoanalysis, 86*, 1099–1131.

10 Alliance Supervision to Enhance Client Outcomes

Matthew Bambling

Overview

Clinical supervision has traditionally been considered an important part of the training and professional development of therapists, being rated highly in the experience of trainees as well as practitioners in the field (Orlinsky, Botermans, & Ronnestad, 2001; Steven, Goodyear, & Robertson, 1998). However, the evidence base for any supervision approach improving outcomes with clients is lacking (Bambling & King, 2000). In this chapter an alternate non-approach bound model of supervision is presented that has preliminary evidence for enhancing client outcomes in brief psychological treatment. The focus of this Three-Stage Alliance Supervision (TSAS) prioritises the interpersonal process of counselling as an independent factor as well as the core construct through which all technical interventions should be given. Below is an introduction to the supervision model used in the first empirical investigation of supervision and client outcome (Bambling, King, Raue, Schweitzer, & Lambert, 2006). While this chapter does not constitute the supervision manual it will provide the reader with sufficient knowledge to adopt an alliance focus in their supervision practice.

Introduction

There are many approaches to supervision, some embedded in models of counselling such as psychodynamic or cognitive-behavioural, or independent of therapy model such as a developmental approach. Bernard and Goodyear (1992) found that therapists assessed supervision as an indispensable training activity that increased both self and therapeutic awareness. Further, therapists have rated supervision highly as an educational procedure that develops treatment skills and professional competency (Steven et al., 1998). Supervision is usually considered an important post-training professional activity and is not restricted to the graduate training setting. During supervision, a supervisor and therapist may systematically examine case-specific treatment and process issues as a method of enhancing both therapist awareness and skills necessary to manage the complexities of client work. Within the practice of psychotherapy and counselling, there is the expectation that supervision might enhance the clinical impact of therapeutic intervention. Therefore, a supervised therapist might reasonably expect to achieve greater clinical outcomes in client work than an unsupervised therapist (Steven et al., 1998).

The proposition that supervision is a procedure that can enhance client outcome was an assumption based on its historical importance in the training and practice of psychotherapy. However, the evidence for how supervision might influence the process of therapy

DOI: 10.4324/9781003490067-13

towards positive client outcome until recently has been nearly non-existent (Bambling et al., 2006; Bambling & King, 2000). Empirical research into supervision typically focused on supervisory alliance, therapist approach, confidence, and core skills rather than on clearly defined client outcomes such as client symptom reduction (Bambling & King, 2000; Ellis et al., 1996; Ladany, Ellis, & Fridlander, 1999). The best test of supervision would be to focus on enhancing an outcome mediating construct such as the working alliance between client and therapist.

Why focus on alliance?

The working alliance represented a usable supervision construct because it is a relational process and involves specific interpersonal skills in therapy. The working alliance is measurable and has a robust relationship with symptom improvement and quality of therapeutic work (Horvath & Bedi, 2002; Martin, Garske, & Davis, 2000). Therefore, the effect of supervision might be found in working alliance scores in the treatment of depression, which is particularly sensitive to alliance in client symptom reduction.

To test this proposition further a three stage model of alliance supervision (TSAS) was developed that could be operationalised through two accepted supervision methods, skill and process focuses in brief therapy (Bambling et al., 2006). TSAS was tested in a randomised treatment trial of the treatment of depression using eight sessions of problem-solving therapy with 103 clients. Skill and process foci were derived from two dominant traditions in psychotherapy supervision; however, the focus was on alliance more so than on technique of therapy. In one approach, the supervisor focused on the development of therapist skills thought to enhance alliance based on the CBT tradition (alliance skill focus). In the other, the supervisor focused on therapist awareness of and sensitivity to the therapeutic relationship based on the psychodynamic tradition (alliance process focus).

As demonstrated in Figures 10.1 and 10.2, supervision significantly enhance working alliance ($f(2) = 54.91$, p <01) and symptom outcome ($f(2) = 13.73$, p < .01) for therapists delivering the standardised problem-solving therapy compared with therapists delivering the same treatment without supervision. Of interest is that skill and process focus did not create differential effects, both focuses were similar in effect (MD = 8.36, SE = 4.62,

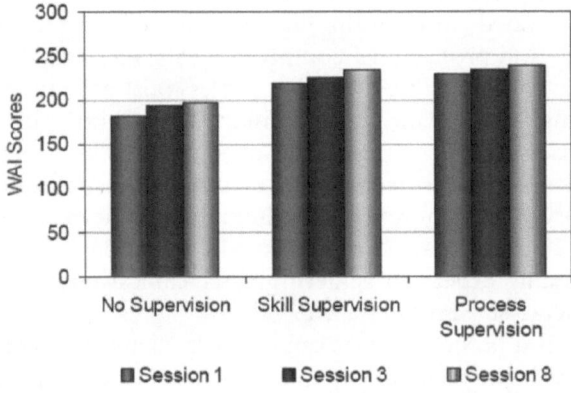

Figure 10.1 Working alliance scores by supervision condition

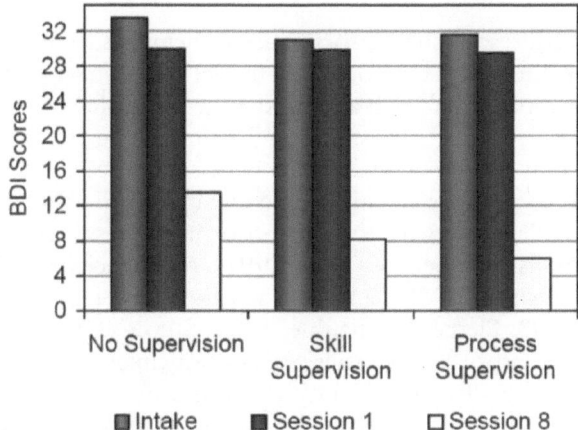

Figure 10.2 Symptom response BDI scores by supervision condition

p = .221). The finding of no effect for supervision approach means that it is likely that the effectiveness of TSAS rests in common supervision mechanisms. Clients receiving the supervised problem-solving therapy were more likely to complete the full treatment compared to the no supervision control ($\chi2$ (2, n = 103) = 23.83, p < .01). Treatment retention is an important outcome factor as failure to complete therapy means no treatment effect.

The most interesting and unexpected finding of this research was that the supervision had an effect from the first session of therapy. In the supervision conditions therapists met with supervisors prior to their first treatment session and were given some basic training in the TSAS model to be used in supervision with either skills or process procedures. Simply being aware of the alliance model presented in this chapter seemed to give therapists an advantage over their colleagues in the control conditions. It is likely that those therapists in the control condition were more focused on the technical delivery of the standardised problem-solving therapy whereas the supervised therapists prioritised relational interventions. This first session finding suggests a training effect for the TSAS supervision manual when used with therapists. Indeed, the model is now used as part of the therapist training curriculum at two prominent Queensland (Australia) universities. The TSAS model is presented below without the skill and process procedures, which will be available in the full treatment manual at a later date.

Three-stage alliance supervision

Introduction

The Three-Stage Model of Alliance Supervision (TSAS) presented here is exactly as used in the randomised clinical trial to test supervision and client outcome (Bambling et al., 2006). The TSAS model was developed by integrating some of the psychotherapy theoretical and empirical constructs of Bordin (1980, 1983), Luborsky, Singer, and Luborsky (1975), and Safran et al. (1990). In this chapter, the TSAS model is described in an applied form with case examples that highlight the application of the model. Client and therapist names and some details in the clinical examples have been changed to ensure confidentiality.

TSAS is designed to provide procedures for supervisors to assist therapists to recognise and manage the working alliance in therapy. Therefore, this model has a strong educational focus that relies on supervisor capacity to teach and model the principles of alliance management to supervisees. To assist supervisees in achieving TSAS learning outcomes a priority is given to developing a positive supervisory alliance with supervisees. A strong supervisory alliance has been shown to enhance (a) supervisee engagement in the supervision process, (b) preparedness to collaborate with the supervisor in the tasks and goals of supervision, (c) capacity to learn skills (Lambert & Ogles, 1997), (d) capacity to model supervisor skills (Schacht, How, & Berman, 1989), and (e) capacity to use learned skills in client work (Bambling & King, 2000; Pierce & Schauble, 1971; Steven, Goodyear, & Robertson, 1998). Therefore, if supervisors aim to utilise TSAS principles to maximise supervisee perception of the supervisory alliance, learning outcomes may be enhanced and the behaviours experienced, observed and learned in supervision will be more likely applied to client work.

TSAS

TSAS combines three approaches that may be considered pan-theoretical. The first stage of this model is adapted from the work of Bordin (1980), being bond, task and goals of therapy, and is conceptualised as a series of collaborative tasks. The bond, task and goal components of alliance are particularly relevant to early engagement in therapy. The second stage is adapted from the work of Luborsky et al. (1975). The alliance is conceptualised as having features that may be considered developmental and occurs as two types. The first alliance type, referred to as type 1, relates to the therapeutic bond and early collaboration. The second alliance type, referred to as type 2, relates to the work stage of therapy. From the TSAS perspective, alliance types provide a framework to understand therapeutic process and appropriateness of interventions. The third stage of the TSAS model is adapted from research into alliance rupture management to provide a set of techniques for addressing or avoiding alliance problems (Safran, Muran, Samstag, & Stevens, 2001). Therefore, the working alliance is conceptualised as a process that requires active therapist management which is explicitly and implicitly negotiated between client and therapist. This explicit and implicit negotiation provides a procedure for therapists to match alliance behaviours to client idiosyncratic preferences for alliance behaviour to enhance client perception of working alliance in therapy (Bambling & King, 2001).

Stage 1 of TSAS: early engagement

Bordin (1994) proposed a definition of the working alliance that contains three component behaviours. This position emphasised the client's positive attachment and collaboration with the therapist against self-defeating thoughts and behaviour. The bond, task and goal components require little modification for use as a supervision construct. The concept of the bond represents the system of positive attachment between the client and therapist and includes the development of trust, acceptance and confidence. The key questions a client asks when developing the bond component is *Will I be safe and can I work with this therapist?* The therapeutic bond may be defined as the mutual liking, respect, and trust between the client and therapist; it is characterised by therapist genuineness, warmth, and understanding, and by client confidence in the therapist. Skills that may demonstrate the quality of the bond include tone of voice, degree of comfort towards a client discussing difficult issues, therapist non-defensiveness, therapist empathy, and the value both participants each place on the others' contribution (Bordin 1976 [a] & [b], 1980, 1989). The primary means of assessing the bond in TSAS is to assist the supervisee assess how the client views the bond by understanding their feelings about each other in therapy.

Tasks are global therapeutic strategies or methods that refer to counselling behaviours, interventions and cognitions that form the counselling process. Supervision offered from the TSAS approach focuses on ensuring that the techniques of the therapy or the strategies developed make sense to the client as an appropriate means of working with their problems. When clients define the tasks as relevant, there is greater acceptance and responsibility for undertaking therapeutic tasks in treatment. The key question a client may ask in therapy regarding the task component is, *Do I believe that the way my therapist works with me is the correct way to deal with my problems?* It is useful to assist supervisees to understand task functions by thinking about the client perception of techniques; does it make sense to the client, does the client understand the rationale for the treatment technique and does the client agree? Further, therapist roles are attached to implementing tasks. When therapists use a strategy of exploration they adopt the role of facilitator as they help clients to increase awareness of their own thoughts, feelings, values and needs. Where therapists use a strategy of confrontation or direction, they adopt the role of an expert. Most importantly, active negotiation of the appropriateness of treatment techniques and therapist role and how these apply to the type of problem the client presents are likely to build consensus about the usefulness of therapy to achieve desired goals. The task component of alliance can be assessed in TSAS according to how responsive the supervisee appears to client reaction and acceptance of the technique of therapy. For agreement to be present regarding the task component of alliance, techniques and ensuing therapist roles should be seen as important, appropriate, and clearly understood by both participants.

Goals represent the agreed outcomes and priorities of therapeutic work between the client and therapist. Both must see goals of the session and long-term therapeutic goals as meaningful and relevant. Goals must also be seen as relevant and consistent to interventions or the task component of therapy. Goals may include decrease in symptoms, improvement in interpersonal skills or relationships, awareness of conflicts, development of new ways of thinking and behaving. Often, goals are not made explicit; rather, they are inferred from the topic or focus of the session. The key question a client may ask when defining the goal component of alliance in therapy is *To what degree is my therapist clear about my priorities for change and do we share those priorities?* In TSAS, supervisees should be assisted to become aware of the client's explicit and implicit goals through actively negotiating these early in therapy through the use of strategic questions and feedback. Goals in therapy can be assessed as the extent to which both participants see the goals of therapy as important, appropriate, and clear. Disagreement may be demonstrated through the supervisee/therapist prioritising different goals to those of the client during a session (Bambling, 2014).

Supervisors should give priority to ensuring that therapists negotiate the bond, task and goal components early in therapy with the client, as it will set realistic expectations and build consensus regarding the therapy. More importantly consensus ensures the supervisee/therapist is clear regarding what the client is seeking from treatment. A common cause of early poor alliance is unrealistic or unclear expectations by the client. If there is not adequate clarity supervisee/therapists may find they are working at odds with their client. An additional benefit of early negotiation of task and goal components of the alliance is that it may assist in the development of the bond. Bordin (1980) demonstrated that some attention to the task and goal component in the first session can aid the bond component to develop (see example below). The bond component may be challenging to negotiate in some cases due to client attachment and trust issues. In all cases, it is recommended that attempts be made to actively negotiate the bond in a collaborative non-threatening manner regardless of individual client attachment and trust issues. For example, in most cases it is important to address early concerns about counselling and negotiate early therapeutic boundaries, and give some attention to task and goals. For clients who may have greater difficulty with developing a bond, some extra attention may be given to issues of confidentiality, addressing client anxiety, not imposing unwanted work or direction, working within client immediate priorities, demonstrating empathy without being overly intimate and clarifying client expectations of the counselling relationship (Bambling & King, 2001). The bond, task, and goal component are the primary early engagement strategy in TSAS model. However, they remain useful strategies to use throughout therapy as a method of continually negotiating therapy and developing a system of mutual feedback that will assist in keeping therapy matched to client preference.

Case example: Stage one of TSAS, negotiating task, bond and goal to maximise early engagement in therapy in a case of a 25-year-old male presenting with a major depressive episode.

John was a therapist at a community mental health service who was conducting a first session with Mike. Mike had attended a prior intake interview where he was diagnosed with a major depressive episode.

John: What brings you here to see me today?
Mike: I have been feeling very bad, kind of depressed, so many things have been going wrong.
John: Sounds like you have a lot on your plate; can you tell me what has been happening to make you feel depressed?
Mike: I have been feeling so depressed, I am having trouble getting out of bed, I am worried about my job, my relationship, you know it reminds me of when I was a kid and my father never had regular work, I feel insecure about everything now.
John: There are a lot of things here. How long have you been feeling so bad?
Mike: Since work started downsizing…about a month, I think. I have to work more hours now, but I am really worried that this job will finish, you know my girlfriend and I are thinking about buying a house.
John: I can see why you are feeling depressed at this time. Ok, I will tell you a bit about the way I work here and see if working with me interests you. The approach I use makes an assumption that there is a link between the problems you are having and your feelings of depression. What do you think?
Mike: Well yeah, that seems kind of logical.
John: Ok then, in that case would you agree that if we could work on some of the problems you mentioned it might be likely to improve the way you feel?
Mike: Yeah, I think it could.
John: How we work with depression here is for you and I to work out what we can do about your problems as a team. However, the therapy is for your benefit and

therefore you get to identify what you want to work on and the most realistic plan of getting you from where you are now a bit closer to where you would like to be. So we mostly work in the here and now of what is going on for you and apply a systematic approach to solve problems. We normally provide around six sessions here if needed. How does that sound?

Mike: Yeah that would be good, as I want to sort this stuff out and feel confident again.

John: Ok, you can be sure that therapy is confidential and I won't release any information about our work without your express permission or instruction. I am interested if you have any concerns about counselling or if there are things I should know that will help our work, or help me avoid making you uncomfortable?

Mike: Privacy worries me a bit so I am glad it is confidential. The way we will work together sounds fine. I haven't had counselling before, so don't really know what to expect…I am not sure how comfortable I will feel about talking about personal stuff. Maybe I need to test things out a bit as we go?

John: Sounds very reasonable, how about I check with you from time to time to see if we are on track or not moving too quickly? I would like you to feel free to let me know if things are not progressing the way you would like or you are not happy about anything we are doing. That is the best way we can ensure that this process will be of most use to you.

Mike: Sounds good.

John: Ok, perhaps we can identify which problems are most pressing and which problem is worrying you the most today out of all the problems you told me about. You mentioned your job, right?

Mike: Well actually, my biggest worry today is my relationship; my mood is really grating on my girlfriend…she must be getting sick of it.

John: So out of all the problems you mentioned if we worked on your relationship concerns today, would that be your choice?

Mike: Yeah, that would be great.

TSAS-FOCUSED SUPERVISION INSIGHTS

In this first session scenario with Mike, John asked orientating questions to get a general sense of Mike's problems and general interest in change and goals for counselling. John then specifically addressed task issues with Mike by explaining the approach used in collaborative language, basic rationale, and length of treatment to develop consensus and interest in proceeding. Some general attention was then given to bond issues by explaining confidentiality and asking Mike about his concerns. John responded to Mike's concerns by negotiating a feedback process.

Finally, goals were made more explicit for the purposes of the session. John's notion of what Mike wanted to work on was not correct. Mike had prioritised a different session goal to what the therapist assessed as a priority, his relationship with his girlfriend. John willingly accommodated and negotiated Mike's goal for the first session discussion. John had actively negotiated the bond, task, and goal aspects of alliance to best match them to Mike's immediate needs and perceptions. Mike was likely to have experienced John as being sensitive and in tune with his needs as well as feeling understood. In this scenario early engagement was maximised by use of bond, task and goal behaviours and a strong early alliance would be likely formed.

Stage 2 of TSAS: developmental features of alliance

Luborsky (1976) defined working alliance as dynamic and as occurring in phases. Two types of alliances were identified and the strength of both these alliance categories was related to positive treatment outcome. The beginning stage of therapy is marked by type 1 alliance that is based on the client experiencing the therapist as supportive and helpful. Type 2 alliance; the work stage of therapy, is typical of later phases of treatment. Type 2 provides a sense of working together, shared responsibility and collaboration in achieving treatment goals. Assisting supervisees to identify alliance type in therapy provides a basis for matching therapeutic interventions to the alliance that may minimise strains and ruptures. The following two examples demonstrate how to use these ideas in the supervisory context.

Case example: a type 1 alliance issue

Jim was an experienced therapist at a university clinic and had seen Tom, a very depressed student for the second session. Tom was not improving and complained of feeling worse and stated that he was experiencing a strong desire to bring a gun to the university and go on a shooting spree and then kill himself. Tom then said to Jim, *but this information is between you and me, and I don't want you to tell anyone what I am thinking about doing.*

TSAS SUPERVISION INSIGHTS

In this situation, Jim felt that Tom had engaged in a therapeutic process as he had returned for a second session and was talking to about his concerns and possible actions. However, evaluating the therapy from the perspective of alliance type, Tom had not begun therapeutic work. Tom was unsure if he could work with Jim or if therapy could help him and was looking for some indication of boundaries and containment to begin to define the bond, task, and goals of therapeutic work. If therapy were to succeed in this extreme example, before any therapeutic work could occur, type 1 issues must be addressed. Jim would need to demonstrate to Tom that he was able to deal with his difficulties and extremes. Jim decided that he should let Tom know that he took his threats seriously and described clearly what measures he would take to ensure both Tom's and others' safety and then negotiated a therapeutic contact in the form of a contract and management plan between sessions.

Integrating stages 1 and 2 of TSAS

Case example, type 2 alliance; integrating bond, task, and goal into type-based alliance thinking; a context for intervention

Jennifer was seeing Mark, a client who was depressed, and she began to wonder if his depression was secondary to a narcissistic personality disorder. Mark would complain that his wife and children did not respect him or do what he said. It was clear to Jennifer that Mark was aggressive and dominating with his wife and children and felt very under appreciated. Whenever, Jennifer tried to discuss the impact of Mark's behaviour on his family he would become angry and accuse her of not understanding or respecting him. Jennifer would become scared and withdraw.

In supervision Jennifer discussed this apparent therapeutic impasse. Examining this case from an alliance perspective revealed several issues. Firstly, a bond had developed, or type 1 alliance was achieved. Mark kept his appointments and would take the trouble to dress nicely, so contact with Jennifer was important to him. There was some idea of a goal as Mark was committed to dealing with family problems. However, type 2, the work stage of therapy, had not yet developed, there was no understanding or agreement between Mark and Jennifer regarding how his goal would be achieved. The block to moving to type 2 alliance in therapy was that the task component of alliance had not been adequately negotiated with Mark.

Using Jennifer's insights about Mark's narcissism it was clear he experienced confronting questions as insults and as siding with his perception of disrespectful family members. It was clear that if therapy was to be effective that this impasse had to be confronted. However, given Mark's sensitivities, confrontation needed to be couched in an alliance-appropriate form as not to rupture the relationship and risk termination. Jennifer decided she would confront Mark using collaborative and supportive language so as not to injure his narcissism and match her intervention to alliance type 1. Jennifer felt this intervention would invite Mark to engage in the work stage (type 2) by negotiating how the communication and feedback tasks of therapy should be conducted around difficult issues.

In the following session Jennifer said to Mark that she wanted to raise an issue with him because she both respected him (using Mark's language as a reference point) and valued their work together. Jennifer said she was concerned that if she didn't raise this issue it would affect their mutual work on his goal of sorting out family issues. Jennifer told Mark that sometimes she would react to what he said and would like to honestly respond to him but held back because she was concerned that he would become angry and upset with her and may discontinue counselling. She said she knew that because respect was important to him he would not like this to be the case and would want to negotiate how she could talk to him more honestly and openly. Mark expressed concern and said he wanted honest responses but knew he could get angry easily. Jennifer and Mark contracted a process for communicating and feedback. In the next supervision session Jennifer reported that the intervention was successful and also she had noticed greater engagement and Mark had begun to do work in therapy indicating that type 2 alliance was developing.

Stage 3 of TSAS: rupture management

A considerable body of research suggests that in successful therapy it is relatively common for the working alliance to go through a series of ruptures and repairs, or become strained (Horvath & Symonds, 1991; Safran et al., 1990; 2011). Strains and ruptures often are the result of clients dealing with problematic issues and difficult patterns of behaviour. If therapy is to be successful alliance rupture must be repaired. Unrepaired alliance ruptures are related to treatment dropout (Safran et al., 2002). The quality of early alliance is particularly important to later successful rupture management as it assists clients to deal with the strains of therapeutic work. The ability of a therapist to directly intervene to address problems in the therapeutic relationship is a key intervention that has been shown to repair ruptures, improve working alliance and reduce early treatment termination

(Safran et al., 2011). The final stage of the TSAS model focuses on managing strains and ruptures through assisting supervisees to focus on conflictual or potentially problematic relationship patterns in therapy. Interventions are then created to correct alliance ruptures to improve overall client engagement and total quality of alliance in therapy.

Stage 3 of TSAS: rupture management and integrating stages 1 and 2

Case example: The third stage of the TSAS model, integrating rupture management with alliance type and bond, task, and goal aspects of alliance.

Mary was a therapist who was seeing Wendy, a 45-year-old woman who was depressed. Wendy lived an isolated life and found intimacy difficult and struggled with the early working alliance. Wendy identified some goals for change in the first session relating to her relationships with adult siblings, yet spent the following three sessions talking about her family of origin experiences. Eventually, Mary felt that Wendy should start working on these issues according to her expressed goals. A subtle conflict developed between them regarding the goals and tasks of therapy. Wendy did not appear interested in the therapeutic interventions Mary provided or the strategies used in counselling to achieve stated goals. Eventually Wendy implied she would terminate therapy as she was not getting anything out of treatment, at which point Mary sought supervision.

TSAS SUPERVISION INSIGHTS

Wendy's difficulties with interpersonal relationships made it difficult for Mary to identify alliance development. Mary had doubts whether Wendy was doing any work in therapy. However, Wendy had in fact progressed to the type-2 work stage alliance. From an alliance point of view, the difficulty was that Mary was working with a set of goals originally contracted with Wendy. Wendy had implicitly changed her goals over a number of sessions stating to Mary that she was finding the exploration of family-of-origin issues for the first time in her life very useful. The tendency for Wendy to evoke power issues in others resulted in loss of empathy reducing awareness of the alliance rupture or need to repair the alliance. A serious alliance rupture had occurred that involved bond, task, and goal issues and dropout was likely without intervention. Mary decided to confront the relational issues directly to address the alliance rupture and renegotiate the bond, task and goals of therapy. Wendy missed her next session and Mary made a follow-up telephone call. Mary told Wendy she had thought about their prior session and she was concerned that she was off track with Wendy's needs and not giving her the freedom to explore issues that were important to her. Mary renegotiated the tasks and goals of the therapeutic work with Wendy. Wendy was clearly pleased and returned to therapy. Mary found that as communication had improved there was opportunity to give and receive feedback that assisted her to keep therapy matched to Wendy's needs and preferences. In this case Mary had identified an alliance rupture and intervened directly to repair the rupture. Addressing relational problems by validating and accommodating Wendy's view of the therapy and renegotiating the task and goals also had a positive impact on the bond. Mary reported that Wendy seemed to connect more with her after alliance was repaired and there was a sense of greater energy in the type 2, the work stage of alliance.

Conclusion

TSAS provides an intuitively appealing simple model that supervisors can integrate into their practice that has demonstrated efficacy. As TSAS is founded in a pan-theoretical framework it should be possible for supervisors of all approaches to integrate it into their practice. The significant effects found for a pre-treatment session of TSAS suggest that this mode of supervision provides an important educational experience for supervisees assisting them to develop sensitivity to the alliance. In summary the TSAS supervisor assists the supervisee to understand, establish, manage, and repair the working alliance with their client during treatment. TSAS supervisors prioritise developing a positive supervisory alliance with their supervisee and actively model working alliance principles and provide feedback as key learning strategies.

TSAS is the first supervision model to have proved to be an effective agent to enhance client outcome through directly impacting on the quality of therapist work. However, the message of TSAS is that it is not the specific techniques of supervision but rather the focus of supervision that has an impact, which suggests that there is much yet to be learned about how supervision influences client outcome. Therefore, this new evidence for supervision in brief therapy should be regarded as preliminary and clearly more research is needed to better understand the mechanisms by which supervision achieves benefits for clients.

Educational questions & activities

1. What are the key principles of TSAS?
   a. Understanding therapeutic process from an alliance perspective
   b. A focus on treatment techniques
   c. Managing the working alliance with clients in therapy
   d. Dealing with client resistance in therapy
   e. a and c
   f. All of the above
2. What does a TSAS orientated supervisor do in supervision?
   a. Models TSAS skills for their supervisee
   b. Develops a positive supervisory alliance with their supervisee
   c. Teaches the TSAS model to supervisees
   d. Provides regular evaluation and feedback to supervisees
   e. a and c
   f. All of the above
3. Why might a focus on working alliance be more important than a focus on delivering the techniques of therapy in supervision?
   a. Working alliance between client and therapist predicts treatment outcome whereas therapy technique does not
   b. Working alliance as rated by clients mediates their response to therapy regardless of treatment approach
   c. Working alliance as rated by clients predicts engagement and retention in counselling
   d. All of the above

4. If your supervisee reports they are stuck in therapy with a client what should you do from a TSAS perspective?
   a. Revisit the treatment plan
   b. Confront the client about the impasse
   c. Provide more skilful techniques to address the impasse
   d. Examine the issues existing in the working relationship between therapist and client
5. What are the 3 components that constitute the TSAS model?
   a. Bond, task, goal; stages of alliance; managing strains and ruptures in the working alliance
   b. Education, learning goals, and experience level
   c. Understanding defences, transference, and the unconscious processes in therapy
   d. Developing individualised treatment plans, teaching therapeutic skills, and measuring symptom reduction

References

Bambling, M. (2014). Creating positive outcomes in clinical supervision. In C. Edward Watkins, Jr. & Derek L. Milne (Eds.), *The Wiley Blackwell International Handbook of Clinical Supervision* (1st ed., pp. 445–457). Chichester, England: John Wiley & Sons.

Bambling, M., & King, R. (2000). Supervision and the development of counsellor competency. *Psychotherapy in Australia, 6*(4), 58–63.

Bambling, M., & King, R. (2001). Therapeutic alliance and clinical practice. *Psychotherapy in Australia, 8*(1), 38–47.

Bambling, M., King, R., Raue, P., Schweitzer, R., & Lambert, W. (2006). Clinical supervision: its impact on working alliance and outcome in the treatment of major depression. *Psychotherapy Research, 16*(3), 317–331.

Bernard, J., & Goodyear, R. (1992). *Fundamentals of Clinical Supervision*. Boston: Allyn & Bacon.

Bordin, E. S. (1980, June). *Of human bonds that bind or free*. Paper presented at the Annual Meeting of the Society for Psychotherapy Research, Pacific Grove, CA.

Bordin, E. S. (1983). A working alliance based model of supervision. *The Counseling Psychologist, 11*(1), 35–42.

Bordin, E. S. (1994). Theory and research on the therapeutic working alliance: New directions. In A. O. Horvath & L. S. Greenberg (Eds.), *The Working Alliance: Theory, Research, and Practice* (pp. 13–37). New York: John Wiley.

Ellis, M. V., Ladany, N., Krengel, M., & Schult, D. (1996). Clinical supervision research from 1981 to 1993: A methodological critique. *Journal of Counseling Psychology, 43*(1), 35–50.

Horvath, A., & Bedi, R. (2002). The alliance. In J. C. Norcross (Ed.), *Psychotherapy Relationships That Work* (pp. 37–69). Oxford, UK: Oxford University.

Horvath, A., & Symonds, B. D. (1991). Relation between working alliance and outcome in psychotherapy: A meta-analysis. *Journal of Counseling Psychology, 38*(2), 139–149.

Ladany, N., Ellis, M., & Fridlander, M. (1999). The supervisory alliance, trainee self-efficacy, and satisfaction. *Journal of Counselling and Development, 77*, 447–455.

Lambert, M., & Ogles, B. (1997). The effectiveness of psychotherapy supervision (Chapter 24). In C. Watkins, Jr. (Ed.), *Handbook of Psychotherapy Supervision*. New York: John Wiley & Sons.

Luborsky, L. (1976). "Helping alliances in psychotherapy: the groundwork for a study of their relationship to its outcome." In J. L. Cleghorn (Ed.), *Successful Psychotherapy* (pp. 92–116). New York: Brunner/Mazel.

Luborsky, L., Singer, B., & Luborsky, L. (1975). Comparative studies of psychotherapies: Is it true that "everybody has won and all must have prizes"? *Archives of General Psychiatry, 32,* 995–1008.

Martin, D. J., Garske, J. P., & Davis, M. K. (2000). Relation of the therapeutic alliance with outcome and other variables: A meta-analytic review. *Journal of Consulting and Clinical Psychology, 68*(3), 438–450.

Orlinsky, D., Botermans, J., & Ronnestad, M. (2001). Towards an empirically grounded model of psychotherapy training: Four thousand therapists rate influences on their development. *Australian Psychologist, 36,* 139–148.

Pierce, M., & Schauble, G. (1971). Graduate training of facilitative counsellors: The effects of individual supervision. *Journal of Counselling Psychology, 17,* 210–215.

Safran, J., Crocker, P., McMain, S., & Munay, P. (1990). Therapeutic alliance rupture as a therapy event for empirical investigation. *Psychotherapy, 27,* 154–164.

Safran, J. D., Muran, J. C., & Eubanks-Carter, C. (2011). Repairing alliance ruptures. In J. C. Norcross (Ed.), *Psychotherapy Relationships That Work: Evidence-Based Responsiveness* (2nd ed., pp. 224–238). Oxford University Press.

Safran, J. D., Muran, J. C., Samstag, L. W., & Stevens, C. (2001). Repairing alliance ruptures. *Psychotherapy: Theory, Research, Practice, Training, 38*(4), 406–412. https://doi.org/10.1037/0033-3204.38.4.406

Safran, J., Muran, C., Samstag, S., & Winston, A. (2002). *A comparative treatment study of potential treatment failures.* Paper presented at the Society for Psychotherapy Research Annual Meeting June, Santa Barbara, CA.

Schacht, J., Howe, E. Jr., & Berman, J. (1989). Supervisor facilitative conditions and effectiveness as perceived by thinking- and feeling-type supervisees. *Psychotherapy, 26,* 475–483.

Steven, D., Goodyear, R., & Robertson, P. (1998). Supervisor development: An exploratory study in changes in stance and emphasis. *Clinical Supervisor, 16*(2), 73–88.

11 Solution-Focused Supervision

Ann Moir-Bussy

Introduction

During the past thirty years, Solution-Focused Supervision (SFS) has gained increasing Western interest as a transformative therapeutic process for professional supervision (Briggs & Miller, 2005; Edwards & Chen, 1999, p. 350). Described as both a competency- and strength-based approach, it has departed 'from the medically modelled tradition that focuses on assessment of deficits or problems, and prescribes a remedy to the *ailing* client by the *expert in charge*' (Edwards & Chen, 1999, p. 350). Described as spaciously simple, and having 'restfully clear' simplicity, SFS is founded on respect, and 'is about collaborating in a partnership that pays attention to, and develops, the interests, best intentions, and goals for supervisees' work' (Waskett, 2006, p. 1). The supervisor takes a '*not-knowing*' position, directs questions appropriately, stays curious, maintains respect, and accommodates/wombs the other (Waskett, 2006). The prime area of focus is the supervisees strengths and preferred goals, and through the use of scales to measure progress, noticing movement, and complimenting, these aspects of growth are freely investigated (Waskett, 2006). '[S]olution-focused clinical supervision...offers a simple yet profound philosophy and structure for the supervisory relationship' (Fowler, Fenton, & Riley, 2007, pp. 30–31).

SFS adapts to a wide range of workplace- and clientele-contexts (Kilminster & Jolly, 2000, p. 829; Wetchler, 1990), and has cross-cultural applicability (Chang, Tong, Shi, & Qifeng, 2005; Cheung, 2001; Kim, Franklin, Zhang, Liu, Qu, & Chen, 2015; Lim, Lim, Michael, Cai, & Schock, 2010). Founded upon traditional Chinese/Taoistic concepts, its emerging contemporary designs result from Eastern and Western amalgamations that recognise, embrace, and promote the development of non-hierarchical supervision (Edwards & Chen, 1999; Hsu, 2009; Moir-Bussy, 2008). The quasi-modern, constructivist concepts of SFS theory 'are easily learnt' and easily integrated into other styles of supervision (Britton, Goodman, & Rak, 2002, p. 34; Briggs & Miller, 2005, p. 200; Cheung, 2001), being 'flexible enough for use with a variety of theoretical orientations' (Wetchler, 1990, p. 129).

The simple definition of the term 'supervision' is *often poorly understood* (Hawkins & Shohet, 2000), being greatly complicated by its capacity to contain a variety of meanings, and therefore, applications (Moir-Bussy, 2008). General definitions such as 'counsellor,' 'teacher,' 'consultant,' 'monitor,' and/or 'evaluator' (Hart & Nance, 2003; Sweitzer & King, 1998) broadly refer to the prescriptive 'promotion of supervisee growth and development as a competent clinician and professional' (Haynes et al., 2003, p. 6). Particular emphasis is placed upon achieving protection of clients (Yontef, 1997, p. 7). Pearson

DOI: 10.4324/9781003490067-14

(2006, p. 241) described clinical supervision 'as an intervention provided by a more senior member of a profession to a more junior member' (Bernard & Goodyear, 2004, p.8), where the focus is on 'the supervisee's clinical interventions that directly affect the client, as well as those behaviors related to the supervisee's personal and professional functioning' (Bradley & Kottler, 2001, p. 5). Characteristics of a good supervisor include having a sound clinical knowledge, being an experienced clinician, having good relationship skills, being accepting/non-judgemental, being keen to impart supervision, knowing each supervisee's developmental level, being constructive when giving feedback, and being empathic, flexible, and available (Moir-Bussy, 2008).

A historic consequence of seniority-based supervisory systems has been the establishment of hierarchical professional relationships and interactions between the supervisor and the supervisee (Wetchler, 1990). According to SFS theory, supervision structured on unequal power relationships characteristically forms unclear relational boundaries that fluctuate between 'closeness and distance' (Collins, 1993). This breeds uncertainty, and inhibits, discourages, and undermines supervisee self-confidence (Kilminster & Jolly, 2000, pp. 833–834). '[T]he hierarchical nature of the supervisory relationship in which supervisors tell supervisees how to do therapy places trainees in one-down, complementary relationships which may reinforce their sense of inadequacy' (Wetchler, 1990, p. 131).

Within a traditional social-work context, Smith (1997) describes supervision as hierarchical and managerial in both administrative and educational supervisory positions, and concedes that the elimination of power differences in supervision is impossible. According to Knight (2003),

> Unfortunately, the demands of contemporary clinical practice often work against a strengths-based orientation...Agency policies, legal mandates, heavy workloads, and the requirements of third party payment pull therapists in subtle and not-so-subtle ways towards a diagnosis and problem-oriented approach to treatment
>
> (p. 154)

As a result of increasing regulation and litigation, supervisors feel a pressure of responsibility for the development of the supervisee, and for the safety of both the client and the profession (Driscoll, 2007; Falvey, 2002). The traditional hierarchical methodology provides a sense of having a safety-net towards ensuring these needs are met and regarding this, the term 'gate-keeper' is one that is often used to describe this aspect of the supervisory role. Comparatively, SFS promotes non-hierarchical supervision within which the afore-mentioned concerns of public safety and institutional responsibility are able to be supported without the exponential pressures that restrictive, task-oriented, conditional, objectifying, and de-valuing methodology imbue.

Supervisory relationships

The primary research outcome in Kilminster and Jolly's (2000) metanalysis of literature regarding effective supervision in practice settings was that '[t]he supervision relationship is probably the single most important factor for the effectiveness of supervision, more important than the supervisory methods used' (p. 827). The strength of the relationship between the supervisor and the supervisee is key to the supervisee's successful professional development, and this is empirically supported in research by Koob (2002). While unconditional positive regard, empathy, respect, and concepts appreciating the idealised state of self-actualisation are well-integrated features throughout client-centred professions, debilitating features inherent in hierarchical supervision have been found to be the single greatest impediment to supervisory success, including to the goal that supervisees develop a sense of competence towards gaining and developing a sense of courageous self-responsibility (Koob, 2002). Hierarchical supervisory superiority inadvertently compounds supervisees' tendency to be their own worst critics, and to become increasingly prone to self-deprecation, and experience heightened anxiety regarding their competence (Briggs & Miller, 2005, p. 200). Desire to learn is over-powered by a system-induced focus on qualifying, which potentially renders them feeling powerless and incapacitates their sense of creative competence. According to Koob (2002), '[t]raditional supervision models have been ineffective in developing positive perceived self-efficacy in therapists.'

Dialogic conversation

Dialogic conversation blends the supervisor's and the supervisee's personal and professional knowledge and qualities to collaboratively build broader, larger, enhanced, and creatively inspired potentials in mutual learning (Kilminster & Jolly, 2000; Moir-Bussy, 2008; Wetchler, 1990). Reliance on reciprocated perspectives within an *I–thou* relationship enables the interviewee (*I*) and the interviewer (*thou*) to form a personal relationship rather than a hierarchical one (Moir-Bussy, 2008; Wu, 1997). The supervisee is not objectified as a *student* lacking skills, but is instead viewed with equity as a co-member of a communicative partnership (Moir-Bussy, 2008). This design presents a significant shift from previous supervisory methodologies, and is supported in research by Kilminster and Jolly (2000), who found that dialogue between supervisor and supervisee enabled reciprocal feedback (i.e., both parties partook in providing and receiving feedback), and that doing so developed greater clarity of comprehension, both in detail and intention. They also found that 'supervisee input into and control over the supervisory process is an essential feature of SFS' (p. 827). Hsu (2009) describes SFS as a process of two people meeting with the aim of enhancing both the personal development and professional development of the student who is studying counselling. This was a sentiment echoed by other authors (Gordon & McBride, 1996; Sweitzer & King, 1998). It is designed to develop self-confidence and achieve a sense of personal and professional self-actualisation through mutually open dialogic exchange, and by enabling ongoing collaborative instruction, skill-, and knowledge-development (Kilmnister & Jolly, 2000; Thomas, 1996).

Dialogic conversation is a two-way process between the supervisor and supervisee (Hsu, 2009). Generating mutually shared conversation, open sharing, and discussion of ideas and views makes 'audible and visible the real…and phenomenal depths of the individual subject' under discussion (Moir-Bussy, 2008). Dialogic conversation is the essential, core component of SFS that differentiates it from monologic therapeutic styles. Rather than operating as the expert, the supervisor holds a position of *not-knowing* (Waskett, 2006). Anderson (2008) speaks of going by a *way of ignorance* in order to come to a place of knowing. The SFS supervisor 'defines the goals, directions, and options with the therapist to construct a participatory experience through consensus and teamwork. Supervision proceeds as a future-oriented endeavour, setting up positive expectations and building on the unique assets of the therapist' (Thomas, 1996, p. 131). There is no right and wrong in SFS, only learning and development, which encourages supervisors to trust in the current and developing competencies of the supervisee, and allows and encourages supervisees to place trust in themselves (Hsu, 2009; Wetchler, 1990). 'The branch will tell me how to carve it…Each piece of wood has its own shape, which you must respect…In each… branch lies a flute; [my] job is to find it' (Thomas, 1996).

During SFS dialogue, the supervisor utilises narrativism to find out about the stories that the supervisee has developed, their contexts, what they inform about clients, and how the supervisee can shift the story and build a new one that creates satisfying outcomes (Skarp, 2012). The SFS supervisor also uses reflection to establish what is happening for the supervisee (Skarp, 2012). Using a solution focus helps to focus on what works, identify solutions, and transform problems into goals (Skarp, 2012). Solution-focused supervisors help supervisees identify times/situations when the problem was less invasive, or didn't exist. In other words they look for positive exceptions (Skarp, 2012).

Personal development

SFS supervisees are engaged in both professional and personal development (Hsu, 2009). Any new situation in a person's life may lead to a new positioning of perspective for that person (Hermans, 2004). The internship process places supervisees in a position where they must engage in the external dialogue within the socio-cultural context in which they find themselves, which inadvertently activates their internal dialogue in which information processing between the *many selves* that comprise the composite of their being-self intrinsically occurs (Herman, 2004). Piaget (1977) describes development and learning as resulting from interactions between cognitive structures and inputs received from external environments (Wetchler, 1990).

It may be said that detrimental outcomes resulting from hierarchical supervision are paradoxical to the good intentions inherent in their purpose. Nevertheless, since supervision is intended to develop the supervisee's abilities and 'alleviate clinical confusion,' any potential to leave supervisees so confused and self-doubting as to render them clinically incompetent (Wetchler, 1990, p. 131) could be academically incompatible with evidence-based practice. According to Koob (2002), '[t]raditional supervision models have been ineffective in developing positive perceived self-efficacy in therapists' (p. 161), and the debilitating effect of consequent clinical confusion, self-doubting, and professional dissatisfaction result in a significant amount of staff burnout along the entire career trajectory or both supervisees and supervisors.

Specialised foci

Present versus past

Medina & Beyeback (2014, p. 181) stated that 'no successful sporting coach anywhere in the world would allow players on his/her team to focus excessively on their worst games, greatest failures, and worst fear, and realistically expect a good performance.' SFS is present-focused, strengths-focused, and goal-focused, rather than past-focused on deficits in skill and performance (Koob, 2002; Selekman & Todd, 1995). 'It is not necessary to know the cause or function of a complaint in order to resolve it' (Thomas, 1996, p. 132). While SFS actively acknowledges the relevance of past events in the supervisee's experience, it refrains from over-expending attention upon sourcing factual and subjective meanings regarding their relevance and instead maintains a present-focused view to finding solutions to current issues (Britton, Goodman, & Rak, 2002; Thomas, 1996). Present-focused resolution of present issues potentially resolves parallel, co-related issues that remain upon the supervisees' historic past-timeline, so by dissipating and dissolving the detrimental influences upon the present experience, and future experiences, many lingering peripheral historic issues may be resolved also (Thomas, 1996). This enhances the expedient power of SFS.

Goal versus problem

According to Sweitzer and King (1998), '[s]upervision should provide an extending experience that blends personal knowledge and personal qualities' (p. 88). However, '[m]ost traditional supervision has paralleled conventional counselling, looking for what the supervisee was doing incorrectly or not doing enough of, mostly in the area of technique, and attempting to devise remedial solutions' (Edwards & Chen, 1999, p. 350). SFS is committed to working with supervisees to identify and promote their strengths and successes instead of focusing on areas of error/mistakes, and to acknowledge that successful methodology is egalitarian, contains individual personality, and expends its greater focus on the supervisee rather than on the supervisees clients (Koob, 2002). A major assumption in the SFS model 'is that therapists have the resources and abilities to create their own solutions' (Marek et al., 1994, p. 60). Wetchler (1990) states that the freedom to vocally articulate the areas of 'their clinical work that are effective,' and the fact that areas of success are celebrated, and encouraged to be applied into similar situations, develops positive schemas from which to confidently work (p. 131; Moir-Bussy, 2008). Combined with the affirmative power of hearing their own voice during positive-oriented supervision, the informal, conversational dialogical nature of SFS supervision brings forth greater depth of meaning within the narrative enquiries that open up and give rise to a 'dialogical interplay of voices in which meaning itself is heard' (Shotter, 1994, p. 5). Every positive, dialogic interchange between the supervisor and the supervisee develops a clinical schema based on success and competency for not just the supervisee, but for the supervisor also on his or her own personal journey of learning, and accomplishments (Wetchler, 1990).

> The focus is never placed on what is the correct situation, but rather what seems to be working for a supervisee with a particular case. As supervisors take the stance of being curious about even the smallest exceptions which are successful, their supervisees are allowed to examine he solutions and their strengths
>
> (Wetchler, 1990, p. 132)

By comparison, problem-focused supervision within a hierarchical infrastructure sustains prolonged focus upon identifying and advising and correcting problems and mistakes, which potentially serves to confirm feelings of inadequacy and confusion about how best to improve oneself (Wetchler, 1990).The author continues that focusing on the problem can maintain confusion for the supervisee, whereas a focus on positive aspects allows the supervisee to develop and organise schemas and to grow in self-confidence.

The SFS supervisor participates in each session as a professional equal, so does not behave as the supervisee's superior (Hsu, 2009). Instead, the supervisee is considered the expert on his/her life (Anderson & Goolishian, 1992), while the supervisor sidestep[s] hierarchy in favour of co-constructing ideas with those supervised (Edwards & Chen, 1999, p. 351). This *being* in a state of dialogic equality demonstrates that other ways of knowing, comprehending, and understanding become apparent during SFS (Hsu, 2009). Together they provide the possibility of shared meaning – understanding, comprehending, knowing, that is comparatively tranquil and exponential for growth in comparison with hierarchical-oriented supervision modalities. 'Being' in this way surpasses verbal language. Sullivan (1989) argues that it is a more feminine approach that emerges from '*not-knowing*' ... experiencing and maintaining a focus on the Being, rather than the Doing. When our focus is on this possibility of shared meaning, the 'body is capable of knowing and so is psyche' (Puhakka, 2000, p. 18).

Specialised techniques

A number of useful concepts in the counselling profession highlight features of SFS. The concept of symmetrical voice says that students who are allowed to experience their own voice self-generate a personal therapeutic meaningfulness, resulting in there being no need for a supervisor to take on an 'authority' position (Moir-Bussy, 2008; Wetchler, 1990).

Second is competence: finding out what supervisees have succeeded in. When outcomes have seemed unsuccessful, finding exceptions and emphasising strengths and successful interventions builds self-respect and confidence, willingness to learn regarding areas of inter-personal weakness, and provides a chance to learn more about the client (Moir-Bussy, 2008; Wetchler, 1990).

SFS sessions may start with goal-setting, and during the course of the session, the supervisor may notice exceptions to problems that appear to impede the achievement of goals (Marek et al., 1994, p. 60). Scaling questions provide supervisees with opportunities to rate, and discuss on a 1–10 scale, how they are feeling – satisfaction with the therapeutic supervision experience, their goals, and their confidence in being able to meet them (Marek et al., 1994, pp. 61–62). By asking miracle questions, and suppose questions, exception questions, relationship questions, coping questions, complimenting, normalising, and reframing the supervisor encourages the supervisee to verbalise self-evaluations and self-discover areas of success, and how to reconstruct goals (Hsu, 2009, p. 476). Additional creative techniques, such as sand-tray therapy, may also be included to overcome unique communication difficulties (Koob, 2002).

Wu-Wei and Cross-Cultural Utility

Origins of SFS lie in Chinese/Taoist philosophy which is suggestive of its cross-cultural applicability. Western SFS is informed by Wu-Wei teachings, and dynamic amalgamations of overall principles are easily developed (Wu, 1997). According to Edwards and Chen (1999) the Wu-Wei 'model of supervision potentiates the person-of-the-counselor' (p. 349). 'Wu Wei...translates as 'effortless action' or 'without action,' and offers 'a non-violent, non-authoritative way of doing supervision' (Skarp, 2012). According to Edwards and Chen (1999),

> [t]he usefulness of wu-wei is that it relies on the naturalness of life, thus 'arriving at decisions spontaneously, decisions which are effective to the degree that one knows how to let one's mind alone, trusting it to work by itself. This is wu-wei, since wu means 'not' or 'non' and wei means 'action,' 'making,' 'doing,' 'striving,' 'straining,' or 'busyness.'
>
> (p. 349)

In Wu-Wei, 'the issue is not in the *doing*, or *action*, or *intervening*, but in how much the... supervisor...holds on to his or her version of truth' (Edwards & Chen, 1999, pp. 349–350).

Wu-Wei describes people as being naturally dialogical, whose identities and perceived realities are social constructs formed within each second by a myriad of co-occurring states that influence their present being. Thus, Wu-Wei coaching acknowledges its inability to control another individuals outcomes (Skarp, 2012).

Using his/her knowledge, skills, personality, and identity for making the emerging dialogue itself transparent, but without using formal methodology, the Wu-Wei coach guides supervisees to follow their path of least resistance, finding what successes the supervisee and encouraging those (Skarp, 2012). Since futures are unknown, outcomes cannot be predicted, so the Wu-Wei coach allows the session to unfold, and encourages the supervisee to flow with that unfolding so that changes in thinking and perspective become visible (Skarp, 2012). This makes the process of naturally unfolding change *effortless.*

Skarp (2012) describes the Wu-Wei coach as being expert on previously learned contemporary methodology, and able to use explorative conversation. He further describes the coach as being creative, self-reflecting, mindful/aware, not-knowing/humble, able to work with ambiguity, and be compassionate yet able to be fearless within the session. He/she does not diagnose, and when something in the session doesn't work, it is changed. The idea of multiple voices creates a capacity to consider multiple views or perspectives simultaneously while upholding a 'not-knowing' mind (Edwards & Chen, 1999). Effortless actions empower the client/supervisee to be his/her own expert (Skarp, 2012).

Research further demonstrates the utility of SFS across cultural variation. Moir-Bussy (2008) noted in her research with a group of Chinese Master of Counselling students that SFS was influential towards their becoming more conscious of their abilities and therefore more professionally and personally confident. These students had trained under Western programmes which they then integrated into their lives in Hong Kong (Moir-Bussy, 2008). Students reported that through the dialogic process, an outcome of creative transformation of the self and of professional knowledge had occurred (Moir-Bussy, 2008). They reported being more conscious of their cultural values and knowledge, spirituality, and professional goals after SFS, so that weaving what they had learned from the Western training was transformed for practice in Hong Kong. The informal, conversational dialogue within supervision provided a more equal relationship than one of direct questioning from supervisor to supervisee would have had, and this reportedly enhanced the depths of meaningful discussion that took place (Moir-Bussy, 2008). The dialogic relationship became one in which 'one's own meanings and meanings of others [were] engaged in conversation...transforming...resulting in new creation' (Gergen, 1999, p. 144).

Conclusion

In conclusion, SFS is gaining empirical support as a method-of-choice for supervision. Evidence gained from research studies indicates that positive outcomes far-outweigh any potential negative outcomes. SFS is gentle, accommodating, respectful, present-focused, and highly expedient as a goal-driven process. Expediency will always equate to cost-reductions, and cost reductions will always appeal in terms of socio-economic benefits.

It can be said that dialogue is like a reliable recipe: three parts listening and one part talking. In dialogue, you have to listen to what the client is saying, what you are saying, and what is happening in your silent, inner dialogue.

As Bruce Lee, American Hong Kong martial artist and philosopher, is attributed as saying:

> Be like water making its way through cracks. Do not be assertive, but adjust to the object, and you will find a way around or through it. If nothing within you stays rigid, outward things will disclose themselves. Empty your mind: be formless, shapeless, like water. If you put water into a cup, it becomes the cup. You put water into a bottle and it becomes the bottle. You put water in a teapot – it becomes the teapot. Now water can flow or it can crash. Be water, my friend.

Educational questions & activities

1. A historic consequence of seniority-based supervisory systems has been the establishment of hierarchical professional relationships and interactions between the supervisor and the supervisee (Wetchler, 1990). According to SFS theory, supervision structured on unequal power relationships characteristically forms what, and leads where?
2. During SFS dialogue, the supervisor utilises narrativism to find out what?
3. True or false? The focus is always placed on what is the correct situation, and not what seems to be working for a supervisee with a particular case. As supervisors take the stance of being curious about even the smallest exceptions which are successful, their supervisees are allowed to examine the solutions and their strengths.
4. What are three focuses of SFS?

References

Anderson, H. (2008). *Conversation, language, and possibilities: A post-modern approach to therapy.* New York: Basic Books.

Anderson, H., & Goolishian, H. (1992). The client is the expert: A not-knowing approach to therapy. In S. McNamee & K. Gergen (Eds.), *Therapy as social construction* (pp. 25–39). London: Sage Ltd.

Bernard, J. M., & Goodyear, R. K. (2004). *Fundamentals of clinical supervision* (3rd ed.). Boston, MA: Allyn & Bacon.

Bradley, L. J., & Kottler, J. A. (2001). Overview of counselor supervision. In L. J. Bradley & N. Ladany (Eds.), *Counselor supervision: Principles, process, and practice* (3rd ed., pp. 3–27). Philadelphia, PA: Brunner-Routledge.

Briggs, J. R., & Miller, G. (2005). Success enhancing supervision. *Journal of Family Psychotherapy, 16*(1–2), 199–222.

Britton, P. J., Goodman, J. M., & Rak, C. F. (2002). Presenting workshops on supervision: A didactic-experiential format. *Counselor Education & Supervision, 42,* 31–39.

Chang, D. F., Tong, H., Shi, O., & Qifeng, Z. (2005). Letting a hundred flowers bloom: Counseling and psychotherapy in the People's Republic of China [Abstract]. *Journal of Mental Health Counseling, 27*(2), 104–116. doi: http://dx.doi.org/10.17744/mehc.27.2.hxfupdhht26b30a6

Cheung, S. (2001). Problem-solving and solution-focused therapy for Chinese: Recent developments. *Asian Journal of Counselling, 2001, 8*(2), 111–128.

Collins, P. (1993). The interpersonal vicissitudes of mentorship: An exploratory study of the field supervisor–student relationship. *Clinical Supervisor, 11*(1), 121–136.

Driscoll, J. (2007). *Practising clinical supervision: A reflective approach for healthcare professionals.* Amsterdam: Elsevier Health Sciences.

Edwards, J. K., & Chen, M.-W. (1999). Strength-based supervision: Frameworks, current practice, and future directions. A Wu-Wei method. *The Family Journal: Counselling and Therapy for couples and Families, 7*(4), 349–357. doi:10.1177/1066480799074005

Falvey, L. (2002). *The Buddha's gospel: A Buddhist interpretation of Jesus' gospel.* Adelaide: Institute for International Development.

Fowler, J., Riley, J., & Fenton, G. (2007). Using solution-focused techniques in clinical supervision. *Nursing Times, 103*(22), 30–31.

Gergen, K. (1999). *An invitation to social construction.* London: Sage Publications.

Gordon, G. R., & McBride, R. (1996). *Criminal justice internships: Theory into practice* (3rd ed.). Cincinnati, OH: Anderson Publishing.

Hart, G., & Nance, D. (2003). Styles of counsellor supervision as perceived by supervisors and supervisees. *Counselor Education and Supervision.* 3 December.

Hawkins, P., & Shohet, R. (2000). *Supervision in the helping professions.* Milton Keynes: Open University Press.

Haynes, R., Corey, G., & Moulton, P. (2003). *Clinical supervision in the helping professions: A practical guide.* Pacific Grove, CA: Brooks/Cole-Thomson Learning.

Hermans, H. J. M. (2004). The innovation of self-narratives: A dialogical approach. In L. Angus and J. McLeod (Eds.), *Handbook of narrative and psychotherapy: Practice, theory, and research* (pp. 175–192). Thousand Oaks, CA: Sage.

Hsu, W. (2009). The components of solution-focused supervision. *Bulletin of Educational Psychology, 41*(2), 475–496.

Kilminster, S. M., & Jolly, B. C. (2000). Effective supervision in clinical practice settings: A literature review. *Medical Education, 34*, 827–840. doi:10.1046/j.1365-2923.2000.00758.x/pdf

Kim, J. S., Franklin, C., Zhang, Y., Liu, X., Qu, Y., & Chen, H. (2015). Solution-focused brief therapy in China: A meta-analysis. *Journal of Ethnic & Cultural Diversity in Social Work, 24*(3), 187–201. doi:10.1080/15313204.2014.991983

Knight, J. (2003). Reflections of the therapist–supervisor relationships. In J. Weiner, R. Mitzen, & J. Duckham (Eds.), *On supervised and being supervised – A practice in search of a theory* (pp. 34–48). Basingstoke: Palgrave Macmillan.

Koob, J. J. (2002). The effects of solution-focused supervision on the perceived self-efficacy of therapists in training. *The Clinical Supervisor, 21*, 161–183. doi: 10.1300/J001v21n02_11

Lim, S. L., Lim, B. K. H., Michael, R., Cai, R., & Schock, C. K. (2010). The trajectory of counseling in China: Past, present, and future trends. *Journal of Counseling Development, 88*(1), 4. Retrieved from: http://search.proquest.com/openview/58f8cc61f107116f9c503eaa8ea8a4c2/1?pq-origsite=gscholar

Marek, L. I., Sandifer, D. M., Beach, A., Coward, R. L., & Protinsky, H. O. (1994). Supervision without the problem: A model of solution-focused supervision. *Journal of Family Psychotherapy, 5*(2), 57–64. doi: 10.1300/j085V05N02_04 [Taylor & Francis Online].

Medina, A., & Beyeback, M. (2014). How do child protection workers and teams change during solution-focused supervision and training? A brief qualitative report. *International Journal of Solution Focused Practices, 2*(1). doi: http://dx.doi.org/10.14335/ijsfp.v2i1.17

Moir-Bussy, A. (2008). The counselling education and supervision process – Dialogue and transformation. *Counselling, Psychotherapy and Health, 4*(1), 1–16.

Pearson, Q. M. (2006). Psychotherapy-driven supervision: Integrating counseling theories into role-based supervision. *Journal of Mental Health Counseling, 28*(3), 241–252. doi: http://dx.doi.org/10.17744/mehc.28.3.be1106w7yg3wvt1w

Piaget, J. (1977). *The development of thought: Equilibration of cognitive structures.* New York: Viking Press.

Puhakka, K. (2000). Invitation to authentic knowing. In T. Hart, P. L. Nelson, & K. Puhakka (Eds.), *Transpersonal knowing: Exploring the horizon of consciousness*. Albany: SUNY Press.

Selekman, M. D., & Todd, T. C. (1995). Co-creating a context for change in the supervisory system: The solution-focused supervision model. *Journal of Systemic Therapies, 14*(3), 21–33.

Shotter, J. (1994). Conversational realities: From within persons to within relationships. Paper prepared for The Discursive Construction of Knowledge Conference, University of Adelaide, Feb. 21–24, 1994.

Skarp, A.-P. (July 2, 2012, Monday). Wu Wei coaching: An introduction. Complexity, counselling, Wu Wei coaching [Web log post]. URL unknown.

Smith, M. K. (1997). The function of supervision. *The encyclopedia of informal education*. Last update: January 28, 2005. Retrieved 31/10/06 from: www.infed.org/biblio/functions_of_supe rvision.htm

Sullivan, B. (1989). *Psychotherapy grounded in the feminine principle*. Wilmette: Chiron.

Sweitzer, H. F., & King, M. (1998). *The successful internship – Transformation and empowerment*. Pacific Grove, CA: Brooks/Cole.

Thomas, F. N. (1996). The coaxing of expertise. In F. N. Thomas, S.D. Miller, M.A. Hubble, & B.L. Duncan (Eds.), *Handbook of solution focused brief therapy* (pp. 128–151). San Francisco: Jossey-Bass

Waskett, C. (2006). The pluses of solution-focused supervision. *Healthcare Counselling & Psychotherapy Journal, 6*(1).

Wetchler, J. L. (1990). Solution-focused supervision. *Family Therapy, 17*(2), 129–138.

Wu, K. M. (1997). *On Chinese body thinking – A cultural hermeneutic*. Leiden, The Netherlands: Brill.

Yontef, G. (1997). Supervision from a Gestalt perspective. In E. Watkins (Ed.), *Handbook of psychotherapy supervision* (pp. 147–163). New York: John Wiley & Sons.

12 Processes and Interventions to Facilitate Supervisees' Learning

Keithia Wilson and Alf Lizzio

Overview

This chapter seeks to answer the fundamental question: What supervisory processes and interventions can be used to support the learning of supervisees? Three types of interventions will be considered: contracting and relationship building, supervisor meta-competencies for facilitating learning, and specific supervisory learning activities.

Supervision is a complex intervention which is best conceptualised as an interpersonal exchange (Bernard & Goodyear, 2004). Thus, any meaningful consideration of supervisory interventions needs to be contextualised within the supervisory relationship. There is strong evidence to indicate that the quality of supervision in the formative stages of professional development has a longstanding effect on supervisees (Barnett, Doll, Younggren, & Rubin, 2007; Milne & Westerman, 2001), and findings from a range of studies indicate, collectively that supervision is a powerful process with the potential for both enhancing, as well as stunting the growth of supervisees (Barnett, Cornish, Goodyear, & Lichtenberg, 2007; Gazzola & Theriault, 2007). The empirical evidence indicates that the quality of the supervisory relationship is both a foundational intervention goal in its own right, and enabling of more specific supervisory methods and interventions used (Kilminster & Jolly, 2000; Lizzio & Que, 2009).

Given that the origins of supervision lie in the helping professions, it is not surprising that supervisory methods and processes have traditionally been conceptualised using counselling frameworks. However, the increasing generality of the process to a wider range of professions has facilitated the broadening of the construct from a counselling to an educational orientation (Carroll, 1996; Lizzio & Wilson, 2002). This is leading to a greater emphasis on understanding professional supervision as a learning relationship (Lizzio, Stokes, & Wilson, 2005).

Facilitating supervisees' learning can be conceptualised as a scaffolded process (see Figure 12.1). At the most foundational level the process of contracting is used to establish a working alliance that optimises supervisees' development and self-regulation. The learning potential of the supervisor-supervisee alliance is then realised through the meta-processes of critical reflection on the supervisees practice and the provision of quality developmental feedback. These meta-processes are inherent facets of the commonly used supervisory interventions of case study, observation and role play.

Thus, this chapter is structured in three parts. The first part focuses on meta-process interventions, in particular contracting, that can contribute to a positive supervisory working alliance. The second part focuses on the learning processes (for instance, facilitation of reflective practice and the provision of constructive feedback) which underpin the

DOI: 10.4324/9781003490067-15

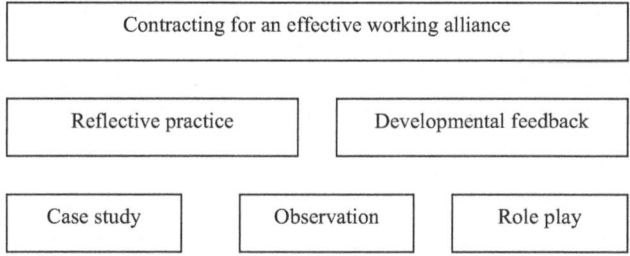

Figure 12.1 The structure of supervisory interventions

effectiveness of the supervisory interventions. The third part focuses on the use of specific interventions (for example, case study, observation, role plays) in supervision.

Establishing an effective working alliance

The quality of the supervisory relationship is the basis for learning in supervision and makes a critical contribution to both positive processes and outcomes (McMahon & Simons, 2004; Worthen & Mc Neill, 1996). At its best, a strong supervisory working alliance prevents the development of supervisor–supervisee conflict, and at worst it mitigates supervisor–supervisee differences and difficulties (Bordin, 1993; Nelson, Barnes, Evans, & Triggiano, 2008). As Watkins (1997) eloquently states, the supervisory relationship is 'a necessary ingredient to the making, doing, and being of the supervision process itself and seemingly facilitates or potentiates whatever takes place within that process' (p. 4). Despite the importance of quality supervisory relationships, the experience of relationship difficulties is relatively common. Negative supervision experiences have been reported from a number of authors (e.g., Ellis, 2001; Barnett et al., 2007). For example, Galante (1998) found 47 per cent of trainees in their study had experienced at least one ineffective supervisory relationship. Thus, at a meta-process or macro-level, a positive supervisory working alliance can be considered the most potent intervention for promoting effective personal and professional development in supervisees.

So, what are the qualities of an effective supervisory relationship? There is reasonable consensus that a trusting and collaborative relationship is a prerequisite for success, and that supervisors need to create a safe learning environment in which supervisees can openly discuss their work, raise concerns about their competence and personal limitations, and have permission and support to experiment with new strategies, techniques, and behaviours (Barnett & Barber, 2005; Ellis, 1991; Ladany, Ellis, & Friedlander, 1999; Wulf & Nelson, 2000). Moreover, there is strong evidence to indicate that timing is important in the development of an effective supervisory relationship. The quality of supervision in the formative stages of professional development has been shown to have a longstanding effect on supervisees (Milne & Westerman, 2001). Thus, interventions which build a trusting, collaborative, and safe working relationship at the outset of supervision are critical to learning success.

A potent early intervention for building an effective supervisory working alliance is contracting. The *content* purpose of contracting is to establish a clear working agreement regarding the goals, roles, and processes of the supervisee–supervisor relationship. The failure to establish such shared expectations from the outset has been identified as a key source of conflict between supervisees and supervisors (Nelson et al., 2008). Beyond this, not surprisingly, more effective outcomes are reportedly achieved when supervisees are engaged as active partners (e.g., conjoint goal setting, process review) in the supervisory process (Sheikh, Milne, & MacGregor, 2007) and have some input into and control over the supervisory process (Kilminster & Jolly, 2000). Thus, the *process* purpose of contracting is to establish supervisees as empowered co-creators of the supervisory process. Some regulatory boards in North America, Europe, and Australia require supervisors to outline their beliefs about, and orientation to, supervision (e.g., the supervision model that informs their practice, modalities typically employed). Such transparency can be thought of as a 'supervisor's epistemological declaration' (Liddel, 1988, p. 157) and the accountable disclosure of the professional and organisational elements within the supervision context (Magnuson, Norem, & Wilcox, 2000). Thus the *ethical* purpose of contracting is to provide the supervisee with the basis for informed choice. There is also considerable literature that supports the importance of goal setting in learning (Brookfield, 1986). For example, learning contracts have been demonstrated to result in stronger engagement with learning processes, and more effective learning outcomes (Knowles, 1984). Thus, the *educational* purpose of contracting is to optimise the relevance and effectiveness of supervisees' learning.

So what are the key areas of contracting in supervision? Contracting involves both supervisor and supervisee discussing the following types of questions:

- What learning goals shall we pursue?
- What approach to learning suits our circumstances?
- What type of relationship do we wish to have?
- What management processes do we wish to establish?

We propose that a capacity to formulate and set explicit and meaningful goals is not only a key part of the contracting process, but also the foundation for a mutually empowering and systematic learning process for both supervisor and supervisee. Thus, the process of contracting is in fact the primary or meta-intervention in supervision. The core learning goal or capability which enables a professional to continue to develop and direct themselves outside the context of supervision is proposed as a capacity for self-management and self-regulated learning – a set of meta-skills which enable more specific skills to be appropriately and strategically applied. Thus, used reflectively and interactively, these agenda setting or contracting processes are in essence interventions to facilitate supervisee self-regulation.

What learning goals shall we pursue?

There is strong agreement that effective supervision is goal focused and outcome-oriented (Kilminster & Jolly, 2000). A supervisor and supervisee having a 'shared map' or 'common language' about the range of goals and outcomes they might achieve together in supervision provides a number of benefits: facilitating the coordinated setting of goals, and making clearly discussable the developmental nature of supervision, and the fact that priorities will necessarily change over time. There are a range of approaches to identifying learning goals (e.g., from structured checklists to open-ended discussions) and use will vary depending on personal preferences, career stage, and the requirements of regulatory authorities. The following is one approach to conceptualising the potential domain of learning goals for supervision (Lizzio & Wilson, 2002):

- Self-regulation: capacity to independently self-reflect on practice and learn from experience.
- Systemic competence: understanding and managing the context of professional practice, working relationships and organisational dynamics.
- Role efficacy: managing the expectations and requirements of one's formal role or position (e.g., work standards, practices and accountabilities).
- Conceptual competence: conceptualising practice and explicating underlying principles that inform interventions.
- Ethical judgement: accountably addressing the issues and dilemmas stimulated by practice.
- Technical competence: mastery of the techniques and strategies for intervention and service delivery.
- Personal development: awareness and management of the personal aspects of professional practice.

What approach to learning suits our circumstances?

There is a well-established distinction in the educational literature between didactic and collaborative/facilitative pedagogies (Smerdon, Burkam, & Lee, 1999). Didactic approaches involve a teacher-controlled process of knowledge transmission (Vaill, 1996) and emphasise the learner's need for instruction, support and guidance in decision-making (Corno & Snow, 1986). Facilitative approaches involve the learner's active involvement (Järvelä & Salovaara, 2004) and emphasise an interactive reflection on the learner's experience. Thus, for example, in the context of professional supervision, a supervisor providing advice on how to address a specific issue could be said to be employing a didactic approach. In the same situation if the supervisor helped the supervisee develop their own judgement on the issue they would be exemplifying a facilitative approach.

Our research conducted with graduates undertaking mandated professional supervision to gain registration as psychologists found that supervisor's approaches to supervision were similarly understood by supervisees in terms of facilitative and didactic approaches to learning (Lizzio et al., 2005). Importantly, supervisors' use of a facilitative approach reduced supervisees' anxiety and resistance and increased their sense of professional self-regulation. Similarly, Couchon and Bernard (1984) found that in supervision sessions conducted before a counselling session, supervisors tended to be more directive and prescriptive with supervisees, but that little of this was able to be translated into practice by the supervisee. In contrast, however, supervisor's behaviour was more facilitative following a counselling session, with resulting high levels of transfer of learning by the supervisee into their counselling practice. These findings do not suggest that supervisors should not engage in direct instruction where appropriate, but rather that 'teaching' should be delivered within a broader facilitative approach.

In addressing the question of 'What approach to learning best suits our circumstances?' the supervisor and supervisee might usefully discuss:

The *process of learning* in supervision

- When and how might the supervisor use facilitative and reflective methods of learning?
- When and how might the supervisor use teaching or information transmission methods?

The *content of learning* in supervision

- To what extent might the supervisor focus on theory?
- To what extent might the supervisor focus on practical techniques?

What type of relationship do we wish to have?

The relational style of a supervisor has been defined as the distinctive and consistent manner of engaging with supervisees and implementing the process of supervision (Fernando & Hulse-Killacky, 2005; Kennard, Stewart, & Gluck., 1987). There is strong empirical support for the conceptualisation of the supervisory relationship as comprising the three relationship factors of support, challenge, and openness (Lizzio & Wilson, 2008). *Support* can be operationalised as the extent to which the supervisee feels adequate and affirmed as a result of their interactions with their supervisor. *Challenge* can be operationalised as the extent to which the supervisee feels challenged and stretched as a result of their interactions with their supervisor. *Openness* can be operationalised as the extent to which the supervisee feels their supervisor relates to them openly and non-defensively in regard to their background, limitations, and opinions.

Achieving an optimal balance of support and challenge is essential to effective supervisee and client outcomes. This has been identified not only as one of the most frequent sources of conflict in supervision, but also as one which can be readily resolved (Moskowitz & Rupert, 1983). Overall, a supervisor's goal is to provide sufficient challenge to stimulate growth and development, with enough support to enable the supervisee to adequately respond to the learning opportunity without retreating.

Research into high-quality supervision has identified a key aspect of openness as the supervisor's willingness to surface and discuss potential or actual issues and to actively problem solve them. Thus, openness has been related to effective conflict management in supervision (Nelson & Friedlander, 2001).

In addressing the question 'What type of relationship might we wish to have?' supervisor and supervisee might usefully discuss:

- What type and level of support might be valued? What forms of support might be counterproductive?
- What type and level of challenge might be valued? What forms of challenge might be counterproductive?
- What type and level of supervisor openness or disclosure might be appropriate?

What management processes do we wish to establish?

There are also a range of practical management processes that need to be explicated as part of the working supervisory contract:

- Purpose: To what extent is supervision for purposes of professional development and/ or monitoring of quality and accountability?
- Boundary management: What boundaries conditions (e.g., confidentiality, dual relationships) need to be discussed?
- Preparation: What level or type of preparation is expected between sessions?
- Feedback: How will the supervisory process be reviewed and evaluated?

Both supervisors and supervisees might use the contracting framework to inform critical self-reflection about their current and preferred approaches.

Supervisor reflection

- What is your current approach to contracting? How systematically and explicitly do you use contracting as an intervention process?
- Which intervention domains (e.g., learning goals, learning processes, relationship profile, and management procedures) are under or overemphasised in your practice?
- How do you use contracting to facilitate supervisees' capacity for self-regulation?
- Do you have a supervisory resume or position that summarises your approach to supervision?

Supervisee reflection

- To what extent are you willing to share responsibility for the management of the supervisory process?
- What are your needs and preferences across the various intervention domains (e.g., learning goals, relationships)?
- What conditions will optimise your learning in supervision?

Initial contracting

- How might you as a supervisor educate about and empower your supervisee in the contracting process?
- How might you as a supervisee educate and empower yourself in the contracting process?
- What type of 'working agreement' do you both wish to have?

Ongoing review

- How might you as a supervisor educate your supervisees about the developmental nature of supervision, and the fact that their priorities will necessarily change over time as their confidence and skills develop?
- How might you as a supervisee take responsibility for letting your supervisor know when you would like to discuss possible changes to ways of working?
- What ongoing processes might be used to review personal development and goal achievement in individual sessions and in supervision overall?

Supervisory meta-competencies

There are a number of well-established supervisory methodologies to develop supervisees' capability (e.g., case studies, role plays, observation of practice). While these will be discussed in a subsequent section of this chapter, it is firstly important to understand that their effective use is underpinned by two supervisory meta-competencies: providing supervisees with constructive feedback and facilitating supervisees' reflection of their practice. The central role of these meta-competencies is well acknowledged in the supervision literature (Hill, Stahl, & Roffman, 2007; Lambert & Arnold, 1987; Milne & James, 2000).

Processes for Constructive Feedback

Effective supervisors have been found to not only establish a non-threatening and supportive learning environment, but relatedly, to provide constructive feedback to their supervisees (Kilminster & Jolly, 2000). There is evidence to suggest that while the provision of feedback is generally perceived positively by trainees (Kadushin, 1992; Holmwood, 1993), critical and negative feedback from supervisors has been associated with increased anxiety and decreased sense of self-efficacy by supervisees (Larson & Daniels, 1998). Clearly, the quality of supervisor feedback would seem to be a key mediator of supervisees' ability to learn from experience.

At the level of general strategy there is a fair degree of consensus that feedback perceived to be effective evidences two key features. Firstly, effective feedback should provide specific information regarding the perceived gap between current and perceived performance (Butler, 1993; DeNisi & Kluger, 2000). Secondly, effective feedback should allow the recipient to participate or be actively involved. De Nisi and Kluger (2000) argue that feedback that causes the recipient to focus less on the task and more on the self (a dynamic termed meta-task processing) is more likely to attenuate or reduce performance. The idea here is that focusing on self or identity related issues (e.g., 'What will my supervisor think of me? What is going to happen to me at work if I do not perform well?' or 'Am I cut out to do this work?') occupies cognitive resources that could otherwise be used to improve task performance. Providing opportunities for supervisees to 'have a voice' has been found to mitigate self-oriented or meta-task processing when receiving negative or developmental feedback (Lind & Tyler, 1988; Lizzio, Wilson, & McKay, 2008).

Forms of participation and voice

While supervisee participation is clearly beneficial to the feedback process, it can be operationalised in a variety of different ways. The various forms of bilateral participation employed include: value-expressive or process control (the opportunity to express versions of events or rebut alternative versions, Greenberg, 1986); outcome control (the chance to contribute to the final decision or evaluation); general involvement (equitable proportion of airtime, Cawley, Keeping, & Levy, 1998), and self-appraisal (opportunities to self-assess prior to external feedback, Kanfer, Sawyer, Earley, & Lind, 1987). While all of these modes of participation have been found to enhance the effectiveness of feedback, it is expressive participation (the opportunity for the recipient to present their personal viewpoints or reactions to feedback) that consistently evidences the stronger association with positive (Cawley et al., 1998).

The timing and nature of opportunities for supervisees' voice or participation are important considerations in the construction of a feedback intervention. Findings to date indicate that both inviting a supervisee to react or respond to feedback – a process of facilitating 'voice' subsequent to supervisor feedback (i.e., 'I'm interested to hear your opinions of what I've said.'), and providing opportunities for self-appraisal – a process of facilitating 'voice' prior to the supervisor feedback (i.e., 'Are there any issues from your point of view that would be useful for us to discuss?') (Lizzio et al., 2008; Sharlicki & Folger, 1997) are effective strategies for reducing supervisee reactance. However, an invitation to respond to supervisor feedback is perceived most positively by supervisees, perhaps because this strategy provides opportunities for *feedback correctability* (Sharlicki & Folger, 1997), and on a symbolic level may provide a stronger signal about the valuing of supervisees.

The optimal protocol for giving feedback has been found to combine a sequence of strategies: invitation to self-appraise positive feedback, developmental feedback, and invitation to respond to the feedback. This strategy is consistently evaluated as more effective, and as less risky (reducing supervisees' feelings of confusion and anxiety) (Lizzio et al., 2008). This evidence-based protocol for providing constructive developmental feedback is presented below:

1. Invite and facilitate the supervisee to self-review using open-ended questions (e.g., *How do you think you went with...?*)
2. Express appreciation for their efforts (e.g., *You really tried to...*), acknowledge their achievements (e.g., *You were able to...*) and show awareness of the context (e.g., levels of complexity or difficulty) (e.g., *What I thought was particularly challenging was...*)
3. Provide data-based feedback on 'performance gaps'
   • be timely (give the feedback close to the event),
   • be specific and concrete,
   • provide data-based examples, and
   • indicate the consequences of the behaviour/strategy/technique used for the client/system/supervisee.
4. Invite their response to your feedback and discuss their reactions (in terms of ability, motivation, opportunity, learning) (e.g., *I very much want to get your perspective on this. What is your first reaction?)*
5. Invite their ideas for practice improvement or change (e.g., *What do you think might be useful...*)
6. Provide comment on their ideas, adding in any additional ideas you may have as the supervisor
7. Invite their response to your ideas
8. Collaboratively plan the supervisee's practice development and future learning (achievement, improvement, enabling)
9. Briefly review the feedback process for the supervisee's perceptions of fairness, effectiveness (e.g., *I would value your feedback on this feedback process...*)
10. Invite follow-up on the feedback at the next contact/session (e.g., *Would it be useful to revisit this at a later date to see if...?*)

Facilitating reflective practice

Supervisees commonly report that the greatest impetus for their change or learning comes from actual events or critical incidents which are outside of their control, experience and understanding (Kilminster & Jolly, 2000). Clearly frameworks and interventions which are able to facilitate the extraction of *learning from experience* and the development of *confidence from crisis* are foundational components of a supervisor's repertoire. Not surprisingly, *reflection on practice* has been proposed as the defining focus of supervisory practice (Booley, 1997; Fish & Twinn, 1997; Fisher, 1996; Paterson, 1994), and more recently we have seen the emergence of systematic training programs to develop reflective practice as a core learning mechanism in supervision (Sheikh et al., 2007).

Simply framed, supervisors are involved in assisting supervisees to learn from their experience. A practical understanding of experiential learning is central to the success of this enterprise. The experiential learning model is widely acknowledged as particularly appropriate for adult learning contexts such as supervision (Milne & Westerman, 2001).

There is both theoretical argument (Hager, 1999) and empirical evidence (Kember & Leung, 2005; Lizzio & Wilson, 2004) to indicate that didactic strategies rarely contribute to generative or metacognitive learning outcomes. The tacit nature of key aspects of professional knowledge (Stenberg & Horvath, 1999) means that they are more likely to be developed through reflection on action (Marsick & Watkins, 1996). In this sense metacognitive skill is developed through the process of reflecting on performance in context.

We argue that one of the fundamental goals of supervision should be developing the capacity for professional judgement: the ability to confidently act in *no right answer* (Schon, 1983), or *unfamiliar and changing* circumstances (Stephenson & Weil, 1992). In this regard it is important to distinguish the learning goals of *developing competence* (a capacity to routinely apply previously acquired knowledge) and *developing capability* (a capacity to generatively question the assumptions that inform current practice) (Stephenson, 1998). These goals respectively reflect Argyris and Schon's (1974) classic distinction between the processes of single and double loop learning.

The act of reflection, in itself, does not necessarily engender learning. Supervisors need to be able to scaffold supervisees' efforts at reflection to create a zone of proximal development (the gap between the quality of unassisted reflection and what can be potentially achieved with guidance or structure) (Vygotsky, 1978) is particularly relevant in this context. Supervisees critical thinking will be enhanced if they are purposely engaged and supported in three related practices: examining their assumptions, considering evidence from multiple perspectives, and taking responsibility for making a considered conclusion based on their reflections (King & Kitchener, 2004).

The ways in which people make sense of or represent the world (their mental models, personal theories, guiding values, theories in use) (Senge, 1990) is the primary focus or content of these reflective processes. As Dall'Alba and Sandberg (1996) demonstrate, the way in which practitioners understand professional practice (e.g., their underlying ideas and schemas about what they should be trying to achieve as a professional in a particular situation) is the basis for how they perform. In Argyris and Schon's (1974) terms, peoples' *governing values* drive their *action strategies.*

Thus, in essence, the process of problematisation or critical reflection involves making previous tacit aspects of situational appraisal (taken-for-granted beliefs and assumptions) explicit and subject to conscious scrutiny (Claxton, 1999). The guiding tenet is that awareness of assumptions is key to effectiveness. Untested assumptions (e.g., what we might construe others' motives to be in a situation), by definition, have a greater probability of contributing to ineffective outcomes. In this sense, effectiveness is a function of the degree of match or congruence between our espoused theory (what we think or say we believe and do) and our theory in use (what we actually believe and do) (Argyris & Schon, 1974). As Dall'Alba (2004) argues, it is the exploration of assumptions that facilitates a richer description of the interdependency of professionals and their practice.

A simple shared framework can be particularly helpful in facilitating critical reflective dialogue between supervisor and supervisee. The reflective practice cycle (see Figure 12.2) can be used to aid supervisees engage in structured planning or prospective analysis (*What might I do in this situation?)* or retrospective reflection (*What did I do in this situation?).* The framework can be used to scaffold reflection from *multiple points of entry*. Thus, for example, a supervisee might commence a discussion by reporting their intentions (*What they want to achieve*). The supervisor can help the supervisee explore their thinking by

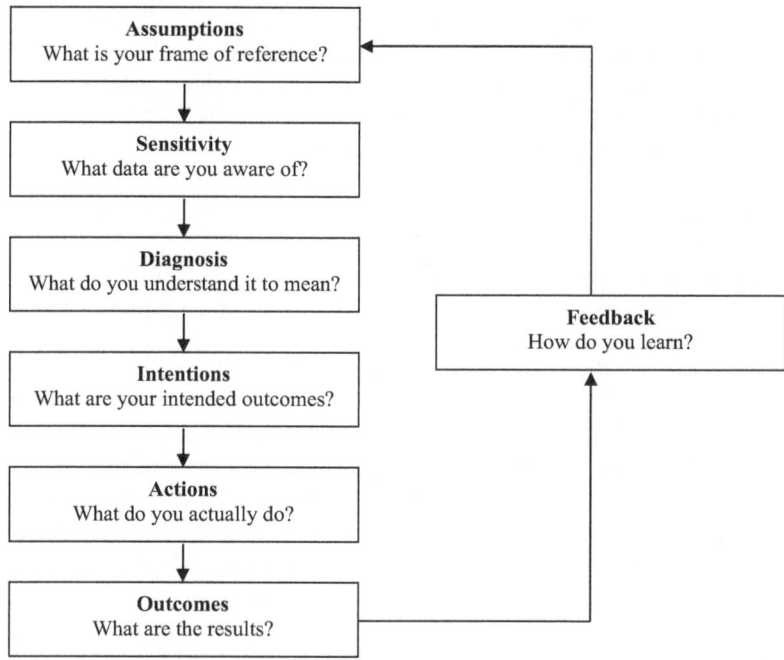

Figure 12.2 The reflective practice cycle in supervision

inviting either backward reflection (e.g., *What diagnosis are these intentions based on? What data informs your diagnosis?*) or forward reflection (e.g., *What might you actually do? What might be likely consequences?*).

The framework is particularly useful for helping supervisees reflect on potential gaps or discontinuities in their practice. The most common forms of these are:

- What is the level of congruence between what I observe (data or evidence) and the meaning I make (diagnosis)? To what extent does the data support my conclusions?
- What is the difference between what I planned to do (intentions) and what I actually did (actions)? How do I explain this?
- What is the match between the outcomes I expected from my actions (intended consequences) and what actually resulted (unintended consequences)?

Specific supervisory methodologies

In this section we review three well-established methodologies for evaluating and enhancing supervisees' practice: case studies, observation of practice, and role plays or modelling (Hill et al., 2007). Each of these methodologies emphasises different learning modes: case discussion, involving feedback and theorising can be seen as employing more 'symbolic' processes; observation of practice generally through videotaped sessions is more directly 'iconic'; and role-play and the use of learning exercises make use of 'enactive' processes (Milne & Westerman, 2001). The purposeful combination of these methodologies provides a means through which supervisees can translate and evolve their declarative knowledge (*knowing about something*) to procedural knowledge (*know how to do something*) and strategic knowledge (*knowing when and why to do something*) (Furr & Carroll, 2003).

How might a supervisor know when and what methodology to use? Choice of methodology is determined by a number of factors relevant to both the supervisor and the supervisee. Borders and Leddick (1987) elaborate six considerations in matching method to context: the supervisee's learning goals, level of experience and developmental needs, and learning style; in combination with the supervisor's theoretical orientation, goals for the supervisee, and personal goals for the supervisory experience. It is also important to note that their complementary nature means that these methodologies can be usefully combined in a particular supervision session. Thus, for example, a case study discussion or the processing of a videotaped session may evolve to include role playing particular aspects of the counsellor/supervisee's intervention.

Case studies

Case studies are most widely used for skill development, and are the most popular format for individual and group supervision (Holloway & Johnston, 1985). The commonly espoused goals of this methodology are to develop supervisees' skills in case conceptualisation, diagnosis, and intervention. It is generally recognised that while behavioural skills can be developed relatively quickly with supervision, skills in conceptualising cases and the ability to make treatment decisions develop more slowly and require the direct facilitation by a supervisor (Holloway & Neufeldt, 1995; Kilminster & Jolly, 2000). The case study method is well suited for this purpose.

There is some evidence regarding the factors which facilitate or inhibit the efficacy of the case study as a learning tool in supervision. Nolan, Hawkes, and Francis (1993) found both the development of an effective working alliance and supervisory process competence to be particularly important factors facilitating change in supervisee's thinking and behaviour. Case studies were experienced as more effective when supervisors adopted an outcome orientation (reflection with a specific purpose or outcome in mind), and actively facilitated the level and quality of data (e.g., making timely observations).

The case study method is typically initiated either through supervisee relatively informal verbal *self-report* or the more formal presentation of *case/process notes*. The more preparation of a case study by the supervisee prior to the session the more likely the process is to be of value. Written documentation is particularly helpful in that it provides a clear focus for discussion in the session and allows the supervisor to more readily assess the supervisee's level of cognitive processing and understanding of the case. In fact, Goldberg (1985) argues that the major value of the case study is that it allows the supervisor to work with the supervisee's current level of functioning. From a psychosocial perspective, placing control for the presentation of case material in the hands of the supervisee may reduce perceived threat levels and the possibility of their engaging in defensive self-presentation or meta-task processing with the supervisor. In this regard case studies may be an optimal early intervention for novice supervisees who may feel threatened by more direct forms of supervision.

There are several available formats to guide supervisees in the structuring of process notes in preparation for a supervision session (e.g., Schwartz, 1981). The following protocol, adapted from Bernard and Goodyear (2004), is a fairly typical approach to reflecting on a counselling session:

1. What were your *goals and strategies* for this counselling session?
2. Did anything happen *during* the session that caused you to re-consider either your goals or your strategies? How did you resolve this?
3. What was the major focus or *theme* of the session?
4. What are your current *hypotheses?*
5. Describe the *interpersonal or relationship dynamics* between you and the client during the session?
6. What was achieved in the session? How *successful* was it from yours and the client's perspective?
7. What did you *learn* about yourself and the helping process from this session?
8. What are your *goals and strategies* for the next session?
9. What *questions* or concerns do you want to raise with your supervisor?

Beyond reflection of *set pieces* such as planned interventions or scheduled sessions, unanticipated or critical incidents also provide important opportunities for learning and development in supervision. Incidents outside of the control and experience of the supervisee have been found to be powerful catalysts for change, provided they are processed effectively (Furr & Carroll, 2003), and there is both anecdotal and case study based evidence to support the efficacy of critical incident based methodologies when facilitated expertly (Davis, 2006).

Critical incidents, by definition, involve *a series of imperfect choices made in the light of limited information and pressing concerns*. Thus, a simple *choice-point* format, somewhat akin to Schon's (1992) notion of *manoeuvring in the swamp of practice* may be particularly helpful in capturing the dynamics of unstructured or emergent situations. The sequence of prompts is along the lines of:

- Where were you?
- What did you do?
- What were the immediate consequences? For you? For others?
- Why do you think you did what you did?
- What did other people think about what you did?
- What were the implications of the above?
- How sure are you that you now understand this situation?
- Have you experienced this type of situation previously?
- What do you think you have learnt?
- What do you consider that you still need to learn?

Beyond the higher-order structure of a case study, the style of dialogue between supervisor and supervisee is particularly crucial to the type of learning achieved. Given the goals of self-regulation and independent professional judgement it should not be surprising that supervisors employ Socratic methods of inquiry with the aim for the supervisee to *discover their truth* in the exchange with their supervisor and progressively learn to understand and trust his or her own cognitive and emotional personal process. These are noble aims, but the success of this method hinges on the capacity of the supervisor to question out of the supervisee's, rather than their own, theoretical and personal frame of reference (Glickhauf-Hughes & Campbell, 1991).

While the case study methodology has a figural role in supervisee development its effective use requires a particular sensitivity to context. Firstly, Holloway (1988) cautions that the case study methodology may require complex cognitive processing beyond the capacity of some supervisees. This suggests the importance of judicious pace and depth of inquiry to minimise feelings of supervisee incompetence and allow the incremental development of conceptual complexity. Secondly, Bernard and Goodyear (1992) observe that case notes can provide a way for the supervisee to control, and thus limit, the type of information presented on their practice for supervisor reflection. Thus, some clinicians only recommend exclusive reliance on case study presentations with advanced supervisees (Goldberg, 1985). Finally, there is a widely endorsed view that while the use of case notes is a valuable practice, it needs to be supplemented by other interventions, particularly more direct observation of practice (Kilminster & Jolly, 2000; Milne, Pilkington, Gracie, & James, 2003).

Finally, it is worth noting that the supervisory process itself can offer a 'living case study' or parallel process of the supervisee's functioning in similar contexts (Glickauf-Hughes & Capmbell, 1991). The value of parallel process is based on the assumption that a supervisee's difficulties with learning in supervision can often reflect similar difficulties between the supervisee as counsellor and their client. In order to effectively process these dynamics a supervisor needs to be both empathically connected with the supervisee, and able to disengage from his or her own emotional reactions.

Observation

Observation is perhaps the only form of direct supervision of practice, and typically implemented via one of three forms: audiotapes, videotapes, and live observation. The added benefit of this methodology beyond case notes is the wider range of available data on the supervisee's interpersonal, therapeutic, and process skills. All three observational modes have been found to produce learning outcomes. There is no empirical evidence that videotape is superior to audiotape as a means of enhancing supervisee performance or skills, and audiotape remains the most practical means of observation in supervision (Bernard & Goodyear, 1992). The strategic combination of observation and structured feedback (e.g., the rehearsal of microcounselling skills supplemented by supervisory feedback from audio or video-taped sessions) has been demonstrated to produce, not only enhanced counsellor skills, but also improved clinical outcomes for clients such as attendance and resolution of problem behaviours (Blashki, Hickie, & Davenport, 2003). Contrary to popular opinion, observational methods are not associated with high levels of supervisee anxiety (Ellis, Krengel, & Beck, 2002).

Context setting (providing the supervisee with a rationale), planning (establishing a protocol for the review, and selection of practice samples) and contracting (negotiating a mutually suitable process) are central to the effective use of observation as a learning methodology. As a general principle, because of the time intensive nature of this methodology, more productive outcomes may result from sessions with an identified *point of focus*. Bernard and Goodyear (1992) suggest that useful criteria for identifying points of focus from a supervisees' perspective include: the most *productive* or important part of the session, the part of the session in which they feel the most challenge or sense of struggle or confusion. In addition, supervisors may also choose to bring supervisees' attention to parts of the session where there is apparent incongruence or where dynamics appear potently therapeutic or unfortunately strained or where recurring themes are well illustrated.

Actively managing the presentation of a practice sample will facilitate both time efficiency and learning outcomes. Apart from the basic requirement of selecting a particular tape segments in advance of the session, the supervisee can set the context for the supervisor by providing their reason for selecting this particular sample, briefly summarising relevant history (*session to date*), explaining their intentions or goals in the practice sample, and asking for specific help.

Perhaps the most widely used methodology for processing videotapes is Interpersonal Process Recall (IPR) (Kagan, 1980). The process of IPR has been well documented and is relatively simple. The supervisor and supervisee together watch a pre-recorded video counselling session. Both supervisor and supervisee are empowered at any point to stop the tape to explore what is happening. The particular rationale underlying Kagan's (1976) process is the safe exploration of issues that seem to be unaddressed in the session, for example, a supervisee's frustration, confusion, uncertainty, or incongruence. The supervisor responds in the enquirer role using open-ended questions to facilitate the supervisee exploration towards some resolution (insight, understanding). The supervisor facilitates the supervisee to surface, explore and understand their internal processes in response to the client and the counselling session. The particular value of the IPR process is the potential to identify 'psychological barriers to communication' for supervisees as counsellors and therapists (Kagan, 1980). Given that this is a time consuming process, preparation is critical, to ensure that the most salient events or interactions are processed.

Role play

Experiential learning through role play is a well-established method for training counsellors in both micro-counselling skills and interventions, and can also be used as an effective means for developing diagnostic and conceptualisation skills (Lizzio, Wilson, & Gallois, 1993). There is evidence that while simple counselling skills can be learned didactically, more complex skills such as empathy, and timing of confrontation require more complex teaching methodologies, especially role play and modelling (Lambert & Arnold, 1987). There is strong empirical support for the efficacy of role play in counselling and clinical training (Glickauf-Hughes & Campbell, 1991; Rabinowitz, 1997), with the strongest level of skill development occurring when combined with modelling (O'Toole, 1979; Teevan & Gabel, 1978). Early career practitioners, in particular, report role play in combination with modelling and feedback as an effective learning mechanism in supervision (Rabinowitz, 1997).

A contextual model for role play

The complexity of professional practice necessitates supervisors employing approaches to role play that take account of the context of behaviour. The simple use of role-play to rehearse or shape behaviour (e.g., assertion) without enhancing awareness of its situational appropriateness or interpersonal consequences is mechanistic training rather than genuine professional development. The following seven-step model can be used in both individual and group supervision. For a detailed description, see Lizzio et al. (1993).

1. *Identifying the focus.* The supervisor and supervisee briefly discuss the 'focal situation' or 'focal task' (the supervisee wanting to develop more functional responses to previous, current, or anticipated situations). This 'background briefing' (the setting, the people involved, the supervisee's typical behaviour and feelings) sets the scene for the role play. For example, a female supervisee (call her Anita) may select a situation where she feels

that she 'goes out of her way' to support a male client and receives what she believes is unfair criticism from him on the effectiveness of her counselling. Anita apologises but feels hurt, angry and resentful.

2. *Specifying tentative goals*: The supervisee nominates his or her learning goals (What I want to do differently and how this might be helpful to me). In the present example, Anita may have the initial goal of defending herself from what she perceives as unfair criticism from her client. It is important to remember that initial goals must be set with a tentative spirit and will be reviewed after further situational analysis.

3. *Enacting present behaviour*: The supervisee role plays his or her present behaviour (this is how I responded or am likely to respond in this situation). The purpose is to provide a sample of behaviour in context to inform a discussion about responses, likely reactions of others, assumptions, and the broader context. In the present example, Anita enacts her typical way of responding, while the supervisor, another person (if in a group supervision context) or an empty chair can take the role of the 'ungrateful client.'

4. *Analysing the situation*: The aim here is to produce a rich description of the dynamics of the situation so as to well- inform new responses that have a good chance of being both effective (likely to work better than the current response) and feasible (likely to be enacted). A rich description of the situation is likely to include some consideration of:

- *Personal issues*, including the supervisee's assumptions, self-statements, anxieties, and interaction style;
- *Interpersonal issues*, including the nature and history of the relationship and typical patterns of interaction between the supervisee and others involved (e.g., manipulative strategies involving anger or guilt used by either person);
- *Situational or contextual issues*, including the relevant social rules and goals in the situation, the perception of other people, the organisational culture, social supports the supervisee can use, the nature of the task, the influence of gender, culture, or professional status.

Beyond simple discussion, the processes that can be used to heighten the supervisee's awareness and training relevant behaviours in this step are as varied as the supervisor's skills and creativity. Some commonly used strategies include feedback from the supervisor to the supervisee, self-analysis by the supervisee, and group reaction and feedback in a group supervision context. The supervisor's input at this stage can include any number of activities such as:

- Inductive questioning eliciting the supervisee's perceptions of their choices and alternatives;
- Interrupted role play, where the action is stopped at crucial points during the enactment of typical behaviour in the situation and the dynamics of the situation are interpreted with the supervisee;
- Group reaction and feedback, or eliciting the perceptions of other people in a supervision group about the situation, as a way of introducing and reinforcing new perspectives on the situation;
- Role reversal, in which the supervisee takes the role of the other person (e.g., client), either in imagination or actual behaviour and tries to see the world from that person's point of view. The process of role reversal is intended to develop skills in

meta-perception (Argyle, 2013), sensitise supervisees to the impact of their behaviour on clients, and make them more aware of their obligations as opposed to their rights in the situation; or

- Modelling, in which the supervisor takes the role of the supervisee in the situation and models alternative strategies.

5. *Reassessing goals:* The outcome of a well-conducted situational analysis is the supervisee is better able to formulate well-informed goals (What I think is going on here is... The type of response that I would like to work towards is... This will be helpful to all concerned because...).

6. *Developing the preferred strategy:* The situation is role played again with the supervisee attempting to enact their preferred strategy through a process of 'successive approximations' (behaviour rehearsal and feedback).

7. *Planning for action:* The session can be usefully concluded with a discussion of the challenges related to transfer of learning ('doing this for real') and processes for self-management or support.

Conclusion

This chapter has focused on the supervisory processes and interventions that can be used to support learning and development in supervision. We have argued that, because all supervision depends on the quality of the working relationship between supervisor and supervisee, contracting and relationship-building are necessary and foundational supervisory interventions. We framed clinical supervision as a learning relationship and proposed the supervisory meta-competencies of facilitating reflection and providing constructive feedback as underpinning the effectiveness of supervisory interventions. Finally, we considered how specific supervisory interventions (i.e., case study, observation, role plays) contributed to learning outcomes.

Educational questions & activities

1. Describe, using the contracting framework presented, your preferred supervisory working relationship. You may do this from either the perspective of a supervisor or supervisee.
   - What learning goals do you wish to emphasise?
   - What approach to learning suits you?
   - What type of relationship do you wish to have?
   - What management processes are important for you?
2. Identify two situations:
   - Where you felt that you received constructive feedback?
   - Where you felt that you received ineffective feedback?
   Can you identify:
   - What did you do that helped or hindered the feedback process?
   - What did others do that helped or hindered the feedback process?
   - How might your reflections be relevant to enhancing feedback processes in supervision?

3. Use the evidence-based protocol for giving developmental feedback to construct a feedback message to a supervisee.
4. Identify a critical incident or interaction and use the reflective practice cycle to critically review the choices you made.
5. Identify a critical incident or interaction and use the role play model to develop new responses or strategies.

Selected references for further reading

Lizzio, A., & Wilson, K. (2007). Developing critical professional judgment: the efficacy of a self-managed reflective process. *Studies in Continuing Education, 29*(3), 277–193.
McMahon, M., & Patton, W. (2002). *Supervision in the helping professions.* Frenchs Forest: Pearson.

Selected Internet Resources

Professional supervision for counsellors
www.theaca.net.au

Professional supervision for psychologists
www.psychology.org.au/study/working/registration_boards

Professional supervision for rehabilitation counsellors
www.asorc.org.au/

Professional supervision for school counsellors
www.asorc.org.au//

Professional supervision for social workers
www.aasw.asn.au

References

Argyris, C., & Schon, D. (1974). *Theory in practice: Increasing professional effectiveness.* San Francisco: Jossey-Bass.
Barnett, J. E., Doll, B., Younggren, J. N., & Rubin, N. J. (2007). Clinical competence for practicing psychologists: Clearly a work in progress. *Professional Psychology: Research and Practice, 38*(5), 510–514.
Barnett, J. E., Erikson Cornish, J. A., Goodyear, R. K., & Lichtenberg, J. W. (2007). Commentaries on the ethical and effective practice of clinical supervision. *Professional Psychology: Research and Practice, 38*(1), 268–275.
Barrett, M. S., & Barber, J. P. (2005). A developmental approach to the supervision of therapists in training. *Journal of Contemporary Psychotherapy, 35*, 169–183.
Bernard, J. M., & Goodyear, R. K. (1992). *Fundamentals of clinical supervision* (2nd ed.). Boston, MA: Allyn & Bacon.
Bernard, J. M., & Goodyear, R. K. (2004). *Fundamentals of clinical supervision* (3rd ed.). Boston, MA: Allyn & Bacon.

Blashki, G., Hickie, I. B., & Davenport, T. A. (2003). Providing psychological treatments in general practice: How will it work? *The Medical Journal of Australia, 179*(1), 23–25.

Booley, S. (1997). The supervisory role in the fostering of critical self-reflection capacity in social workers. *Social Work, 33*(2), 110–119.

Borders, L. D., & Leddick, G. R. (1987). *Handbook of counseling supervision.* Alexandria, VA: Association for Counselor Education and Supervision.

Bordin, E. S. (1993). A working alliance based model of supervision. *The Counseling Psychologist, 11*(1), 35–42.

Brookfield, S. D. (1986). *Understanding and facilitating adult learning.* San Fransisco: Josey-Bass Publishers.

Butler, R. (1993). Effects of task- and ego-achievement goals on information-seeking during task engagement. *Journal of Personality and Social Psychology, 65,* 18–31.

Carroll, M. (1996). *Counseling supervision: Theory, skills and practice.* London: Cassell.

Cawley, B. D., Keeping, L. M., & Levy, P. E. (1998). Participation in the performance appraisal process and employee reaction: a meta-analytic review of field investigations. *Journal of Applied Psychology, 83,* 615–633.

Claxton, G. (1999). *Wise up: The challenge of lifelong learning.* London: Bloomsbury.

Corno, L., & Snow, R. E. (1986). Adapting teaching to individual difference among learners. In M. C. Wittrock (ed.), *Handbook of research on teaching* (pp. 605–629). New York: Macmillan.

Couchon, W. D., & Bernard, J., M. (1984). Effects of timing of supervision on supervisor and counsellor performance. *The Clinical Supervisor, 2,* 3–21.

Dall'Alba, G. (2004). Understanding professional practice: investigations before and after an educational program. *Studies in Higher Education, 29,* 679–692.

Dall' Alba, G., & Sandberg, J. (1996). Education for competence in professional practice. *Instructional Science, 24,* 411–437.

Davis, P. J. (2006). Critical incident technique: a learning intervention for organisational problem solving. *Development and Learning in Organisations: An International Journal, 20,* 13–16.

DeNisi, A., & Kluger, A. N. (2000). Feedback effectiveness: can 360-degree appraisals be improved? *Academy of Management Executive, 14,* 129–139.

Ellis, M. V. (1991). Critical incidents in clinical supervision and in supervisor supervision: assessing supervisory issues. *Journal of Counseling Psychology, 38*(3), 342–349.

Ellis, M. V. (2001). Harmful supervision, a cause for alarm: comment of Gray et al. (2001) and Nelson and Frielander (2001). *Professional Psychology: Research and Practice, 48,* 401–406.

Ellis, M. V., Krengel, M., & Beck, M. (2002). Testing self-focused attention theory in clinical supervision: effects of supervisee anxiety and performance. *Journal of Counseling Psychology, 49,* 101–106.

Fernando, D. M., & Hulse-Killacky, D. (2005). The relationship of supervisory styles to satisfaction with supervision and the perceived self-efficacy of master's-level counseling students. *Counselor Education and Supervision, 44*(4), 293–304.

Fish, D., & Twinn, S. (1997). *Quality supervision in the healthcare professions. Principled approaches to practice.* Oxford: Butterworth-Heinemann.

Fisher, M. (1996). Using reflective practice in clinical supervision. *Professional Nursing, 11*(7), 443–444.

Furr, S. R., & Carroll, J. J. (2003). Critical incidents in student counselor development. *Journal of Counseling and Development, 81,* 483–489.

Galante, M. (1998). Trainees' and supervisors' perceptions of effective and ineffective supervisory relationships. *Dissertations Abstracts International, 49,* 933B.

Gazzola, N., & Theriault, A. (2007). Relational themes in counseling supervision: broadening and narrowing processes. *Canadian Journal of Counseling, 41*(4), 228–243.

Glikauf-Hughes, C., & Campbell, L. (1991). Experiential supervision: applied techniques for a case presentation approach. *Psychotherapy, 28*(1), 625–635.

Goldberg, D. A. (1985). Process notes, audio, and video tape: modes of presentation in psychotherapy training. *The Clinical Supervisor, 3,* 1–13.

Greenberg, J. (1986). Determinants of perceived fairness of performance evaluations. *Journal of Applied Psychology, 71,* 340–342.

Hager, P. (1999). Finding a good theory of workplace learning. In D. Boud & J. Garrick (eds.), *Understanding learning at work* (pp. 65–82). London: Routledge.

Hill, C. E., Stahl, J., & Roffman, M. (2007). Training novice psychotherapists: helping skills and beyond. *Psychotherapy: Theory, Research, Practice, Training, 44*(4), 364–370.

Holloway, E. L. (1988). Instruction beyond the facilitative conditions: A response to Biggs. *Counselor Education and Supervision, 27,* 252–258.

Holloway, E. L., & Johnston, R. (1985). Group supervision: Widely practiced but poorly understood. *Counselor Education and Supervision, 24*(4), 232–240.

Holloway, E. L., & Neufeldt, S. A. (1995). Supervision: Its contributions to treatment efficacy. *Journal of Consulting and Clinical Psychology, 63*(2), 207–213.

Holmwood, C. B. (1993). The gentle art of feedback. *Australian Family Physician, 22*(10), 1811–1813.

Järvelä, S., & Salovaara, H. (2004). The interplay of motivational goals and cognitive strategies in a new pedagogical culture. *European Psychologist, 9,* 232–244.

Kadushin, A. (1992). Social work supervision: A research update. *The Clinical Supervisor, 2,* 9–27.

Kagan, N. (1976). *Influencing human interaction.* Washington, DC: American Association for Counseling and Development.

Kagan, N. (1980). Influencing human interaction – eighteen years with IPR. In A. K. Hess (ed.), *Psychotherapy supervision: theory, research and practice* (pp. 262–286). New York: John Wiley.

Kanfer, R., Sawyer, J., Earley, P. C., & Lind, E. A. (1987). Fairness and participation in evaluation procedures: Effects on task attitudes and performance. *Social Justice Research, 1,* 235–249.

Kember, D., & Leung, D. Y. P. (2005). The influence of active learning experiences on the development of graduate capabilities. *Studies in Higher Education, 30,* 155–170.

Kennard, B. D., Stewart, S. M., & Gluck, M. R. (1987). The supervision relationship: Variables contributing to positive verses negative experiences. *Professional Psychology: Research and Practice, 18,* 172–175.

Kilminster, S. M., & Jolly, B. C. (2000). Effective supervision in clinical practice settings: A literature review. *Medical Education, 34,* 827–840.

King, P. M., & Kitchener, K. S. (2004). Reflective judgment: Theory and research on the development of epistemic assumptions through adulthood. *Educational Psychologist, 39,* 5–18.

Knowles, M. S. (1984). *The adult learner: A neglected species.* Houston, Texas: Gulf.

Ladany, N., Ellis, M. V., & Friedlander, M. L. (1999). The supervisory working alliance, trainee self-efficacy and satisfaction. *Journal of Counseling and Development, 77,* 447–455.

Lambert, M. J., & Arnold, R. C. (1987). Research and the supervisory process. *Professional Psychology: Research and Practice, 18*(3), 217–224.

Larson, L. M., & Daniels, J. A. (1998). Review of the counseling self-efficacy literature. *The Counseling Psychologist, 26,* 179–218.

Liddel, H. A. (1988). Systemic supervision: Conceptual overlays and pragmatic guidelines. In H. A. Liddel, D. C. Breunlin, & R. C. Schwartz (eds.), *Handbook of family therapy training and supervision* (pp. 153–171). New York: Guilford.

Lind, E. A., & Tyler, T. R. (1988). *The social psychology of procedural justice.* New York: Plenum Press.

Lizzio, A., Stokes, L., & Wilson, K. L. (2005). Approaches to learning in professional supervision: Supervisee perceptions of process and outcome. *Studies in Continuing Education, 27,* 239–257.

Lizzio, A., & Wilson, K. L. (2002). Outcomes in professional supervision. In M. McMahon & W. Patton (eds.), *Supervision in the helping professions: A practical guide* (pp. 27–42). Sydney: Pearson Education.

Lizzio, A., & Wilson, K. L. (2004). Action learning in higher education: An investigation of its potential to develop capability. *Studies in Higher Education, 29,* 469–488.

Lizzio, A., Wilson, K. L., & Gallois, C. G. (1993). Training assertive communication in its social context. In K. L. Wilson & C. G. Gallois (eds.), *Assertion and its social context* (pp. 155–169). London: Pergamon.

Lizzio, A., Wilson, K., & McKay, L. (2008). Managers and subordinates' evaluations of feedback message components. *Journal of Applied Social Psychology, 38*, 919–946.

Lizzio, A., Wilson, K., & Que, J. (2009). Relationship dimensions of professional supervision: supervisees' perceptions of processes and outcomes. *Studies in Continuing Education, 31*(2), 127–140.

Magnuson, S., Norem, K., & Wilcoxen, S. A. (2000). Clinical supervision of prelicensed counselors: Recommendations for consideration and practice. *Journal of Mental Health Counseling, 22*(2), 176–188.

Marsick, V. J., & Watkins, K. (1996). *Informal and incidental learning in the workplace.* London: Routledge.

McMahon, M., & Simons, R. (2004). Supervision training for professional counselors: an exploratory study. *Counselor Education and Supervision, 43*(4), 301–309.

Milne, D., & James, I. (2000). A systematic review of effective cognitive-behavioural supervision. *British Journal of Clinical Psychology, 39*, 111–127.

Milne, D., & Westerham, C. (2001). Evidence-based clinical supervision: rationale and illustration. *Clinical Psychology and Psychotherapy, 8*, 444–457.

Milne, D. L., Pilkington, J., Gracie, J., & James, I. (2003). Transferring skills from supervision to therapy: A qualitative and quantitative N = 1 analysis. *Behavioural and Cognitive Psychotherapy, 31*, 193–202.

Moskowitz, S. A., & Rupert, P. A. (1983). Conflict resolution within the supervisory relationship. *Professional Psychology: Research and Practice, 14*, 632–641.

Nelson, M. L., Barnes, K. L., Evans, A. L., & Triggiano, P. J. (2008). Working with conflict in clinical supervision: Wise supervisors' perspectives. *Journal of Counselling Psychology, 55*(2), 172–184.

Nelson, M. L., & Friedlander, M. L. (2001). A close look at conflictual supervisory relationships: The trainee's perspective. *Journal of Counseling Psychology, 48*, 384–395.

Nolan, J., Hawkes, B., & Francis, P. (1993). Case studies: Windows into clinical supervision. *Educational Leadership, 51*(2), 32–36.

O'Toole, W. M. (1979). Effects of practice and some methodological considerations in training in counseling, interviewing skills. *Journal of Counseling Psychology, 26*, 419–426.

Paterson, B. (1994). The view from within: Perspectives of clinical teaching. *International Journal of Nursing Studies, 31*(4), 349–360.

Rabinowitz, F. E. (1997). Teaching counselling through a semester-long role play. *Counselor Education and Supervision, 36*, 216–223.

Schon, D. (1983). *The reflective practitioner: How professional think in action.* New York: Basic Books.

Schon, D. A. (1992). The crisis of professional knowledge and the pursuit of an epistemology of practice. *Journal of Interprofessional Care, 6*(1), 49–62.

Schwartz, R. (1981). The conceptual development of family therapy trainees. *American Journal of Family Therapy, 2*, 89–90.

Senge, P. (1990). The *fifth discipline: The art and practice of the learning organisation.* Australia: Random House.

Sheikh, A. I., Milne, D. L., & MacGregor, B. V. (2007). A model of personal professional development in the systematic training of clinical psychologists. *Clinical Psychology and Psychotherapy, 14*, 278–287.

Skarlicki, D. P., & Folger, R. (1997). Retaliation in the workplace: The roles of distributive, procedural and interactional justice. *Journal of Applied Psychology, 82*, 434–443.

Smerdon, B. A., Burkham, D. T., & Lee, V. E. (1999). Access to constructivist and didactic teaching: who gets it? Where is it practiced? *Teachers College Record, 101*, 5–34.

Stephenson, J. (1998). The concept of capability and its importance in higher education. In J. Stephenson & M. Yorke (eds.), *Capability and quality in higher education.* London: Kogan Page.

Stephenson, J., & Weil, S. (1992). *Quality in learning: A capability approach to higher education.* London: Kogan Page.

Sternberg, R. J., & Horvath, J. A. (1999). *Tacit knowledge in professional practice.* Mahwah, NJ: Lawrence Erlbaum.

Teevan, K. G., & Gabel, H. (1978). Evaluation of modeling, role playing, and lecture-discussion techniques for college student mental health professionals. *Journal of Counseling Psychology, 25,* 169–171.

Vaill, P. B. (1996). *Learning as a way of being.* San Francisco: Jossey Bass.

Vygotsky, L. S. (1978). *Mind in society: The development of higher psychological processes* (M. Cole, V. John-Steiner, S. Scribner, & E. Souberman, eds. and trans.). Cambridge, MA: Harvard University.

Watkins, C. E. Jr. (1997). Defining psychotherapy supervision and understanding supervisor functioning. In C. E. Watkins Jr. (Ed.), *Handbook of psychotherapy supervision* (pp. 3–10). New York: John Wiley.

Worthen, V., & Mc Neil, B. W. (1996). A phenomenological investigation of 'good' supervision events. *Journal of Counseling Psychology, 43,* 25–34.

Wulf, J., & Nelson, M. L. (2000). Experienced psychologists' reflections or predoctoral internship supervision and its contributions to their development. *Clinical Supervisor, 19*(2), 123–145.

13 A Common Oversight

Supervision of Christian Counsellors

Shannon Hood and Tracey Milson

'Here is a trustworthy saying: Whoever aspires to be an overseer desires a noble task.' So says St Paul, in the first verse of chapter 3 from a letter he wrote to his friend and work-mate Timothy (circa 65AD) taken from the New Testament of the Christian Bible (1 Tim 3:1). Counselling supervision in essence oversees counselling work. In this brief chapter, we outline often overlooked aspects of Christian counselling supervision.

Christian counselling supervision

This chapter is written for the clinical supervisor who finds themselves providing supervision (or over-sight) of a Christian counsellor. The role of supervisor/overseer is an ancient idea that is at the core of the Christian worldview.

The original Greek text quoted above utilises the word 'epi-scopos' which is comprised of two words: 'epi' (over, above) and 'scopos' (sight, perspective). Whilst most English translations of the Bible use the word 'overseer,' it could equally well be translated as 'Super-visor.' It is this word that was translated as bisceop in Old English and bishop in today's vernacular.

The importance of the role of overseer is emphasised by the high standards expected from those who occupy it. According to the Christian Bible (1 Tim 3:2–3) overseers are to be 'above reproach.' Examples of what this means include being 'temperate, self-controlled, respectable, hospitable, able to teach, not given to drunkenness, not violent – but gentle, not quarrelsome and not a lover of money.' This list serves as a reminder to all of us involved in Supervision that who we are is as important as what we do.

This chapter begins with an exploration of what a Christian counsellor is – observing that having this well-defined will be essential for the supervisee. This definitional work will help classify Christian counsellors into four broad types. One of these – the professional Christian counsellor will be explored in more detail as it is supervision of this type of counsellor for which this chapter is most relevant. Specifically, we focus on some of the unique challenges likely to be faced by the professional Christian counsellor particularly in their work with Christian clients, and on how the supervisor can help navigate these challenges. It will include a brief discussion on the closely related topic of pastoral supervision.

Whilst the chapter is written specifically for supervision of Christian counsellors, it is hoped there are elements that can be adapted to support supervisors who are overseeing supervisees of other faiths. It is inevitable the faith journey of the supervisee will emerge as an important topic of supervision.

DOI: 10.4324/9781003490067-16

Table 13.1 Definition of Christian counselling

Collins (1979)	Hood (2018a)
Counselling is a relationship between two or more persons in which a person (the counsellor), seeks to advise, encourage or assist, another person/s (the counselee[s]) to deal more effectively with the issues of life.'	Christian counselling is a relationship between two or more persons in which a Christian (the counsellor), in partnership with the Holy Spirit, seeks to advise, encourage or assist, and/or accompany another person/s (the counselee[s]) to deal more effectively with the journey of life.'

Christian counselling

Many authors have observed the lack of an agreed definition of Christian counselling (McMinn, 2011; McMinn et al., 2010; Sutton et al., 2016). However, if we are to discuss supervision of the Christian counsellor, we must define what a Christian counsellor is so we can 'spot one when we see one.' We begin this process with a definition of counselling provided in 1973 by Collins (2007), which has stood the test of time to the extent that it is still being utilised by leading contemporary authors such as Tan (2011). Alongside Colin's definition we have provided a working definition of Christian counselling. The unique aspects of Christian counselling are highlighted in Table 13.1 These will be expanded individually below because they draw attention to some unique elements of Christian counselling.

A Christian

This definition suggests that Christian counselling can (and should) only be done by someone who is a Christian themselves. It is far beyond the scope of this chapter to endeavour to provide a failsafe measure to evaluate whether another is a Christian, but for our purposes if a supervisee self-identifies as being a Christian that will probably suffice. What we are seeking to challenge is the alternate suggestion that a person of any (or no) faith persuasion can provide Christian counselling with integrity.

In partnership with the Holy Spirit

Every adherent to the Christian faith will acknowledge a special relationship with the Holy Spirit. The vastly different views on how and when this connection happens must be appreciated but is beyond the scope of this chapter. The Bible refers to the Holy Spirit as a 'paraclete' (e.g., variously in John 14–16) – one who is called to come along side. This is variously translated as 'helper' (English Standard Version) or even 'counsellor' (Revised Standard Version). For the Christian counsellor, the function of the Holy Spirit will extend beyond their personal lives and into their professional practice. For each supervisee this will be described differently but words such as 'help,' 'encouragement,' 'inspiration,' 'reve-lation,' 'vision,' 'nudge,' and 'prompting' are often used when discussing the operation of the Holy Spirit. As a Supervisor it can be helpful to ask the Christian counsellor if they feel their work is done in partnership with the Holy Spirit, and if so, how that operates for them. The value in this supervision discussion is not for the supervisor to assess the appropriateness of the supervisee's answer but more for the supervisee to take the time to explore the answer for themself.

To accompany…on the journey of life

Collins' initial definition restricted the activities of the counsellor to 'advise, encourage and assist…in dealing with the problems of life.' The initial definition reflects the common experience of counselling being utilised exclusively to resolve a specific problem or issue and then terminated once this is done. Christian counselling is often quite different. Although the client will typically begin with some kind of presenting issue, the Christian counselling journey can quickly become one of two pilgrims on a shared journey – where assistance morphs into accompaniment.

The supervisor should be attuned to the difference, as many supervisees can struggle with the transition from issue resolution to 'accompaniment' and the associated need to recontract. Recontracting might be formal or informal, but it is important the supervisee and their client agree that the nature of the relationship changes when the counselling relationship moves from 'assistance in dealing with problems' to 'accompanying on the journey of life.' Problem (or solution) focused methods and interventions within a structured counselling plan may need to be set aside for a relationship that is a little more reactive and 'day-to-day.' The conversation can include a lot more celebration of joys as well as dealing with problems. The goal focused supervisee can struggle with this transition and the inexperienced supervisors can struggle to encourage it. Of course, this 'accompaniment' phenomenon occurs elsewhere but in Christian counselling it is far more prevalent.

Types of Christian counselling

Previously published research has identified four types of Christian counselling (Hood, 2018a). Enormous benefit can be found when supervising Christian counsellors by exploring these types to see which (if any) the supervisee identifies with and even whether they find themselves moving between types depending on the context and client/s. The types are discussed below in order of most to least likely to present for supervision. Whilst the discussion will explore elements of supervision unique to each type, it should be noted that all that has been said so far in this chapter is relevant to all types that follow.

Professional Christian counselling

This is the professional counsellor[1] who intentionally incorporates their 'Christian-ness' into their practice. Whilst these professionals encounter all the 'normal' challenges of their colleagues, there are some unique challenges they encounter that are likely to emerge in supervision. Space only permits exploration of five of these that have been identified through the experience of both authors.

A. The use of Spiritual and Religious Interventions (SRIs) within the counselling conversation is perhaps the most uniquely challenging aspect of Christian counselling.

In 2015, the Psychotherapy and Counselling Federation of Australia (PACFA) commissioned a Literature Review into the effectiveness of Spiritual/Religious (S/R) interventions in psychotherapy and counselling. This review concluded 'Overall, the literature provides ample evidence to support the integration of a client's S/R beliefs and practices as part of good counselling and psychotherapy practice' (Kennedy, Macnab, & Ross, 2015, p. 2). Whilst the Literature review provided several examples of S/R Interventions, it did not provide a wider definition nor guidance on their use.

The most common examples of SRIs in a Christian context are Prayer,[2] Reference to Scripture, meditation/mindfulness and Forgiveness (Aten et al., 2011; Hawkins & Clinton, 2015; McMinn, 2011; Ohlschlager, 2013; Thompson, 2018; Vasiliauskas & McMinn, 2013). It is highly likely SRIs will be requested by the Christian client or may be seen to be useful by the Christian counsellor for a specific client situation, and the supervisor should be prepared for a conversation about the ethical use of SRIs by the professional Christian counsellor including informed consent. Rather than explore each of these examples in detail, it is helpful to have a framework for approaching the use of any intervention which can then be applied to SRIs broadly and any one of the examples specifically. The Hexethogram is one such framework that has been developed for this purpose and used extensively by these authors.

The application of an SRI to a specific client in their unique context will of course be made on a case-by-case basis. However, there are six broad principles that can be helpful in guiding both counsellor (and by extension their Supervisor) in determining suitability of use. These are described as the Hexethogram. Like an effective playground fence, the boundaries represented by the six sides of the Hexethogram give permission for exploration and discovery within the confines of a fence that is clearly designed to keep everyone safe.

i. The context of the counselling situation is a critical consideration for the suitability of using SRIs. In a recent survey of counsellors, 23 per cent of those who were directly employed and 25 per cent of those who worked as sub-contractors for an agency felt they did not have permission to include spirituality in their work (Hood, 2018b).

Counsellors who work as employees are subject not only to their professional code of ethics but also to that employer's policies and procedures. Occasionally these place explicit expectations and/or limitations on the counsellor's practice and at times these expectations or limitations may be undocumented.

In some ways Christian counsellors who work as sub-contractors for agencies can face the greatest ambiguity. Generally speaking, it would be unwise and inappropriate for any professional counsellor to be utilising SRIs when working for an independent agency contracted (say) to a commercial enterprise or a Government Department – even where the client might hold to a Christian worldview. But what about (for example) the context in which a Christian counsellor responds to a tragedy at a Christian School as a contractor employed by Catholic Care or The Salvation Army? Answers to questions like this are often not easy to come by, which is why they are often (and appropriately) raised in supervision. Simply asking the supervisee to consider the full breadth of the counselling context (policies, procedures, inclusion and diversity statements, reasonable expectations of clientele, physical location, advertising/marketing content) can often prove invaluable in helping evaluate the contextual suitability of SRIs.

ii. Informed consent from the client is essential before considering any intervention (Martindale et al., 2009; Sullivan et al., 1993). Provided below is a three-fold strategy that supervisees may be encouraged to consider:

1. For the sake of transparency, practice information forms might openly declare one's own religious affiliation whilst being clear that no client will be discriminated against

based on gender, race, sexuality or religious worldview. This information should be provided to every client and may often be included with other introductory documentation such as the fee structure, confidentiality agreements and the like, and in their practice marketing and advertising.

2. It is typical for client information (intake) forms to ask a series of questions (marital status, current medication, next of kin, etc.). Therefore, inclusion of questions such as 'Do you wish your spirituality to be included in counselling?' or when they add their religious affiliation 'Would you like spiritual interventions used in sessions?' can be quite natural. Any client who answers 'No' would not be questioned further and would be deemed unsuitable for S/R Interventions. If a client answers 'Yes' the counsellor might enquire about the client's spiritual background and ask what they imagine it might look like if spirituality or S/R Interventions were included in their counselling experience. This client-centric approach then guides the process.

3. If the outcome of the discussion above is that they would like Christian 'Spiritual Practices' such as prayer, meditation, reference to the Bible, etc. included in their counselling experience then asking the client to sign a separate consent form to this effect can be useful.

iii. The client worldview must be respected (Christian Counsellors Association of Australia, 2020) and affirmed (Australian Counselling Association, 2012). A client's spirituality and religion are a key component of their worldview. The Counsellor must be careful not to impose their own worldview upon the client but only offer interventions that they know are supportive of the client's worldview.

iv. Evidence informed principles of practice should be applied. PACFA intentionally encourages evidence informed (as opposed to evidence based) practice (Psychotherapy and Counselling Federation of Australia (PACFA, 2019). The subtle but important challenges of an evidence based (comparted to evidence informed) approach is noted by (Kumah et al., 2019). Epstein (2009) observes that an evidence informed approach enables practice that is 'enriched by prior research but not limited to it.' With respect to using SRIs the counsellor (and by extension the supervisor) must be aware of the evidence relating to the efficacy and risks associated with any potential intervention and allow this evidence to inform decisions of suitability. Generally speaking, the evidence supporting the efficacy of introducing spirituality into the counselling conversation is strong and growing stronger (Captari et al., 2018; Gubi, 2011), however, this does not permit complacency when discerning the suitability of a specific intervention to a particular client situation.

v. Counsellor competence and integrity is a key issue to consider when determining suitability of using SRIs. The demand for counsellors to operate within their training and competence is normative and deeply engrained in most codes of practice and conduct. Yet challenges to counsellor integrity are often not so well considered. There is insufficient space to do justice to the importance of counsellors operating with integrity to themselves but suffice to say there is nothing in the ethical codes to suggest that concepts of integrity, dignity, and respect for worldview in the counselling relationship apply only to the client. With regard to SRIs this means (for example) a Muslim counsellor should not feel obliged to pray to a Christian God, a Jewish counsellor should not feel obliged to treat the New Testament scriptures as sacred and a Christian counsellor should not feel obliged to lead a Buddhist client in Eastern meditation. Within the Christian counselling context, these challenges of integrity even occur within different denominational expressions of their shared Christian faith between client and counsellor. If a client requests interventions that are beyond the integrity of the counsellor and this cannot be resolved, then referral is an option that should be considered.

vi. Client best interest completes the 'fence-line' of the Hexethogram. Even if all of the five prior conditions are met, the ethical concept of beneficence (Psychotherapy and Counselling Federation of Australia, 2017) demands that an intervention only be applied if it is in the Counsellor's best professional judgement that no other intervention is likely to be better for the client. Just because an intervention can be done does not mean it should be. Overwhelmingly the preferred way of navigating this ethical boundary is by emphasising that consent must be informed. Where there are a number of interventions that may support the client, it is generally best practice to explain these to the client including the risks and possible benefits and allowing the client to decide which they would prefer.

B. The purpose of the counselling journey is slightly nuanced for most people seeking Christian counselling and must be appreciated by both Counsellor and supervisor. In Christian counselling the principles of client centeredness are upheld including the Rogerian assumption that clients have 'vast potential for understanding themselves and resolving their own problems without direct intervention' (Corey, 2016, p. 165). However, these assumptions are held in tension with the equal assumption that 'True Christians are people who acknowledge and live under the Word of God. They submit without reserve to the Word of God' (Packer, 1993, p. 116)

This idea of living 'under the word of God' (i.e., in accordance with the teachings of the Bible) may represent the most difficult aspect of Christian counselling for the atheist supervisor to work with.[3] Paradoxically, the upervisor who comes from an alternate faith background (e.g., Islamic, Jewish, Buddhist) will often be comfortable with the idea of submitting one's life to an external set of religious teachings – they may not agree with the choice, but they can resonate with the idea. However, this idea that an external set of teaching provides the primary source for practical solutions to life's challenges can be seen to be far removed from the Rogerian idea that clients should seek answers to their questions from within themselves.

Many clients come to counselling in order to minimise the discomfort they are experiencing in life and maximise life's happiness. Whilst these objectives are not unimportant for the Christian client, the client's greater purpose is often to live in accordance with the teaching of the Bible even if this brings with it discomfort and unhappiness. The Christian counsellor will often find themselves coming to supervision to discuss ways of supporting clients in their desire to endure (not avoid) suffering and persist in discomfort in order to uphold their Christian worldview.

C. Dual relationships are a common issue that need to be managed for the Christian counsellor. Dual relationships are almost inevitable when one is part of a small community. Examples of small communities include a country town, a community of a similar culture or language within a large city, or the active Christian community in any city. When one further divides these 'active' Christians into sub-groups according to denomination or geography, multiple relationships tend to become an inevitability that must be managed rather than something that can be completely avoided. Where a supervisee is challenged by a situation of the possibility of a dual relationship forming the following may be some helpful strategies:

- Referral to another Christian counsellor – alternative delivery modes such as face to screen/online may need to be considered.
- Agreement to put 'on-hold' the 'other' relationship for an appropriate time frame to accommodate the counselling season. This may mean the client or counsellor chooses to temporarily (for example) no longer be part of the choir or they choose to attend Church services at different times.
- Have the counsellor explain that if they inadvertently 'bump-into' the client (e.g., at the coffee queue) the counsellor will make no reference to the counselling connection, and recommend the client refrains from doing so or engage in lengthy, social conversations.
- Encourage regular check-ins within the counselling journey to specifically discuss the management of any dual relationship.

D. Self-Disclosure is often more prevalent in Christian counselling. Many Christian counsellors will indicate that they find themselves engaging in noticeably more self-disclosure when supporting Christian clients who have requested Christian counselling. This is perhaps not surprising when one enters the paradigm of being on a shared journey of Christian living with a fellow pilgrim. In Christian parlance the notion of Discipleship is often referred to – where the counsellor and the counselee share a common journey of the Christian life with its struggles and joys. The Supervisor should not necessarily be concerned if they sense a level of self-disclosure that might otherwise be surprising in other settings.

Professional counselling by a Christian

The second type of Christian counselling is professional counselling by a Christian (Hood, 2018a). According to a recent Australian Census, 52 per cent of Australians self-identify as having a Christian Religious Affiliation of some form (Australian Bureau of Statistics, 2017). Thus, every supervision session conducted in Australia has a better than even chance of a Christian overlay. It is inevitable that this Christian worldview will shape the counsellor's understanding of good and evil, will influence the lens through which they view their clients, will be part of how they make sense of personal and relationship broken-ness and will underpin their deepest understanding of the meaning and purpose in life. It is equally true and inevitable that the counsellor's own gender identification, marital status, sexuality, and racial association (to name a few) will shape the counsellor's worldview. However, the experienced, person-centred counsellor will often develop strategies to conceal their worldview from the client experience. This will often mean suppressing their own views particularly when supporting a client whose views, gender, sexuality, values, marital status, etc. are different to their own. Some mental health professionals (MHPs) have become so well-schooled in this approach that they find it hard to conceive of any alternative.

For the sake of definition, we label this type of Christian counselling as professional counselling by a Christian (Hood, 2018a). Usually, this situation occurs by the counsellor's choice. In these instances, challenges such using SR Interventions and self-disclosure discussed earlier rarely come to the surface for the counsellor and therefore rarely present in supervision. Ironically, whilst the professional Christian counsellor (discussed earlier) is often bringing the question 'How can I ethically express my faith?' to supervision, this new type of Christian counsellor is often asking 'How do I professionally suppress my faith?'

This can be especially challenging where the client has specifically indicated they do not want their spirituality included in their counselling conversation or the counselling context prohibits it, yet the counsellor has a preference to allow their faith to be expressed.

Pastoral counselling

The authors have great regard for the highly effective Christian counselling conducted by religious leaders (pastoral counselling) who provide support for members of their religious community.

It is pleasing that an increasing number of religious leaders (including ordained clergy) are seeking supervision for their pastoral work.[4] Whilst there may be many points of overlap between the practice of clinical supervision of a mental health professional and pastoral supervision (supervision of a religious leader or religious worker), one must be careful not to simply 'cut-and-paste' from one domain to the other.

Barletta provides a helpful definition of clinical supervision as 'a process whereby colleagues of a similar profession…' (Barletta, 2017, p. 6). The Clinical Supervisor who is considering taking on a supervisee who is a religious leader should consider whether they are truly 'of a similar profession,' particularly if they do not share the supervisee's religious beliefs. Having provided pastoral supervision to a number of religious leaders, the authors share a few insights below. The four areas of supervision (Armstrong, 2020, pp. 27–29) still broadly apply but need to be adapted to the supervisee's pastoral context:

1. ***Identifying any mental or emotional issues.*** It has been the experience of these authors that the presence of mental and emotional issues is often more likely in pastoral supervision than clinical supervision of an MHP, due to the pastoral commitment to their people.
2. ***Challenging use of theories, modalities, and ethics.*** Religious leaders and workers tend to face 'situations' rather than 'clients.' Whilst client-specific conversations can tend to occupy the many MHP supervision sessions, it is not uncommon for this to be replaced by discussions of 'situations.' Having said this, asking the pastoral supervisee to identify and refer to codes of ethics (how decisions should be made) and codes of conduct (acceptable behaviours) or their equivalent can lead to equally powerful insight in supervision. Sometimes these codes are explicit and documented but sometimes the supervisee will gain great insight by seeking and exploring 'undocumented codes.' The supervisor from a mental health background must be open to the idea that these codes of conduct in a religious context may not always align with those that they are familiar with. Situations faced by religious leaders can include conflict between two key influential families, moral failure of a key leader, managing the expectations of a needy family who are abusing the congregation's generosity, and challenges to doctrinal teaching. These examples also demonstrate how far-removed pastoral work and mental health work can be that the supervisor must be prepared for.
3. ***Professional development.*** This can often be a fruitful discussion particularly where the supervisee can be supported in their use of systems and processes that exist within the denominational or institutional framework.
4. ***Career development*** may take on a very different perspective where the church is concerned. Where an individual has taken a vow to pursue a 'vocation' and there is only

one 'employer,' navigating one's career is truly unique. This varies dramatically across different denominational settings even within the Christian community.

The above discussion is provided to give a few ideas when supervising a religious leader (even in their Christian counselling work) as well as caution the clinical supervisor considering offering supervision as to whether they are truly 'of a similar profession' and appropriately equipped. It emphasises the much-needed expansion of clinical supervision training for religious leaders by religious leaders that will encompass their Christian counselling work amongst many other aspects of their pastoral and Church worker functions. Many churches have embraced, and more will likely embrace in the future, professional Christian supervision as part of their staff requirements.

Lay Christian counselling

The authors have high regard for the final type of Christian counsellor – the lay person who comes alongside a brother or sister in the faith to advise, encourage, assist or accompany them on the journey of life. If only more of this were done more effectively, perhaps there would be less need for professional help. Whilst this group is affirmed and acknowledged, they are unlikely to present for supervision and are therefore beyond the scope of this chapter.

Professional Christian supervised supervision

So far we have limited our discussion to supervision of Christian counsellors. However, we must also consider supervised supervision. Supervised supervision appears to work best when an effective alliance with an experienced and qualified Christian supervisor of supervisors enables a deeper reflective space and increased learning, resulting in best practice for professional Christian supervisors. It may involve scrutiny and curiosity of clinical supervision practice, ethically and relationally, creating checks and safeguards for the practitioners and their Christian clients. Professional and pastoral Christian supervised supervision may be described as an exponential step up from supervision and it is recommended that professional Christian supervising supervisors be required to demonstrate greater expertise, experience, credentials, training, responsibility, and knowledge of SRIs. In Australia supervised supervision is a counselling association requirement.

Conclusion

The supervision of Christian counsellors will be different depending on the type of Christian counsellor the supervisee identifies as. Exploring the four types of professional Christian counselling provided in this chapter is recommended as beneficial for the supervisee. As noted, the professional Christian counsellor will likely face some unique challenges. When brought to supervision the supervisor needs to be ready and equipped to deal with them knowledgeably, ethically, compassionately, and non-judgmentally. Generally speaking, competent supervisors will be able to provide adequate supervision for the professional counsellor who happens to have a Christian faith. However, supervisors are advised to think carefully about their own suitability for supervising professional Christian counsellors and pastoral Counsellors as colleagues in a similar profession. The need for

Professional Christian supervision and pastoral supervision is expanding and can no longer be a common oversight.

Educational questions & activities

1. As a Christian supervisor how might you gain informed consent to incorporate Spiritual and Religious Interventions (SRIs) in supervision sessions?
2. What might be some contextual situations where the use of SRIs may be considered appropriate in counselling as discussed in supervision?
3. Considering faith-based supervision practices, such as ministry supervision, how might this differ from supervising counsellors?

Acknowledgment

This research was supported by an Australian Government Research Training Program (RTP) Scholarship.

Notes

1 For the sake of this chapter, professional counsellor is an umbrella term that encompasses any mental health professional that utilises counselling. Primary examples include registered counsellors, psychologists, and social workers.
2 The suitable use of prayer in counselling is a topic unto itself and cannot be covered in this chapter. The supervisee should be encouraged to bring to supervision what 'using prayer' might actually look like, as its application can be as range from the counsellor praying before each session begins through to the use of prayer ministry (or prayer counselling) in session, which is specifically prohibited in some codes of conduct (Christian Counsellors Association of Australia, 2017), and countless options in between.
3 A practical, relevant, and often emotive example of this surrounds conversion therapy, which in many places is now illegal. There can be no doubt that people have been harmed by well-intentioned religious groups, and harm must be prevented. This chapter has already outlined the importance of operating within a client's worldview at the subordination of the worldview of the counsellor. However, the Christian counsellor will inevitably encounter various individuals that wish to suppress all types of sexual attraction in order to live a life in accordance with how they interpret the Bible. Just as the counselling relationship must be a safe place for the client to discuss these matters, so the supervision relationship must be a safe and non-judgmental place for Christian counsellors to bring these complex ethical challenges confident they will not be met with simplistic solutions from their supervisor. Similarly, this applies to not converting a client to a faith or religion of the counsellor's preference against their wishes. This dilemma may, however, be discussed openly in supervision to consider informed consent and ethical best practice.
4 This phenomenon is likely this is being driven, at least in part, by recommendation 16.45 emerging from Australia's recent Royal Commission into Institutional Responses to Child Sexual Abuse: "that all people in religious or pastoral ministry, including religious leaders, have professional supervision" (Royal Commission into Institutional Responses to Child Sexual Abuse, 2017).

References

Armstrong, P. (2020). *RISE UP Certificate of Attainment in Group and Individual Supervision Manual* (3rd ed.). Alyciana Pty Ltd.

Aten, J.D., McMinn, M.R., & Worthington, E.L.J. (Eds.). (2011). *Spiritually Oriented Interventions for Counseling and Psychotherapy*. American Psychological Association.

Australian Bureau of Statistics (2017). *Religion in Australia*. www.abs.gov.au/ausstats/abs@.nsf/ Lookup/ by Subject/2071.0~2016~Main Features~Religion Data Summary~70

Australian Counselling Association (2012). *Code of Ethics and Practice* (Issue July). www.theaca.net. au/documents/ACA Code of Ethics and Practice Ver 13.pdf

Barletta, J. (2017). Introduction to Clinical Supervision. In N. Pelling, & P. Armstrong (Eds.), *The practice of counselling and clinical supervision* (p. 446). Samford Valley, QLD: Australian Academic Press

Captari, L.E., Hook, J.N., Hoyt, W., Davis, D.E., McElroy-Heltzel, S.E., & Worthington, E.L. (2018). Integrating clients' religion and spirituality within psychotherapy: A comprehensive meta-analysis. *Journal of Clinical Psychology*, 74(11), 1938–1951.

Christian Counsellors Association of Australia (2020). *Code of Ethics*. https://ccaa.net.au/wp-content/uploads/2018/09/CCAA-CODE-OF-ETHICS-Nov-2020-1.pdf

Collins, G.R. (2007). *Christian Counseling: A Comprehensive Guide*. Thomas Nelson Publishers.

Corey, G. (2016). *Theory and Practice of Counseling and Psychotherapy* (10th ed.). Brooks/Cole Publishing Company.

Epstein, I. (2009). Promoting harmony where there is commonly conflict: Evidence-informed practice as an integrative strategy. *Social Work in Health Care*, 48(3), 216–231.

Gubi, P.M. (2011). In W. West (Ed.), *Exploring Therapy, Spirituality and Healing* (pp. 63–76). Macmillan.

Hawkins, R.E., & Clinton, T.E. (2015). *The New Christian Counselor*. Harvest House.

Hood, S.R. (2018a). Better by definition. *Accord*, 1(Summer), 6–13.

Hood, S.R. (2018b). Practice makes perfect. *Counselling Connections Across Australia*, July, 1–10.

Kennedy, G.A., Macnab, F.A., & Ross, J.J. (2015). *The Effectiveness of Spiritual/Religious Interventions in Psychotherapy and Counselling: A Review of the Recent Literature*. Melbourne: PACFA.

Kumah, E.A., McSherry, R., Bettany-Saltikov, J., Hamilton, S., Hogg, J., Whittaker, V., & van Schaik, P. (2019). Evidence-informed practice versus evidence-based practice educational interventions for improving knowledge, attitudes, understanding, and behavior toward the application of evidence into practice: A comprehensive systematic review of undergraduate student. *Campbell Systematic Reviews*, 15(1–2). https://doi.org/10.1002/ cl2.1015

Martindale, S.J., Chambers, E., & Thompson, A.R. (2009). Clinical psychology service users' experiences of confidentiality and informed consent: A qualitative analysis. *Psychology and Psychotherapy: Theory, Research and Practice*, 82(4), 355–368.

McMinn, M.R. (2011). *Psychology, Theology, and Spirituality in Christian Counseling*. Tyndale House.

McMinn, M.R., Staley, R.C., Webb, K.C., & Seegobin, W. (2010). Just what is Christian counseling anyway? Professional Psychology: *Research and Practice*, 41(5), 391–397.

Ohlschlager, G.W. (2013). Praying the Scriptures within Congnitive/Behavioural/Systems Therapy. In D. W. Appleby, & G. W. Ohlschlager (Eds.), *Transformative Encounters: The Intervention of God in Christian Counseling and Pastoral Care* (p. 388). Downers Grove: InterVarsity.

Packer, J.I. (1993). *Knowing God*. InterVarsity Press.

Psychotherapy and Counselling Federation of Australia (2017). *Code of Ethics*. www.pacfa.org.au/ wp-content/ uploads/2017/11/PACFA-Code-of-Ethics-2017.pdf

Psychotherapy and Counselling Federation of Australia (PACFA) (2019). *Evidence-Informed Practice Statement*. 2. https://doi. org/10.1037//0033-2909.122.3.203.Wampold

Royal Commission into Institutional Responses to Child Sexual Abuse (2017). *Royal Commission into Institutional Responses to Child Sexual Abuse: Final Report Recommendations.*

Sullivan, T., Martin, W.L., & Handelsman, M.M. (1993). Practical benefits of an informed-consent procedure: An empirical investigation. *Professional Psychology: Research and Practice*, 24(2), 160–163.

Sutton, G.W., Arnzen, C., & Kelly, H.L. (2016). Christian counseling and psychotherapy: Components of clinician spirituality that predict type of Christian intervention. *Journal of Psychology and Christianity*, 35(3), 204–214.

Tan, S. (2011). *Counseling and Psychotherapy: A Christian Perspective*. Baker Academic.

Thompson, K. (2018). *Christ Centred Mindfulness*. Acorn Press.

Vasiliauskas, S.L., & McMinn, M.R. (2013). The effects of a prayer intervention on the process of forgiveness. *Psychology of Religion and Spirituality*, 5(1), 23–32.

14 Supervision of Social Work in Australia

The Appropriateness of Including Administration

Rebecca Braid

Supervision of social workers

The Supervision Standards of the Australian Association of Social Workers (AASW) reference authors Davys and Beddoe to define supervision for the profession of social work as:

> Supervision is a forum for reflection and learning...an interactive dialogue between at least two people, one of whom is a supervisor. This dialogue shapes a process of review, reflection, critique and replenishment for professional practitioners. Supervision is a professional activity in which practitioners are engaged throughout the duration of their careers regardless of experience or qualification. The participants are accountable to professional standards and defined competencies and to organisational policy and procedures.
>
> (Australian Association of Social Workers, 2014, p. 2)

The supervision of social workers is becoming increasingly demanding as more and more social workers engage as private practitioners, This is often in conjunction with an employed position as a social worker establishes their private practice, or to bolster an irregular income from private practice. In light of this many social workers are maintaining the standards of private practice and the disconnection a part-time position can engender. As a result, supervision can encompass the responsibilities of private practice, and the isolation this creates.

Components of social work supervision

The three broad components of social work supervision are outlined in the 2014 Standards with reference to Kadushin, these components are Educational, Supportive and Administrative Standards (Australian Association of Social Workers, 2104, pp. 3–4). In these challenging economic and overly administrative times, many social workers are seeing supervision provided internally within their organisations as being overly work-based assessment rather than support or administrative advice. It is certainly not educational in terms of professional development but rather educationally based on the issues of the organisation and its politics. One of the most common anecdotal questions raised in the Supervision Training Courses run at Eden Therapy Services speaks to this issue. These training courses are run under licence issued by Dr Philip Armstrong's private business, Optimise Potential. The question concerns the subordination of supervision to the accountability needs of the place of employment. This issue becomes a dilemma when

DOI: 10.4324/9781003490067-17

accountability becomes the dominant force, rather than one of the three broad functions of supervision being practised. In the workplace this means that social workers are being asked to 'manage' the more junior social workers according to the goals of the organisation at the expense of time being spent on professional supervision. This work would appear to be at odds with the idea of reflection as the information discussed in the supervision could also be used to challenge the social workers standing in the organisation in terms of promotion or accountability.

The following definition includes the idea of the administrative process, the supportive function and the educative function. It's not just about accountability:

> The administrative function describes the practitioners and supervisor's accountability to the policies, protocols, ethics and standards which are prescribed by organisation, legislation and regulatory bodies. The educative function addresses the ongoing professional skill development and resourcing of the practitioner. The supportive function attends to the more personal relationship between the practitioner and the work context
>
> (Davys and Beddoe, 2010, p. 25)

While the AASW Supervision Standards reflect the functions of supervision to be three broad components of social work, it would appear that in the experience of private practice those components need expanding. In private practice the common question from social workers in supervision is rather based on the complex assessment of contracts and the contracts legal implications for their practice. Put another way, what appears to be emerging in private practice is the common question from social workers in supervision about the complex assessment of contracts. Each area that the private practitioner engages in requires a different contractual obligation. For example, the registration with Medicare as a provider, the different government departments such as Veterans Affairs, the Australian Defence Force, Victims Services or the National Disability Insurance Scheme to name a few. Each of these different departments requires different contractual commitments from social workers and different reporting requirements. Increasingly these contracts should be checked by the individual social worker's lawyer for the personal responsibilities the social worker will have to each of these organisations. The individual contracts from each government department may also not reflect the core values of social work.

The management of dual relationships by social workers has long been a touch stone for the profession as a point of difference to other counselling professions such as psychology. Social workers actively engage with managed dual relationships for the best outcome for clients such as inviting a volunteer who has survived and managed domestic violence in the group work intervention of current domestic violence survivors. Some organisational contracts may not allow for the use of dual relationships or even support the idea of volunteer inclusion in interventions and see it as a violation of client confidentiality. Indeed, some contractual agreements may go so far as to see the use of dual relationships as grounds for an internal complaint which the accrediting body of the AASW may have no issue with as dual relationships are often seen as an effective way forward for some clients and augments change for the client who moves on to become a volunteer. The AASW states in its Code of Ethics 2020 that dual relationships 'are not to be exploited to gain personal, material or financial advantage' and that where the dual relationship exists with former clients that the social worker will 'set and enforce explicit, appropriate professional boundaries to minimise the risk of conflict of interest, exploitation or harm' (Australian Association of Social Workers, 2020, pp. 13 & 21).

Changes to social work standards for supervision

It is interesting to note that the social work standards for supervision have changed from Kadushin's original three components of supervision from Educational, Supportive, and Administrative to 5.1 Education, 5.2 Support, and 5.3 Accountability (Australian Association of Social Workers, 2014, pp. 3–4). The reality of administrative tasks in the arena of supervision is vastly different to accountability of social workers. The administrative component of supervision that Kadushin outlines would appear to be important to social workers and should not be transposed into accountability which is a given in the professional conduct of a social worker. Rather, Pelling and Armstrong's definition of supervision is helpful when looking at supervision for the private practitioner and employed social worker. Two types of supervision, the clinical and the administrative are recommended for the private practitioner and employed social worker. Two types of supervisions are recommended, the clinical and the administrative:

> Whereas the focus of clinical supervision is concerned with counselling and aims to be educational the focus of administrative supervision is involved with organisational, managerial and procedural issues. Administrative supervision includes the managing of areas such as service evaluation, financial issue, time considerations, record keeping, role and function, professional development, policy and procedures, resource allocation, information technology and organisational issues
>
> (Barletta, 2017, p. 17)

The area of dilemma for most social workers who are arriving to train in supervision at Eden Therapy Services appears to be in the administration of organisation. Social workers are accountable to their code of ethics and also administratively responsible to the organisation that employs them whether contractually or on a permanent part-time basis. This arena of administrative supervision is an area filled with contractual challenges and uncertainty for the social worker who wishes to also have a private practice. Belonging to their professional association is important. Whilst the 2017 edition of *The Practice of Counselling and Clinical Supervision*, edited by Pelling and Armstrong, omitted to include the 11,000 member AASW in the list of 31 international counselling and psychology organisations presented, Pelling does reference social workers as needing to belong to professional organisations alongside counsellors, therapists, and psychologists (Pelling, 2017, pp. 72–76). It is possible that while other counselling associations are embracing the idea of the administration of practice and the supervision of this administration standard, the AASW is at a point of difference as it has subsumed administration issues into accountability standards.

However, the inclusion of both the clinical and administrative component of supervision would seem timely for today's practising social worker and private practitioner. This acknowledges the need for the social worker to have clinical input to encourage the idea of reflective practitioner widely accepted in the United States as the basis for supervision. It also allowed for the social worker to have administrative input to enable the consideration of 'a new phase of change' in supervision (Davys and Beddoe, 2010, p. 13).

> Two major factors have influenced this change. The first factor is the neoliberal preoccupation with systems of accountability...the second factor is the impact of the 'the risk society' and the concomitant public critique of professional practice. These features

come together in a social trend described as a 'crisis of trust' in professionals...Fear of failure, concern for public safety and a deep fear of public criticism...on the part of government has led to more emphasis on compliance in oversight of professional practice and mandatory and continuous professional development

(Davys and Beddoe, 2019, pp. 13–14)

While mistrust of the professional is certainly culturally relevant to the dominant western discourse, the rise of supervision support for the culturally disadvantaged has also emerged. Hair and O'Donoghue argued for the consideration of the less dominant cultural discourse of the Aotearoa indigenous Maori population could be incorporated into the New Zealand social workers interventions (Davys and Beddoe, 2010, p. 18). Rather Beddoe and Egan stated that the 'supervision process that is grounded in spatial, tradition, and coherent theoretical understandings congruent with a unique worldview' would serve the social worker and their intervention so that 'culture becomes the overarching environment of supervision (Beddoe and Egan, 2010, p. 18). Indeed, in supervising social workers for many years there is a curiosity about religion, spirituality, and faith as assets to client interventions. However, social work has been comfortable with the inclusion of spirituality in our practice particularly when driven by the client centred process. 'Counsellors tend to include a wide range of variables in the assessment process yet are reluctant to ask about a client's religious or spiritual background lest they appear to be imposing their values on the client' (Corey et al., 2010, p. 140). Certainly, the practice-based research done at Eden Therapy Services called for the client's voice on spirituality and its inclusion in social work interventions. The qualitative study revealed that clients did want spirituality, and their spiritual view included in their interventions and social work practice should accommodate this and the view of their minister, pastor, priest, or spiritual director (Braid, 2008, p. 260).

Case example: The changing face of supervision

What does the changing face of supervision mean for the practising social worker in the complex world of contracts, private practice and business administration? What does the emerging view of supervision for both the supervisor and supervisee mean in present practice? A case example has been chosen with a lens of the interaction of supervisor and supervisee. The case example is of a high-risk client who when interviewed initially was clearly eligible for inclusion in the Royal Commission to give evidence on Institutional Sexual Abuse of Children. The following clinical example of just such a case and its interwoven supervisor and supervisee perspectives will highlight the real time issues for a practising social worker, and the role that supervision can play in both clinical revelation and administration of the contracts involved in service provision for this particular client. The following de-identified example is presented with the permission of the client, supervisee, and advocate involved (see Figure 14.1).

The client entered the practice via a Mental Health Referral (MHCP) from her local General Medical Practitioner (GP) after her friend had told her about the help she received from a particular social worker. Like many complex trauma survivors, she had multiple medical needs and multiple medication needs. Her GP was perplexed by her medical presentation and was looking for another view of her patient. The client had always thought that the domestic violence she experienced in her first marriage was her fault and had not linked the institutionalised abuse history to her lack of life skills and parenting ability. This is typical presentation of long-term abuse survivors. The client received no support to

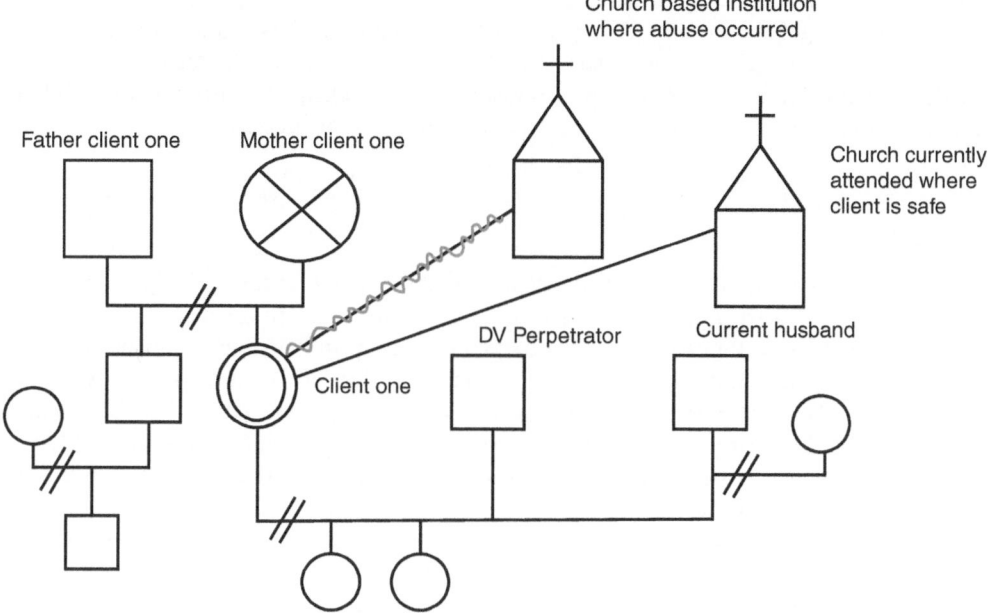

Church based institution
where abuse occurred

Father client one

Mother client one

Church currently
attended where
client is safe

DV Perpetrator

Current husband

Client one

Figure 14.1 Client genogram at time of referral to Eden Therapy Services

return to the care of her biological parent when her time for discharge from the church-based institution came. After another placement she received no support once again when she was returned with her brother to the care of family. She quickly moved toward a relationship in which she married and had two daughters of her own. Typical of most abuse survivors the violence she experienced in her youth followed her into her own choice of relationship patterned on her abuse experiences. The domestic violence she watched her mother go through and the domestic violence she was experiencing in her own marriage decided her on leaving the marriage when her youngest daughter turned one. She went into a refuge, struggled, and as with many domestic violence survivors rented various accommodation, continued to struggle, continued to blame herself and remained isolated. She received some assistance from friends and various church and non-church-based Charites and continued to struggle to raise her daughters. She was drawn out into the community again by her local church where she became more personally buoyant and eventually met a safe man whom she married and who has supported and loved her all the way to the Royal Commission. She states that her faith has been one of the strongest supports for herself and her children. At this point after being in a safe and supportive relationship, her GP referred her to Eden Therapy Services (ETS).

From an initial interview she was quickly assessed as an institutionalised child sexual abuse survivor. At the time of the referral, she was unaware of the Royal Commission and had no idea that she was eligible to utilise the Royal Commission in any redress issues she may wish to pursue. On initial interview she was fragile and tearful and wondering if she could trust ETS as a service provider. What stood out for the social work intervention was the question about the client's fragility and whether this would deny her eligibility to present at the Commission. At the time of initial referral, the Royal Commission had already begun its hearings, and it was unclear whether the client would be able to address the commission at this late stage of its hearings. The client was also eligible for the Victims Services Counselling Scheme and Recognition Scheme and as this would provide more counselling hours free to the client that the MHCP. This was explained to the client and, with assistance, she applied and was registered as a victim of crime with the NSW Department of Justice Victims Support Service. This was a huge step for the client and one that benefited her further into her own personal robustness.

Supervision issue 1

The supervisee took to supervision of the issue that the client was certainly eligible under the Royal Commission to present evidence but was in no state emotionally or physically to present information on a range of perpetrators who may still be living and working in health areas and present a danger to others. Supervisee needed to discuss how well the client fitted with the parameters of the Commission investigation. The supervisee heard that the client's self-determination in regard to applying for Victims Services enabled a view that the client was robust and increasingly becoming aware that services existed to recognise and assist her journey.

Conclusion of supervision was to continue to build trust and see how the client progressed as intervention was in its early stages and to hold the other issues in tension. The clinical discussion had been helpful to contain the supervisee's need to see justice served through the lens of appearing at the Royal Commission and to identify the supervisee's own desires in regard to having the client heard when the client may not benefit from this. This idea was also held in tension. The administrative issues raised by the supervision included the idea that the commission could be approached with the client in session so that the client would be supported, and the supervisee could assess the robustness of the client when speaking to the commission's information line. Here we can see the use of clinical reflection and the administration relating to the supervisees need to become conversant with the terms of reference of the Commission and how this initial approach to the Commission could affect the client's robustness and resilience. Without supervision at this point the need to hold this supervisee's initial enthusiasm about a client being able to contribute to a national discussion may have overwhelmed the need for the client to be safe and held in a self-determined view of her immediate success of being recognised by the funding she received as a victim of crime for her counselling. Supervision at this point can be clinically revelatory as it assists the supervisee to explore the desire to see the possibility of their own needs for a victory in the story of the client. The supervision also refocuses onto the role of the administration of the current services available to the client and whether they are in the best interests of the client at that time.

Case update. Once trust was gained, she began to detail her previous marriage being filled by emotional and physical abuse and the emotional drain that multiple court cases had placed on her and the children. However as with other childhood trauma survivors, her life was pursued by issues of violence ever since the first violation of her as a child. After nearly a year of counselling she began to detail the institutional care she was placed in and only then began to tentatively detail the sexual abuse she suffered by the staff of the church-based facility. The men managing the institution she was placed in systematically abused her over a period of time. She also recounted amazing stories of finding meaning for herself in the respite she would receive from the abusers when she went to church as part of the programme at the institution. She was safe and not harmed in this building and she chose to focus on whatever safety she would seek out or was in her control to enjoy and accept.

Supervision issue 2

The supervisee raised the unusual resilience of this client as she began to prosper under empowerment and feminist models of practice and intervention. Supervision concentrated on a clinical smorgasbord that had been used to empower the client as seen in the research of Pelling in her 2005 and 2006 study of the characteristics and activities of Australian counsellors (Lack and Pelling, 2009, p. 212; Kadushin & Harkness, 2014). The initial empowerment and safety of the counselling, with focused psychological strategies were augmented by the feminist informed theory challenging the false memory debate. (Braid, 1996, pp. 51–54). The further work was informed by advocacy models of practice in group work referencing 'Managing Complex Trauma Through Art' by Cohen, Barnes, and Rankin (1995, p. XV). As indicated by Pelling, the Australian counsellor is offering a broad range of clinical interventions presented by various counsellors which are eclectic in nature (Lack & Pelling, 2009, p. 218). This supervision increasingly became important for discussing clinical interventions to support the improvements seen in the client.

The supervisee was also concerned about the client managing the idea of institutions, the one where she had been abused and the other, the local church where she found social meaning and support. This raised issues of power and politics in light of the Royal Commission and the responses by institutions such as the church to the accusations of covering up abuses and not taking responsibility for the abuses that happened while children were in their care. The management of these issues of power involved supervision being able to allow room for the larger societal view in relation to the effect of the Royal Commission on clients and their healing. This larger societal view is well documented by Josie McSkimming (McSkimming, 2017, p. 127).

Conclusion of supervision was to remain curious and see the unique strengths of this client as the supervisee's desire to see justice in her view as the presentation to the Commission needed to be held in check while resilience was tested and weighed with the client. These ideas were to be discussed with the client as suggestions and possibilities. The supervisee must withhold her expectation of the possible presentation to the commission.

Case Update. At this point the client went through a phone consultation with the Royal Commission in a session while the supervisee was present. This was decided on as a confidential way to check on the client's reactions to being exposed to another institution, such as the commission. The phone contact was useful for the administrative information about the commission's operations for clients and the supportive and sensitive way that the phone call was handled.

Supervision issue 3

Supervisee raised the issue of the recognition payment from the Attorney General's Department for victims of crime. The supervisee had become aware that the eligibility for a recognition payment was high for this client as an institutional sexual abuse survivor. The policy and administrative issues surrounding this recognition payment were explored prior to supervision. The Supervisor knew that the literacy of the client was challenged by dyslexia and her schooling years had not been finished and, according to the client, were unfruitful. The Supervisor wondered about introducing another person to the process of the application for recognition payment in the form of an advocate who would assist her lack of literacy and aid the filling in of the forms relating to the payment. The Advocate Service at Eden Therapy Services had been operating as a programme for several years with the services of an advocate who was an OAM recipient for his services to the disability field and an awarded social reformer in disability and employment. The supervisee also raised concerns about the client's robustness if the recognition payment was knocked back by Victims Services or the meeting of an advocate would be too confrontational to the client.

Conclusion of supervision was to see the introduction of an advocate as a way to further the client's reach into the community and to be heard by another. This advocate would hear parts of her story so that the application would be assisted, and recognition payment gained, plus there was another person hearing and giving veracity to her history as a survivor of childhood sexual abuse. It was useful to hear from the supervisor that if the recognition payment was not forthcoming this would need to be raised with the client and anticipated and reframed as not a failure but rather another attempt for her narrative to be told as the application in itself would be registered with Victims Services. The clinical aim was to increasingly address triggered memories that the client was presenting and work through those for future robustness and health. The clinical revelation was the increasingly tested narrative of the client's exposure to different possibilities. As this emerged as an ongoing strength for the client, the supervisee and supervisor could become more confident in the client's exposer to the administration of government policies and procedures for redress as being empowering for this client. It was also recognised that this experience would not be the same for every client and that the supervisee had case examples usually representing the exact opposite reaction.

Case Update. The successful application to receive a recognition payment was a great encouragement for the client and came at a time when increasing physical limitation due to her health deficits meant her husband was retiring from work to care for her. As a result, the transition for the whole family was made easier by the new narrative in the household that her survival was now acknowledged by the government and was seen in a practical way in the recognition payment. It was not just empty words for this family.

Supervision issue 4

The client was now very robust and had a growing opinion in regard to the political climate surrounding the issue of the Royal Commission and the terms of reference of the commission. The client stated, 'I never want this to happen to another child again' and she wishes to see the terms of reference of the commission expanded to include the survivors and overcomers of any form of child sexual abuse to be included by the commission. The supervisee raised the issue of the attachment felt toward the client and the way this was ameliorating the many years of practice with cases and families where such growth had not been experienced by the client, the client's family or the supervisee. The questions began to be asked about giving the client permission to not 'owe' the supervisee anything and that she may need to branch out with her views into the wider public forum without so much involvement of the supervisee. The clinical revelation was to have the supervisor reassure the supervisee that a very complex case had been managed and that the supervisee's strong feelings of amelioration could be entertained and even enjoyed as the case had been managed well.

Supervision concluded that the celebration of the case was reasonable; the complex nature of childhood trauma rarely afforded the supervisee a 'win' and that in supervision this could be validated and acknowledged. The administration of the supervisee at this point was not only affirming the clinical management of the client but encouraging a view that the case could be very insightful to others in view of the advocacy work and positive engagement with the Royal Commission. As a result, with the client's permission, the case was presented at the AASW Annual Conference in Hobart in 2017. The presentation furthered the experience of the supervisee and the growth of the client who was encountering her story at another level in the teaching of other social workers.

Case Update. The client felt further heard by the knowledge of the presentation of her journey to other professionals. She felt that this furthered her concern that this 'never occur again' and that by educating professionals to this view she had achieved peace for herself.

Conclusion

The addition of the concept of the administration of the supervisee in a complex childhood trauma issue for supervision is pivotal. If this administrative exploration had instead been about the accountability of the supervisee, the gains made in the case may not have emerged. A more conservative case management may have resulted in a cautious reflection on the Royal Commission rather than the successful administration of the government's policies, procedures and recognition payments which the client benefited from and still to this day remains actively around. The clinical revelations would also have been affected by supervision of a one up and one day nature. The sage like approach to supervision would probably caution the use of the current political provision for survivors. Instead, what emerged was a supervised and managed clinical exploration of the unusual robustness of the client and her reaction to the telling of her story. Without supervision the healing of the client would not have been experienced in its fullness for the client and the supervisee.

To quote the client, 'the first thing I want my grandkids to say is, 'Wow, what a different life my grandma or great grandma lived' because I am doing this, so their life doesn't have to have anything to do with abuse' (Braid, 2016, Recorded Interview).

Educational questions & activities

1. How does the AASW define supervision for social workers?
2. What is the basis of the common question social workers have in supervision when in private practice?
3. What does the author, Braid, believe that counsellors are reluctant to do in the assessment process and why?
4. What does the author believe is pivotal in complex childhood trauma?

Acknowledgement

The case example provided was used with the permission of all involved and has been de-identified for publication purposes.

References

Australian Association of Social Workers. (2014). *Supervision standards.*

Australian Association of Social Workers. (2020). *Code of ethics.*

Barletta, J. (2017). Introduction to clinical supervision. In N. Pelling & P. Armstrong (Eds.), *The practice of clinical supervision and clinical supervision* (2nd ed., pp. 5–22). Samford Valley, QLD: Australian Academic Press.

Beddoe, L., & Egan, R. (2010). Social work supervision. In A. Davys & L. Beddoe (Eds.), *Best practice in professional supervision: A guide for the helping professions.* Jessica Kingsley Publications.

Braid, R. (1996). *Our say: Women's response to the false memory debate* [Unpublished Master of Social Work Thesis]. The University of New South Wales.

Braid, R. (2008). *Our healing: An empirical study of the interrelationship between therapeutic intervention and spiritual intervention in a social work private practice* [Unpublished Doctor of Philosophy Thesis]. La Trobe University.

Braid, R. (2016). *Eden Therapy Services: Client royal commission interview.* Magic Squirrel Media Pty Ltd.

Cohen, B., Barnes, M., & Rankin, A. (1995). *Managing traumatic stress through art.* The Sidran Press.

Corey, G., Haynes, R., Moulton, P., & Muratori, M. (2010). *Clinical supervision in the helping professions: A practical guide* (2nd ed.). American Counseling Association.

Davys, A., & Beddoe, L. (2010). *Best practice in professional supervision.* Jessica Kingsley Publishers.

Kadushin, A., & Harkness, D. (2014). *Supervision in social work* (5th ed.). Columbia University Press.

Lack, C., & Pelling, N.J. (2009). Who are Australian counsellors and how do they attend to their professional development. In N. Pelling, J. Barletta, & P. Armstrong (Eds.), *The practice of clinical supervision* (1st ed., pp. 212–221). Australian Academic Press.

McSkimming, J. (2017). *Leaving Christian fundamentalism and the reconstruction of identity.* Routledge.

Pelling, N. . (2017). International counselling and psychology professional organisations and resources. In N. Pelling & P. Armstrong (Eds.), *The practice of clinical supervision and clinical supervision* (2nd ed., pp. 71–83). Australian Academic Press.

Part 4

Professional Counsellors and Supervisors

Part 4, **Professional Counsellors and Supervisors** section, comprises four chapters which are generally oriented toward the more personal dimensions of clinical supervision such as identifying who Australian counsellors are, counselling and supervisory relationships, supervisor development and training, and multicultural counselling supervision. Chapter 15 provides a baseline description of counsellors in Australia, information which has the potential to be used in moves to advance the professionalisation of the group. Chapter 16 is a succinct review of the basic areas relating to the supervisory relationship and is offered in a way the reader will be encouraged to explore at greater length issues for which they have specific interest. Chapter 17 explores the development of supervisors and how supporting them in their work has become more recognised. Supervisors of supervisors and supervisors of therapists, need to address their own personal and relational development, be experienced as therapists, engage in professional training relative to supervision, and also be in supervision themselves. Such reflective practice with clients and supervisees requires lifelong learning. Chapter 18 explores how culture can be honoured in supervision.

Chapter overview

Chapter 15, **Who are Australian Counsellors and How Do They Attend to Their Professional Development?**, by Caleb Lack, Nadine Pelling, and Deah Abbot, provides a state of the (counselling) union glimpse based on recently published comprehensive workforce studies. The chapter ultimately provides the reader with a baseline description of counsellors in Australia, information which has the potential to be used in moves to advance the professionalization of counsellors as a group worthy of, and in need of, some form of statutory recognition.

Chapter themes

In this chapter you will explore the following themes:

- Australian Counselling
- Method
- Comparisons
- Methodology

DOI: 10.4324/9781003490067-18

- Results
- Discussion

Chapter 16, **The Supervisory Relationship**, by Jason Dixon, reviews the nature of the working relationship that is developed between supervisor and supervisee, without which, useful outcomes are unlikely. This chapter examines, albeit in a cursory fashion, the very important concepts of the parallel process and transference, with a useful table which explores the developmental nature of a clinicians' increasing awareness of such issues. An inventory in the form of a list of stimulating questions that supervisors and supervisees could consider will ensure the supervisory relationship and the process of supervision are heading in the right direction.

Chapter themes

In this chapter you will explore the following themes:

- Importance and nature of the supervisory relationship
- Factors affecting the supervisory relationship
- Parallel process, transference and countertransference
- Taking inventory of the supervisory relationship

Chapter 17, **Supervisor Development**, by Nadine Pelling and Elisa Agostinelli, explores the factors that relate to supervisory identity development. The chapter addresses the questions: How does one become a supervisor and what factors relate to supervisory iden-tity development? The Supervisor Complexity Model of Watkins is reviewed as are the personal and relational factors related to supervision. Counselling experience, supervision training, and supervisory experience are then reviewed and presented as having an impact on one's development as a supervisor. If you are a new supervisor you will want to read this chapter as it illustrates common supervisory development factors and the stages of development many new supervisors will encounter as they become more proficient at supervision.

Chapter themes

In this chapter you will explore the following themes:

- Supervisor Development
- SCM stages
- Possible influences on supervisory development
- Personal/relational variables
- Counselling experience
- Supervisory training
- Supervision experience

Chapter 18, **Multicultural Counselling Supervision: Strengthening Learning and Practice Applications**, by Nancy Arthur, explores the impact of culture not just on coun-selling but on the supervisory relationship. With a skilful use of scenarios, the import-ance of culture in the supervisory relationship is demonstrated. The chapter provides information on addressing cultural influences in supervision. Thus, this is a very practical chapter regarding the application of culture in counselling supervision.

Chapter themes

In this chapter you will explore the following themes:

- Multicultural Counselling: Identities, Social Location, and Social Justice
- Multicultural Counselling Competency Frameworks
- Multicultural Counselling Supervision
- Connecting Multicultural Counselling, Advocacy, and Social Justice
- Challenges in Multicultural Counselling Supervision
- Strengthening the Working Alliance in Multicultural Supervision
- Supervision Scenarios
- Tools for Reflective Practice

15 Who are Australian Counsellors and How do they Attend to their Professional Development?

Caleb W. Lack, Nadine Pelling, and Deah Abbott

Introduction

Australian counselling is still a developing profession and four main workforce surveys have been conducted in an effort to identify the characteristics of Australian counsellors and describe their activities. Three published workforce surveys used as their foci members of different Australian counselling organisations, primarily the Australian Counselling Association (ACA) and the Psychotherapy and Counselling Federation of Australia (PACFA) (Pelling, 2005; Schofield & Roedel, 2012; Schofield, 2008). The fourth published workforce survey examined individuals advertising themselves as counsellors in the Australian Yellow Pages (Pelling, Brear, & Lau, 2006). All four studies illustrate methodological strengths and limitations and purport to describe counsellors in Australia. In this chapter we are integrating the newest research with those covered in our previous overview (Lack & Pelling, 2009) to provide the broadest overview of Australian counselling to date.

Results show many similarities among the findings, possibly illustrating a fairly homogeneous group despite the different organisational affiliations/populations used to sample counsellors. It is suggested that a baseline description of Australian counsellors has thus been obtained and it is therefore recommended that counselling organisations in Australia, most notably the ACA and PACFA, work together to advance the profession, as they appear to be representing similar groups of people. Recommendations for future counselling workforce surveys are provided and include a strong suggestion to sample larger amounts of the counselling workforce in Australia. Accurate workforce descriptions can aid supervisors in providing targeted and appropriate supervision to specific groups of supervisees. In addition, results regarding counsellor participation in supervision and professional development activities are also presented.

Australian counselling

Counselling is a developing profession without statutory regulation in Australia. Despite this, or maybe because of it, a number of organisations exist that purport to represent counselling and counsellors in Australia, each with differing educational and general membership requirements (Pelling, 2006; Pelling & Sullivan, 2006; Pelling & Whetham, 2006). For counsellors who do not affiliate with the psychological or social work professions there exist a number of specialty, state, and national counselling organisations. This includes two primary national general counselling organisations: the Australian Counselling Association (ACA) and the Psychotherapy and Counselling Federation

DOI: 10.4324/9781003490067-19

of Australia (PACFA) (Armstrong, 2006; Pelling, 2006; Schofield, Grant, Holmes, & Barletta, 2006). The ACA represents more than 4,100 counsellors and psychotherapists (ACA, 2016) and PACFA is an umbrella organisation that represents various member organisations (Schofield, 2008).

Historically, some have viewed the ACA and PACFA as competitors. However, the ACA and PACFA have worked collaboratively for years to develop a joint register for counsellors to aid in their common goal of having counselling recognised as a profession by the Australian government for the purposes of government health (Medicare) service rebates (P. Armstrong, personal communication, April 28, 2008). To this end, the Australian Register of Counsellors and Psychotherapists (ARCAP) was founded in 2011 (Australian Register of Counsellors and Psychotherapists, 2011). One of the primary obstacles to establishing this register was a disagreement about training standards for inclusion (Schofield, 2012). Despite moving forward with the register, the ACA and PACFA never actually came to a consensus on this matter (Australian Register of Counsellors and Psychotherapists, 2011).

This lack of consensus has resulted in a complicated system, with seven different types of ARCAP registrants who are divided into two separate divisions (Australian Register of Counsellors and Psychotherapists, 2011). The primary purpose of this convoluted structure appears to be to minimize any changes to the membership requirements for the ACA and PACFA as individual organisations. The current standard is that practitioners may register under Division A by meeting PACFA standards or under Division B by meeting ACA standards. There are three different categories of Division A registrants: provisional registrants, clinical registrants, and mental health practitioners. Provisional registrants must have completed an undergraduate degree and graduate degree in a related field (or the equivalent), at least 200 hours of client contact, and 50 hours of supervision (Psychotherapy and Counselling Federation of Australia, 2013) Clinical registrants must have completed all of the requirements of a provisional registrant and plus an additional 750 hours of client contact and 75 hours of supervision over a minimum of two years. Mental health practitioners are clinical registrants who have completed additional training and supervision with a mental health professional (Australian Register of Counsellors and Psychotherapists, 2011). There are four different levels of Division B registrants. Level 1 requires the lowest level of training and experience: a diploma from an ACA accredited course, 25 points of ACA approved professional development per year, and 10 hours of professional supervision per year. Each level progressively requires more training and/or experience with Level 4 requiring a degree from an ACA accredited course of study, a minimum of six years post-degree counselling experience, a minimum 1,000 total client contact hours, a minimum of 100 total hours of professional supervision, ten hours of professional supervision per year, and 25 Points of ACA approved professional development per year. It is important to stress that the ARCAP is simply a self-regulatory body, and that it is not currently recognized by the Australian government.

Our review found that four published studies in the past decade (Pelling, 2005; Pelling, Brear, & Lau, 2006; Schofield & Roedel, 2012; Schofield, 2008) have attempted to identify who is providing service to the Australian public under the term *counsellor*. While all have relied on survey data to reach their conclusions, each has differed in terms of their methodology, sample population, and other factors. The aim of this chapter is to provide a critique of the methods used, describe the differences and similarities of these studies, and provide information to assist in improving such research in the future. Following this methodological comparison, the results of the four workforce studies are compared. The chapter ends with a general description of Australian counsellors and some recommendations for counselling representation and future workforce studies.

Method

Studies that have evaluated what counsellors in Australia do and who they are were identified via searches of the PsychINFO and Medline databases (using the following keywords: Australia, counsellor, counselling), reference lists from those identified articles, and contacting the authors of found articles to see if they were aware of other work which had been published on the topic. This resulted in four identified studies to review (Pelling, 2005; Pelling, Brear, & Lau, 2006; Schofield, 2008; Schofield & Roedel, 2012). Given that Dr Pelling is the lead author of two of the published workforce surveys under examination, it was deemed inappropriate for her to lead the methodological critique, and so Dr Lack and Ms Abbott took the lead on that aspect of this chapter while Dr Pelling focused on the results comparison. The methodological review examined general methodology/ procedure, sample population, and return rates. The results were compared regarding Demographics, Education & Professional Activities, and Work Settings.

Methodological comparisons

Studies will be discussed chronologically, with comparisons afterwards. Pelling's (2005) article focused on self-identified members of the ACA. Using a similar survey to Pelling, Brear, & Lau (2006), this article focused on gathering information from those ACA members who received the journal *Counselling Australia*, although those who received electronic communication from the ACA were also sent the survey. The survey asked about multiple demographic characteristics (e.g., gender, age, racial/ethnic group, religious affiliation, and marital status), training and professional development, provision of services, involvement in professional organisations, and comfort with six topics likely to be encountered by counsellors (i.e., use of electronic means to provide services; sexual orientation issues; service provision to indigenous populations; and comfort treating depression, anxiety, and substance use). The data were collected over a one-month period of time in April of 2004, with no reported follow-ups or reminders to increase the return rate. A total of 241 (out of 1000) responses were received from those who were given the survey through the mail, with only 48 (out of 2000) responses from those who received the electronic communication. Those 48 were excluded from all analyses.

Pelling, Brear, and Lau's (2006) article used a highly similar survey, but did not report questions concerning comfort level with likely encountered issues. For their sample, the responders were drawn from those persons who advertised themselves as counsellors in the Australian Yellow Pages, with a total of 587 surveys sent to a randomly selected portion of all advertised counsellors across the country. These data were collected between March and April of 2004, and utilized a specified reminder procedure to increase return rate (see below). A total of 317 (out of 510 deliverable surveys) were returned to the authors.

Schofield (2008) focused on members of PACFA member associations for her research. All 41 PACFA member associations, approximately 3,000 total persons, were involved in this survey. The survey itself had 48 total questions that covered multiple areas: limited demographic information (i.e., gender and age), priorities for the future of PACFA, experience and training background, involvement in professional organizations, professional development activities, work setting and practices, and information about private practice.

In Schofield's (2008) study, data were also collected during 2004, with the first mailings occurring in January and stretching over the next six months, during which "several email reminders" (p. 6, Schofield, 2008) were sent to the PACFA member associations. A total of 316 (out of over 3,000 reported members) responses were returned, although only 122 identified themselves as counsellors or psychotherapists. Thus a return rate of 10.5%, including the entire sample obtained, was achieved.

Schofield and Roedel (2012) sought to overcome the limitations of prior work that only included members of one association by asking some 50 different associations to invite their members to participate in a survey. Of those, 47 sent out the survey to their members, 37 of which were PACFA member associations and one of which was the ACA. The organisations that participated emailed a link of the online survey to their members, sent reminder emails, and some of them included a link to the survey on their websites. The online survey consisted of 543 items designed to assess demographic characteristics, professional identification and background, qualifications, training, perceived adequacy of training, supervision, membership in Australian professional bodies, career development, and professional organisation. The survey remained open for responses during a six-month period in 2008. This study had 1,025 participants, 1,003 of which were included in in final analysis. This represented around 10% or so of the total target population. Of those that responded, 703 (70%) identified as being counsellors. The researchers did not analyse the data of these participants separately from those who reported being in other professions such as psychotherapists, ministers, and nurses.

As can be seen, all studies focused on self-reported survey data. In addition, three of the studies (Pelling, 2005; Pelling, Brear, & Lau, 2006; Schofield, 2008), despite their varied publication dates, collected their survey data in the first half of 2004. The remaining one (Schofield, 2012) collected data in 2008. Of the four, two (Pelling, 2005; Schofield, 2008) focused on members of a particular organisation, one included members of multiple organisations (Schofield & Roedel, 2012), and only one attempted a random sample of counsellors (Pelling, Brear, & Lau, 2006), although this was drawn from those advertised as providing counselling services in a telephone directory. As such, each of these studies has threats to their ability to generalise to the total population of self-identified counsellors. The low rates of returned surveys for the studies focusing on members of the ACA and PACFA could indicate high rates of self-selection, particularly given the high rates of advanced degrees (Master's or Doctoral; see below) in both samples. Given that counselling is a non-regulated profession, the random sampling method used (Pelling, Brear, & Lau, 2006) likely represents the most accurate assessment of the population in question.

Also concerning in terms of applicability to wider samples and populations is the fact that three of the studies had very low return rates (10% or less of total sample for Pelling, 2005; Schofield, 2008; Schofield & Roedel, 2012), even though the information was requested under the auspices of an organisation to which the persons belonged. The fourth used multiple mailings to gather information and remind people to return the survey, resulting in a much higher return rate (62.2%; Pelling, Brear, & Lau, 2006). Again, this contributes to this study being more likely representative of the counsellor population as a whole. It is also important to note that the Australian Bureau of Statistics estimates the total number of counsellors in Australia to be over 17,500 (as cited by Australian Government Job Outlook, 2012), therefore each study has sampled only a tiny percentage of the total counsellors in the nation, from 0.7% (Schofield, 2008) to 1.4% (Pelling, 2005) to 1.8% (Pelling, Brear, & Lau, 2006) to 4.02% (Schofield & Roedel, 2012). Thus, although all four publications represent workforce surveys, none could be said to truly profile the actual profession of counselling in Australia. Instead, the surveys appear to simply describe, to varying degrees of accuracy, specific sections of the profession.

A last fact concerning the accuracy of these studies on reflecting the counselling population as a whole concerns the types of persons sampled. Each study had widely varying rates of other types of mental health professionals who responded to the survey as a counsellor. For example, Pelling (2005) had 4.1% of her sample comprised of psychologists, while psychologists made up 41.9%, 6.5%, and 16.6% of the other studies (Pelling, Brear, & Lau, 2006, Schofield, 2008, and Schofield & Roedel, 2012, respectively). Also, the Schofield (2008) and Schofield and Roedel (2012) studies included social workers (5.7% and 4.6%, respectively), nurses (9.8% and 3.5%), and medical practitioners (0.8% and 2.7%) in the sample. In addition, the Pelling (2005) and Schofield (2008) studies included students in their sample, at quite different rates (16.6% and 1.7%, respectively). This combined with the differences in rates of regulated professions described above, undoubtedly impacted the findings on educational level, possibly resulting in under (Pelling, 2005) and over-estimation (Schofield, 2008; Schofield & Roedel, 2012) of the average educational qualifications held by counsellors.

In future research, using a randomized sample focusing on all members of the counselling profession (similar to that used by Pelling, Brear, and Lau, 2006) is highly recommended. Going beyond only sampling those who are advertised in the Yellow Pages should definitely be undertaken, as anyone is able to call himself or herself a counsellor due to the non-regulated status of the term. Such work could involve focusing on one particular city or state/territory, starting with those who advertise their services in the phone directories, but also asking those who are advertised if they are aware of any counsellors who do not advertise in the directory. Also, obtaining lists from the city government of all persons listed as having permits to operate within the city in a counselling capacity, if possible, might allow for a wider sampling of people providing counselling services. Surveys of the major counselling organisations (such as ACA or PACFA) should be conducted again, with a focus on getting much higher rates of returned information to gain a better understanding of whom the members are. Alternatively, these organisations could require all members, either joining for the first time or renewing their membership, to complete a survey as part of their application packet. Last, a survey that attempts to gather information from a larger percentage of the total counsellor population should be undertaken, as the current surveys have all surveyed less than 5% of the total populace.

Results

Demographics

In spite of the differences in sampling techniques and populations, much information can be gained by comparing the results of these three studies. Perhaps the most glaring similarity across the studies was the demographic results. For all, a vast majority of the respondents were female (between 70.3% and 78%) and middle-aged (mean ages between 49 and 53 years old). Those studies that reported on other demographics (Pelling, 2005; Pelling, Brear, & Lau, 2006; Schofield & Roedel, 2012) found a majority of the sample to be married or partnered (66.8%, 75.7%, and 72.6%), heterosexual (90.5%, 93.4%, and 97,7%), and living in urban environments (69.3%, 73.8%, and 72.2%) in New South Wales (28.2%, 30.6%, and 34.1%) or Victoria (24.1%, 28.4%, and 28.8%). In terms of racial characteristics, all three studies reported a majority of Caucasians, although Pelling (2005) reported only 14.9% of her sample identifying as such, while the other study reported 86.1% or respondents identifying as Caucasian (Pelling, Brear, & Lau, 2006). Similarly, both Pelling (2005) and Pelling, Braur, and Lau (2006) reported a preponderance of religious affiliations being Christian, at rates of 7.5% and 55.8%. As noted in the methodology section above, the Pelling (2005), Pelling, Brear, and Lau (2006), and Schofield and Roedel (2012) studies provided greater detail regarding the demographic characteristics of the samples than the Schofield (2008) study.

Education & professional activities

Training and education results across the three studies differed significantly. For baccalaureate, Master's, and Doctorate degrees, Pelling (2005) found rates of 34.4%, 18.3%, and 4.6%; Pelling, Brear, and Lau (2006) found rates of 36.9%, 31.2%, and 8.8%; Schofield (2008) found rates of 34.1% and 43.9% (Master's/Doctorate combined); and Schofield and Roedel (2012) found rates of 26.8%, 40.5%, and 8.8%. The lower rates of higher education in the Pelling (2005) study may reflect that fact that over 16% of the sample were students and, thus, may be in the process of completing a degree.

Pelling (2005) and Pelling, Brear, and Lau (2006) studies reported similar rates of engaging in supervision, between 70% and 72%, while Schofield and Roedel (2012) reported somewhat higher rates at 88%. Additionally, the Pelling (2005) and Pelling, Brear, and Lau (2006) studies report that conference attendance and reading books/ journals are the most popular professional development activities, from 65–86% and 89– 96% respectively. The top three journals in both the Pelling (2005) and Pelling, Brear, and Lau (2006) studies remained the same, although their order differed according to study: *Australian Psychologist, Counselling Australia* and *Psychotherapy in Australia*. The Schofield and Roedel (2012) study reported that majority of their participants spent more than 25 hours in the past year in engaging in profession development by reading (67%) or by attending lectures, seminars, courses or conferences (52%).

The average number of years working as a counsellor ranged from a low of 8.6 to a high of 14.8 in the Pelling (2005) and Pelling, Brear, and Lau (2006) studies, respectively. The Schofield (2008) and Schofield and Roedel (2012) studies indicated an average of 13 and 13.7 years, respectively. Given that there was a fairly significant amount of students included in the Pelling (2005) study, once again there appears to be a great deal of similarity among the samples in terms of counselling experience. The studies report participants engaging in very high rates of individual counselling (81–95%) and couple/ family counselling (51–79%). Between 23% and 35% of respondents in the Pelling (2005), Pelling, Brear, and Lau (2006), and Schofield (2008) surveys reportedly engaged in some type of specialised practice.

One glaring difference in the results of the studies was on theoretical orientation. For the Pelling (2005) and Pelling, Brear, and Lau (2006) studies the main theoretical influence was eclectic, with cognitive-behaviour or narrative influences. However, the Schofield (2008) study reported a preponderance of psychoanalytic theorists. The Schofield and Roedel (2012) study found the highest rates of humanistic and interpersonal influences. It is not possible to know why this difference specifically exists, but this may identify a point of real divergence between the samples and thus populations examined. As such, generalizing from any of these samples to the likely theoretical orientation of the counselling profession as a whole in Australia should not be undertaken.

Work setting

Solo private practice was a popular activity with 43–63% of the respondents in the studies working in this setting. Income information was not reported in the Schofield (2008) and Schofield and Roedel (2012) studies. However, Schofield (2008) did state that the sample reported on average holding 1.7 employment positions. The Pelling (2005) and Pelling, Brear, and Lau (2006) studies reported samples which indicated an average salary of $40,000 or less per year, with an average fee between $58 and $80 an hour, respectively.

Discussion

As of 2016, four counselling workforce surveys have been conducted and published in Australia. The current examination shows that these studies sampled only a very small amount of the ABS reported number of counsellors in Australia. The studies themselves vary regarding the sampling procedures used, participants used as the foci for their data collection, and return rate obtained. Nevertheless, great similarities are reported in the results.

Who are Australian counsellors? Generally speaking, Australian counsellors are women of middle-age. They tend to be married or in a partnered relationship, heterosexual, and living in urban environments. In terms of education, most counsellors tend to hold some type of baccalaureate or more advanced degree. Differences in reported post-graduate (master's/doctorate) degrees existed and are likely to be a result of studies including/excluding students, as well as the inclusion of members of government-regulated professions thus seemingly lowering/artificially raising the educational levels reported. A fuller examination of educational level obtained in terms of specific counselling (versus psychological) training and examination of in progress versus obtained degrees could be illuminative in regards to the educational levels held by Australian counsellors, especially those counsellors who do not identify with a different, regulated profession (e.g., psychologists or social workers).

Similarities were also demonstrated between studies in terms of supervisory activities, professional development activities, and experience level. Indeed, counsellors in Australia appear to have a fairly high level of experience in terms of years of practice, with about a decade being fairly standard. Once again, similarities existed in professional activities including the popularity of individual as well as couple/family counselling. Differences were reported in terms of theoretical orientation with eclectic/cognitive-behaviour, psychoanalytic, and humanistic and interpersonal theories being reported as the most frequent across different studies.

Conclusion

Due to the similarities in the findings obtained by the four published Australian counselling workforce surveys, we propose that a baseline description of Australian counsellors has been obtained. As a result, it might be in the best interest of the Australian counselling industry to have the ACA and PACFA to continue working together as what will benefit one group is likely to benefit the other (Australian Register of Counsellors and Psychotherapists, 2011; Pelling & Sullivan, 2006).

Future counselling workforce surveys are encouraged to focus on two main points. First, increasing the return rate obtained possibly by using a multi-mailing or multi-emailing technique, such as that engaged by Pelling, Brear, and Lau (2006) and Schofield and Roedel (2012), is likely to result in higher rates of engagement. Second, a wider sampling of the existing number of counsellors in Australia needs to be obtained in any future survey. Thus, surveys should avoid focusing on one specific association's membership or one limited listing of counsellors, but instead employ a snowballing technique gained to sample a large number of counsellors who could be contacted by various methods. Regardless, Australian counselling can be said to be developing smoothly with a number of published workforce surveys and the two main representative counselling bodies in Australia now working in collaboration.

Educational questions & activities

1. True or False: The three published workplace surveys of Australian counsellors show more similarities than differences.
2. List one main difference found among the three discussed workplace surveys.
3. Is your favourite journal listed among the most popular for Australian counsellors?
4. Describe the general Australian counsellor in terms of demographic characteristics.

Selected references for further reading

Selected internet resources
Australian Counselling Association
www.theaca.net.au
Australian Register of Counsellors and Psychotherapists
www.arcapregister.com.au
Psychotherapy and Counselling Federation of Australia
www.pacfa.org.au

References

Armstrong, P. (2006). The Australian Counselling Association: Meeting the needs of Australian counsellors. *International Journal of Psychology, Special Issue Counselling in Australia, 41*(3), 153–155. doi:10.1080/00207590544000130

Australian Counselling Association (2016). *About the ACA*. Retrieved from www.theaca.net.au/about.php

Australian Government Job Outlook (2012). *Counsellors: Statistics*. Retrieved from http://joboutlook.gov.au/occupation.aspx?search=industry&tab=stats&cluster=&code=2721&graph=EL

Australian Register of Counsellors and Psychotherapists (2011). *The Australian Register of Counsellors and Psychotherapists is a company established by the Psychotherapy and Counselling Federation of Australia and the Australian Counselling Association as an independent, national register of qualified counsellors and psychotherapists*. Retrieved from www.arcapregister.com.au

Lack, C.W., & Pelling, N. (2009). Who are Australian counsellors and how do they attend to their professional development? In N. Pelling, J. Barletta, & P. Armstrong (Eds.), *The practice of clinical supervision* (pp. 212–222). Bowen Hills, Queensland: Australian Academic Press.

Pelling, N. (2005). Counsellors in Australia: Profiling the membership of the Australian Counselling Association. *Counselling, Psychotherapy, and Health, [On-Line Serial], 1*(1), 1–18. doi:10.1080/00207590544000130

Pelling, N. (2006). Professional counselling organisations. In N. Pelling, R. Bowers, & P. Armstrong (Eds.), *The practice of counselling* (pp. 442–453). Melbourne: Thomson Publishers.

Pelling, N., Brear, P., & Lau, M. (2006). A survey of advertised Australian counsellors. *International Journal of Psychology, Special Issue Counselling in Australia, 41*(3), 204–215. doi:10.1080/00207590544000202

Pelling, N., & Sullivan, B. (2006). The credentialing of counselling in Australia. *International Journal of Psychology, Special Issue Counselling in Australia, 41*(3), 194–203. doi:10.1080/00207590544000194

Pelling, N., & Whetham, P. (2006). The professional preparation of Australian counsellors. *International Journal of Psychology, Special Issue Counselling in Australia, 41*(3), 189–193. doi:10.1080/00207590544000185

Psychotherapy and Counselling Federation of Australia (2013). *Individual PACFA Membership.* Retrieved from www.pacfa.org.au/member-associations/individual-pacfa-membership/

Schofield, M. (2008). Australian counsellors and psychotherapists: A profile of the profession. *Counselling & Psychotherapy Research, Special Issue Australian Counselling and Psychotherapy Research, 8*(1), 4–11. doi:10.1080/14733140801936369

Schofield, M., Grant, J., Holmes, S., & Barletta, J. (2006). The Psychotherapy and Counselling Federation of Australia: How the federation model contributes to the field. *International Journal of Psychology, Special Issue Counselling in Australia, 41*(3), 194–203. doi: 10.1080/00207590544000149

Schofield, M. J. (2012). Counseling in Australia: Past, present, and future. *Journal of Counseling & Development, 91*(2), 234–239. doi:10.1002/j.1556-6676.2013.00090.x

Schofield, M.J., & Roedel, G. (2012). *Australian psychotherapists and counsellors: A study of therapists, therapeutic work, and professional development.* Melbourne: La Trobe University.

16 The Supervisory Relationship

Jason Dixon

Introduction to the supervisory relationship

The nature of the relationship that is negotiated, developed and maintained between a clinical supervisor and supervisee is central to effectively engage in clinical work, to promote professional and personal development, and to ensure consistent ethical practice. In this chapter attention is given to the challenges, importance and benefits of the supervisory relationship. The ability to form and sustain relationships in supervision and in clinical practice is more crucial than specific knowledge and therapeutic skills (Dye, 1994). Attention to parallel process, the working alliance, multiple roles, expectations, and acculturative issues are addressed. In this chapter it is assumed that both supervisors and supervisees already have attained the minimum standard of clinical knowledge and skill according to their profession. This is an introduction to some of the most salient issues concerning the supervisory relationship and is a review of concepts and processes discussed in greater depth throughout this textbook. Whether the reader is a trainee supervisor, a practising supervisor, or supervisee, they are encouraged to utilise the references and suggested readings to understand that the nature of supervisory relationship is fundamental to the successful practice of clinical supervision.

Importance and nature of the supervisory relationship

The significance of the supervisory relationship in therapist training and clinical practice is evident by the extensive attention given to it in the scholarly literature (e.g., Bambling, King, Raue, Schweitzer, & Lambert, 2006; Barletta, 2007; Borders et al., 1991; Bordin, 1979; Lampropoulos, 2002; McMahon, 2002; Ronnestad & Skovholt, 1993). The impact on the supervisee's professional identity, clinical skill, self-confidence and relational style are cultivated through the quality of the supervisory relationship. Building on recent literature there is evidence that through the supervisory relationship the attachment styles of insecure trainee therapists can be transformed in their clinical work to an identity of self-confidence and a secure relational style (Bernard & Goodyear, 2004; Renfro-Michel, 2006; Renfro-Michel & Sheperis, 2009). New approaches have been proposed that support the notion that using psychological theory that focuses on the interpersonal relationship, such as attachment theory, is useful to enrich the supervisory working alliance and enhance other approaches to supervisory tasks (Bennett, 2008). Research efforts into the supervisory relationship using interpersonal theories such as attachment theory is still in its infancy, however the results of recent research provide evidence of the importance

DOI: 10.4324/9781003490067-20

and utility of informing the practice of supervision with reference to scholarly research (Wrape, 2015).

The supervisory relationship has been described in different ways each emphasising certain aspects of the relationship. In general terms, supervision involves maintaining relationships while attending to the matters of supervision (McMahon, 2002). It is a relationship of utmost importance with successful supervision experienced as being reciprocal, mutual, and trusting (Safran & Muran, 2000). This relationship provides a container that holds the helping relationship within a therapeutic triad (Hawkins & Shohet, 2000). In Searles's last publication he emphasises the value of both the supervisor's and supervisee's emotional experience of supervision with the therapist and potential importance this may have on the therapist patient relationship (Waugaman, 2015). Within the supervisory relationship specific elements should exist such as empathy, acceptance, openness with confrontation, a sense of humour and appropriate self-disclosure. Supervision is a relationship that constitutes the right balance between support and challenge (Carroll & Gilbert, 2006). This support and challenge is maintained in such a way that supervisees can freely discuss successes and failures, strengths and weaknesses. Open discussion in supervision and the flow of ideas is attained through collaboration, awareness and sensitivity, and is always respectful and non-judgmental (Chiaferi & Griffin, 1997).

Although the purpose, style, and tasks of supervision will vary, the abovementioned issues and preconditions are those that ensure quality, depth and breadth of this important professional relationship.

Factors affecting the supervisory relationship

A factor that is easily attended to, and should be addressed from the outset and readdressed when necessary, is a clear understanding of the roles and expectations of both the supervisor and supervisee. Providing sufficient information on the roles of colleague, counsellor, consultant, teacher, and evaluator, set the way clear for expectations of all parties to be negotiated. Role ambiguity, uncertainty about expectations of performance and evaluation give rise to conflicts, work-related anxiety and dissatisfaction (Olk & Friendlander, 1992). The responsibility to resolve any ambiguity lies with the supervisor to clearly state, or restate, the aspects of multiple roles and be a ready resource to contribute to the induction of the supervisee into the profession. Supervisors in academic settings are more likely to be expected to perform a professional gatekeeping role. It is in this role as gatekeepers, they have the opportunity to have a positive impact on the promotion of successful supervisory relationships by ensuring that supervisees have the necessary characteristics that impact on professional success. When both the work of the supervisor and supervisee are challenging the factors that affect the supervisory relationship can be sources for personal and professional development. Immediacy in attending to ambiguity and clear communication is paramount to a productive supervision experience. Helping supervisees articulate the matters that are affecting the working alliance is sometimes all that is needed to maintain and strengthen the collaborative bond. These are important examples of the commitment supervisors and supervisees should be willing to invest in the supervisory relationship.

Attending to the mechanics of clinical work and to the supervisee's experience of clinical cases can reveal factors that might be affecting the supervisory relationship. For example, a supervisor does well to be concerned if a supervisee only ever presents to supervision with issues related to the experience of clinical work. Exploring and attending to the matters of the supervisee's client casework can reveal any impasse in disclosing these issues and restore balance to the working alliance. A commitment to ensuring that both parties are suitable aligned in the supervisory relationship is an opportunity for both to ensure the supervisory relationship is worthwhile. There requires at the appropriate time, a willingness to offer critical feedback to the supervisor, which the supervisor should be ready to receive and be open to reciprocate. This work is to be carried out in a manner that is appropriate to the supervisee's stage of professional development, and sensitive to specifically address the unique character qualities of a particular supervisee. A supervisory relationship is only possible when the supervisor and supervisee both value the personal capacity to negotiate, engage, and consistently maintain, a collegial relationship that directly promotes the patient becoming well.

Therapy and supervision is serious work with significant implications. While mention of the usefulness and place of humour is few and far between in the literature, there is a lighter side of clinical work. Being able to talk shop and allowing one's sense of humour to emerge (Pearson, 2004), and using humour to facilitate discussion of emotional reactions to clients (Nezu, Saad, & Nezu, 2000) diffuses a stressful environment, is an indication of trust and is an expression of a collaborative spirit. These aspects suggest some of the qualities of a robust collegial and collaborative working alliance at the supervisory level.

It is well documented that there are certain relational conditions between clinician and patient, that when present that account for the outcomes of clinical practice. These include an established working alliance, empathy, goal consensus and collaboration, positive regard, affirmation, congruence and genuineness (Norcross & Lambert, 2011). These account for the largest effect in the outcome of clinical practice, and to a lesser degree and still important are the clinician's adherence to protocol and how the patient rates the competence of a clinician in delivering a treatment (Webb, DeRubeis, Amsterdam, Shelton, Hollon, & Dimidjian, 2011). So despite the many evidence-based interventions available, when the qualities found in a professional helping relationship mentioned above are consistently in place across clinical sessions, the patient stands to gain the most from being engaged in treatment. The author proposes that these relational factors are also necessary for a successful supervisory relationship.

Based on the same research evidence referenced above, it is important to emphasise that to ensure that the above-mentioned factors are in place consistently across treatment sessions, a mechanism for the clinical practitioner to acquire feedback at each session is necessary. Based on the assumption that this would also be true for supervision, then supervisors would also do well to seek feedback from their supervisees about how they rate the supervision provided to them.

Limitations, delimitations, and expectations of the supervisory relationship

As mentioned in the paragraphs above, the initial stages of supervision with a supervisee at the pre-graduate or in the early stages of their career can approach the relationship with more dependent attachment style. The work of the supervisor in establishing an environment where a successful working relationship can emerge can be encouraged by clearly stating the limitations and delimitations of supervision. It is to be expected that a clinician's patients will move and affect them in their during their clinical work, and this is evidence that they are genuinely engaged in the world of their clients (see Yalom, 2001). And there will be times where supervisees will be challenged to the extent that may become impaired by working with some patients. A clear example of this is the vicarious trauma experienced by clinicians working with people challenged by post-traumatic stress disorder. There can also be times when the supervisee is faced with personal problems, that emerge independently to their working life, that are clinically significant. Supervisors do well to advise their supervisees as to when they may introduce a clinical intervention or technique to assist them with challenges they face when their patients affect them, and if they were ever faced with clinically significant personal matters, the supervisor would refer them to seek their own professional help. There is an implied request to the supervisee to trust them with such matters, and as it is in the clinician patient relationship, so it is in supervision, that it is up to the supervisee to give that trust to the supervisor. It is up to the supervisor what he does with that trust.

There are implicit expectations in help seeking behaviour. The patient expects to become well, even in apparently hopeless circumstances, help seeking behaviour is an 'act' of hope. Supervisees expect they will do well in clinical practice, and in so doing expect their patients to become well. Supervisees expect that the relationship with their supervisor also offers some kind of benefit. While researchers such mentioned in this chapter have made the early attempts to answer this question, providing an answer based on scholarly evidence in not practical at this stage. Neither is it possible in the same manner to answer the question of whether or not supervision *makes a difference*. What we can be assured of is that professional bodies and consumers of professional clinical services expect that there is a mechanism of accountability that protects the consumer and ensures a profession maintains reputable standing among public opinion. It is within the supervisory relationship where all the above expectations are grounded.

Transcultural aspects of the supervisory relationship

Culturally and linguistically diverse interpersonal relationships in supervision are an important resource for building a positive supervisory relationship. A supervisor's and supervisee's attitude toward cross-cultural factors in supervision can benefit or hinder professional practice depending on how acculturative factors are negotiated. The cultural factors common to all human cultures must be understood alongside a particular ethnic groups emphasis of certain cultural norms and values compared to another ethnic group. In clinical practice as is the case in clinical supervision, cultural factors are become particularly evident and cause stress, where there is intercultural contact. It is not practical or achievable to gain an extensive multicultural knowledge to the extent of more than one's own cultural background without a considerable investment of time and diverse life experiences. In the least we can be aware that in the course of clinical practice patient disclosure, which is essential to achieving behavioural change associated with treatment, is affected by cultural differences between clinician and patient (Vogel & Webster, 2003). How that occurs interpersonally in the practice of supervision, and how cultural factors promote successful supervisory relationships, in culturally diverse environments, can be explained through acculturation psychology.

Acculturation results when groups of individuals having different cultures come into first-hand contact and over time there are subsequent changes in the original cultural patterns of either or both groups (Redfield, Linton, & Herkovits, 1936). Generally, culturally diverse minority groups appear to engage in four types of acculturative behaviour. *Assimilation* is an abandonment of culture of origin values and norms and an adoption of host cultural values, *integration* is an adoption of host culture values and norms and a retainment of culture of origin values and norms, *separation* is a rejection of host cultural values and norms, and *marginalisation* is an abandonment of the cultural values and norms of both the host culture and the culture of origin (Berry, 1974, 1976, 1980, 1983; Berry, Kim, Young, & Bujaki, 1989).

Although the construct validity of *marginalisation* is questionable, Dixon (2008) demonstrated that attitudes of host culture trainee therapists toward the acculturative strategies of culturally different minority groups could be validly measured. All acculturative strategies are valid, yet supervisees may be biased in that they may expect clients who are culturally different to acculturate to the host culture in a certain way. Exploring this bias and establishing an understanding that all acculturative strategies are valid promotes multicultural competence and sensitivity in the therapeutic triad. Furthermore, cultural differences are an opportunity for learning. Exploring transcultural issues with a supervisor who is culturally different from the supervisee or client conveys respect and value for ethnic identity and is an opportunity to learn the cultural aspects of social norms, and protocols, cultural symbolism, morals, customs, traditions and worldview.

The cultural 'expert' in the triad is independent of the roles in those relationships, or could be shared equally in those relationships. In maintaining a positive supervisory relationship it is important to identify where and between whom the acculturative stress is occurring when formulating best practice in supervision and clinical practice. A patient or supervisee may present with acculturative stress and a particular strategy for negotiating acculturative behaviour depending on whether the stress arises in home, work, or school life. A person of culturally and linguistically diverse background may experience less acculturative stress at work where they are competent biculturally, but at home aspects of the host culture they have integrated as part of their cultural-self maybe at odds with their parents culture and minority group norms. An understanding of the attitudes toward other cultures explained by the acculturative strategies above can predict where and when culturally diverse issues will account for positive outcomes or barriers to treatment.

Parallel process, transference, and countertransference

Parallel process is a replication of the therapeutic relationship in the supervisory context, where supervisees present themselves in a similar way, as do their clients in therapy (Bernard & Goodyear, 2004; Morrissey & Tribe, 2001). Parallel process allows the process of transference and countertransference to be evident in supervision. These concepts are extremely useful regardless of the theoretical orientation adopted. The concept of transference is rooted in the psychoanalytic literature and refers to the projections of the client onto the therapist, while countertransference refers to the needs, feelings, and wishes of the therapist, which are projected onto the client. Bernard and Goodyear (2004) describe transference in simple terms as a phenomenon in which a person transfers to someone in the present, the feelings and responses that have been experienced with someone in the past. Transference reactions are often triggered by something that is familiar in persons in the present, with people in the past, and can be evident in the supervisory relationship. Transference is especially important in supervision when the person in the past is a client, and just as the client has sought some fulfilment of an emotional need in the supervisee, so too the supervisee seeks some fulfilment of these needs from the supervisor. A supervisee who reacts with frustration toward a client who is not perceived as cooperative may also react in a similar manner toward a supervisor who is attempting to encourage autonomy in the supervisee concerning the work with this client. In other words, the supervisor is perceived as being uncooperative and thus transference issues will become evident if they are adequately explored. A useful point of departure in ascertaining if transference is at work in supervision is for the supervisor to think along the lines of where this frustration is 'coming from' (i.e., interactions with the client or perhaps a relationship from the supervisee's personal world).

An example of parallel process is where clients and supervisees experience a halting of the therapeutic process. Supervisees do well when they are aware that both they and their client are stuck and then they seek guidance from their supervisor. Facilitating exploration and awareness of parallel process is dependent on supervisor skill, sensitivity, and approach. Ineffective supervision or conflict can be attributed to unconscious and unrecognised dynamics in the supervisory triad (Pearson, 2000). Encouragement to work with, and not against, exploration and awareness of parallel processes (Gilbert & Evans, 2000) sometimes requires a renegotiation and mending of the supervisory alliance to enable therapist and client to reengage and move with the therapeutic process.

McNeill and Worthen (1989), along with many others, emphasise and regard value of the parallel process as communication and a focus for supervision that is beneficial to both supervisee and client. The goals of working through parallel process and transference issues are to reduce the empathic impairment of the therapist, and to maintain and strengthen the working alliance between all parties in the therapeutic triad (Southern, 2007). This is achieved through a safe and emotionally contained environment where the supervisee can work through conflicts and emotions that impair empathy. There is a sense of catharsis resulting from genuine disclosure that spans both the depth and breadth of the supervisee's experience of clinical work. Supervisees are allowed to be vulnerable during these sessions. Southern points out that inexperienced therapists may be afraid of being vulnerable where an experienced therapist presents as being overconfident and technically proficient, yet lacks self-awareness. Both situations impair empathic interactions and insight. The task rests with the supervisor to be sensitive and aware of such states and respond appropriately to achieve the goals mentioned above.

Table 16.1 is a guide I developed for exploring therapist development, parallel process and transference issues. It can be used when considering the supervisor's approach in dealing with such critical issues. Based on the approach presented below, an experienced supervisee has built the professional capacity to be client(s)-focused. The supervisory relationship requires the supervisor to be supervisee and client/patient focused. However, the challenge for the supervisor is that the client(s) is not available in the moment of the supervision session. These interpersonal factors present during the act of supervision are unique to that environment, but it should be remembered that in some way the supervisee also 'takes' with them elements of the supervisory relationship to the relationship with their patient(s). This describes the supervisory relationship from a trans-theoretical perspective.

Based on the body of research evidence that explains what accounts for the outcomes in clinical practice (Boswell, Kraus, Miller, & Lambert, 2013), and apply it to what we would expect to work in the supervisory relationship should also be best practice. Therefore, supervisors who draw from their specialist knowledge clinical supervision, and engage their supervisees with a commitment to forming a good working supervisory relationship will benefit both the supervisee and their clients. Therefore, we would expect that a supervisory relationship would be successful when there is mutual understanding and consensus, supervisors are congruent and genuine, and they are collaborative. In the

Table 16.1 A guide to therapist development in regards to parallel process and transference in clinical supervision

Therapist Developmental Stage	Therapist Clinical Focus	Status of Parallel Process, and Transference	Supervisory Environment
Therapy Student	Skills and techniques	Unaware	Reassurance, encouragement, facilitate awareness
Emerging Professional	Self-awareness	Conscious and active awareness of feelings	Stimulate and differentiate awareness of client related issues
Professional Therapist	Other-awareness	Conscious awareness of feelings related to self and client	Patience, orientation, exploration of self and others' feelings
Senior Professional Therapist	Comprehensive aspects of therapeutic relationship	Unconscious awareness and immediacy in attending to transferences and feelings	Challenge to stretch therapist's understanding of relationship and client context

course of practicing supervision, the supervisor is responsible for seeking the feedback necessary to maintain these elements within the relationship. When the relationship has moved beyond the initial stages of formation, supervision becomes an environment where supervisees develop professionally, become aware of each clients uniqueness beyond the clinical description of their problems, supervisees are able to stay informed of the best practice clinical knowledge and skills, and maintain the motivation to assist patients in achieving the wellness they seek.

Current research limitations

Research into the models of supervision has attracted considerable attention from scholars at least since the early 1970s (e.g., Ekstein & Wallerstein, 1972). There have also been many proposed theoretical models of supervision, the majority of which have their grounding in psychological treatment theory. There is scholarly evidence that so many systems of psychological treatment are efficacious that it would seem the sensible allocation of research resources should be invested into testing the validity of those models applied to supervision. However, because these models account for so little of the outcome compared to the relationship factors between clinician and patient, it would seem that research efforts into the supervisory relationship should be more resourceful and useful in educating clinicians and as a body of clinical knowledge to inform professional practice. There is very little published research that attempts to explain the factors and conditions necessary in the supervisory relationship to promote best outcomes in clinical practice. If the evidence for what works in the supervisory relationship comparable to the evidence of what works in the therapeutic relationship, then the recommendation for theory informed and feedback informed supervision should also be fundamental to the practice of clinical supervision. Below there are questions that can be used to initiate and maintain a feedback centred approach to the supervisory relationship.

An Inventory of the supervisory relationship

The following is a list of questions that clinical supervisors and supervisees should consider in order to ensure the supervisory relationship and the process of supervision is on track. It is designed to bring attention to both the strengths of the supervisory relationship and the areas for growth that are potentially areas of conflict or threaten the supervisory working alliance.

Questions for the supervisor

- How attentive are you to the dynamics of the relationship with your supervisee? (Not just focused on the mechanics of the supervisee's practice).
- How do you know the extent to which your supervisee is freely able to disclose the experiential and emotional aspects of their work and professional development?
- To what degree is the supervisee disclosing both depth and breadth of their clinical work?
- How does the supervisee challenge you with questions about their work? In what ways do you challenge the supervisee?
- What are the conflicts you have around the goals and processes of supervision? How are they actively dealt with in a timely manner?
- How are you regularly attending to the supervisee's casework, professional development, and personal issues that impact their work?
- Describe the lighter moments in supervision? (i.e., humour)
- In what ways is there a sense of being collegial with your supervisee?
- How are you sensitive to transcultural and acculturative factors with the supervisee and their clients?

Questions for the supervisee

- To what extent do you feel at ease to freely disclose all aspects of your work? What holds you back?
- When do you feel empowered to discuss the success and failures of professional practice?
- To what degree do you feel respected? When do you particularly respect your supervisor?
- How is supervision challenging and edifying?
- How do you know that the supervisor understands the content and context of your clinical work, your personal experience of professional practice?
- How and when do you present ethical dilemmas to your supervisor?
- When are your needs for clinical practice and professional development being met?
- Describe the immediacy you experience in dealing with conflicts that arise with your supervisor?
- How have you identified and informed your supervisor of any transcultural aspects between you and your supervisor/clients? This includes the cultural aspects of social norms, protocols, cultural symbols, morals, customs and worldview.

Concluding statement

This chapter has been written as a concise review of areas pertaining to the supervisory relationship as related to the field of clinical supervision. It is offered in such a way that the reader will be encouraged to explore the issues of how to maintain a supervisory relation-ship from the roll of supervisee or supervisor. The references and selected further reading are an invaluable starting point for any further depth exploration.

The future of our understanding of the supervisory relationship is reliant upon the attention given to this subject through research. The effort to teach the value and import-ance of the supervisory relationship is reliant on clinical educators. The establishment and maintenance of a supervisory relationship that works in service of the supervisee and patient, is reliant upon the supervisor's and supervisee's commitment to the work of super-vision, consistent investment in that relationship, and the wiliness to exchange feedback on how that relationship is going over time. Both the supervisor and supervisee who value and attend to a quality relationship will ensure that insight is clear, strengthen supervisor–supervisee bond, and create an environment where clinical practice is rewarding, patients achieve an improved quality of life and personal and professional development is gained.

Educational questions & activities

1. *Classroom Discussion:* Discuss the implications of supervision of clinical supervi-sion. When and how should supervisors seek supervision for casework related to supervisees? What would be the areas of consideration that would differ from the supervisor–supervisee relationship?
2. *Role Play:* Using the questions from the section *An Inventory of the Supervisory Relationship*, identify and role play scenarios where the selected questions can be answered in such a way that would strengthen the supervisory relationship.

References

Bambling, M., King, R., Raue, P., Schweitzer, R., & Lambert, W. (2006). Clinical supervision: It's influence on client-rated working alliance and client symptom reduction in the brief treatment of major depression. *Psychotherapy Research, 16*, 317–331.

Barletta, J. (2007). Clinical supervision (Chapter 6). In N. Pelling, R. Bowers, & P. Armstrong (Eds.), *The practice of counselling* (pp. 118–135). Melbourne, Australia: Thomson.

Bennett, C. S. (2008) Attachment-informed supervision for social work field. *Clinical Social Work, 36*(1), 97–107.

Bernard, J. M., & Goodyear, R. K. (2004). *Fundamentals of clinical supervision* (3rd ed.). Boston: Pearson.

Berry, J. W. (1974). Psychological aspects of cultural pluralism: Unity and identity reconsidered. *Topics in Cultural Learning, 2*, 17–22.

Berry, J. W. (1976). *Human ecology and cognitive style.* New York: John Wiley.

Berry, J. W. (1980). Acculturation as varieties of adaptation. In A. M. Padilla (Ed.), *Acculturation: Theory, models and some new findings* (pp. 9–25). Boulder, CO: Westview Press.

Berry, J. W. (1983). Acculturation: A comparative analysis of alternative forms. In R. J. Samuda & S. L. Woods (Eds.), *Perspectives in immigrant and minority education* (pp. 65–78). New York: University Press of America.

Berry, J. W., Kim, U., Young, M., & Bujaki, M. (1989). Acculturation attitudes in plural societies. *Applied Psychology: An International Review, 38*, 185–206.

Borders, L. D., Bernard, J. M., Dye, H. A., Fong, M. L., Henderson, P., Nance, D. W., et al. (1991). Curriculum guide for training counseling supervisors: Rationale, development, and implementa-tion. *Counselor Education and Supervision, 31*, 58–80.

Bordin, E. S. (1979). The generalizability of the psychoanalytic concept of the working alliance. *Psychotherapy: Theory, Research and Practice, 16*(3), 252–260. doi:10.1037/H0085885

Boswell, J. F., Kraus, D. R., Miller, S. D., & Lambert, M. J. (2013). Implementing routine outcome monitoring in clinical practice: Benefits, challenges, and solutions. *Psychotherapy Research, 25*(1), 6–19.

Carroll, M., & Gilbert, M. C. (2006). *On being a supervisee: Creating learning partnerships.* Kew, Victoria: PsychOz.

Chiaferi, R., & Griffin, M. (1997). *Developing fieldwork skills: A guide for human services, counseling, and social work students.* Pacific Grove: Brooks Cole.

Dixon, J. M. (2008). *Attitudes toward Acculturative Behaviour Scale: Development, reliability and validity* (Doctoral dissertation, The Ohio University).

Dye, A. (1994). In The Supervisory Relationship. ERIC Digest. Retrieved December 12, 2008, from ERIC Clearinghouse on Counselling and Student Services Web Site: www.ericdigests.org/1995-1/relationship.htm

Ekstein, R., & Wallerstein, R. S. (1972). *The teaching and learning of psychotherapy* (Revised ed.). New York: International Universities Press.

Gilbert, M. C., & Evans, K. (2000). *Psychotherapy supervision: An integrative relational approach to psychotherapy supervision.* London: Open University Press.

Hawkins, P., & Shohet, R. (2000). *Supervision in the helping professions* (2nd ed.). Maidenhead, Philadelphia: Open University Press.

Lampropoulos, G. K. (2002). A common factors view of counseling supervision process. *The Clinical Supervisor, 21*(1), 77–92.

McMahon, M. (2002). Some supervision practicalities. In M. McMahon & W. Patton (Eds.), *Supervision in the helping professions: A practical approach* (pp. 17–26). Frenchs Forest, NSW: Pearson Education.

McNeill, B. W., & Worthen, V. (1989). The parallel process in supervision. *Professional Psychology Research and Practice, 20*(5), 329–333.

Morrissey, J., & Tribe, R. (2001). Parallel process in supervision. *Counselling Psychology Quarterly, 14,* 103–110.

Nezu, A. M., Saad, R., & Nezu, C. M. (2000). Clinical decision making in behavioral supervision. *Cognitive and Behavioral Practice, 7,* 338–342.

Norcross, J. C., & Lambert, M. J. (2011). Evidence-based therapy relationships. In J. C. Norcross (Ed.), *Psychotherapy relationships that work: Evidence-based responsiveness* (2nd ed., pp. 3–21). New York: Oxford University Press.

Olk, M. E., & Friedlander, M. L. (1992). Trainees' experiences of role conflict and role ambiguity in supervisory relationships. *Journal of Counseling Psychology, 39,* 389–397.

Pearson, Q. (2000). Opportunities and challenges in the supervisory relationship: Implications for counselor supervision. *Journal of Mental health Counseling, 24,* 283–294.

Pearson, Q. (2004). Getting the most out of clinical supervision: Strategies for mental health. *Journal of Mental Health Counseling, 26*(4), 361–373.

Redfield, R., Linton, R., & Herskovits, M. J. (1936). Memorandum on the study of acculturation. *American Anthropologist, 56,* 973–1002.

Renfro-Michel, E. L. (2006). *A relationship between counselling supervisee attachment and supervision working alliance rapport* (Doctoral dissertation, Mississippi State University). Dissertation Abstracts International.

Renfro-Michel, E. L., & Sheperis, C. J. (2009).The relationship between counseling trainee attachment orientation and perceived bond with supervisor. *Clinical Supervisor, 28,* 141–154. doi:10.1080/07325220903324306

Ronnestad, M. H., & Skovholt, T. M. (1993). Supervision of beginning and advanced graduate students of counseling and psychotherapy. *Journal of Counseling and Development, 71,* 396–405.

Safran, J. D., & Muran, J. C. (2000). *Negotiating the therapeutic alliance: A relational treatment guide.* New York: Guilford.

Southern, S. (2007). Countertransference and intersubjectivity: Golden opportunities in clinical supervision. *Sexual Addiction and Compulsivity, 14,* 279–302.

Vogel, D. L., & Webster. S. R. (2003). To seek help or not to seek help: The risks of self-disclosure. *Journal of Counseling Psychology, 50*(3), 351–361.

Waugaman, R. M. (2015). Searles's discovery of the parallel process in supervision. *Psychiatry: Interpersonal and Biological Processes, 78*(3), 225–230.

Webb, C. A., DeRubeis, R. J., Amsterdam, J. D., Shelton, R. C., Hollon, S. D., & Dimidjian, S. (2011). Two aspects of the therapeutic alliance: Differential relations with depressive symptom change. *Journal of Consulting and Clinical Psychology, 79*(3), 279–283.

Wrape, E. R. (2015). *Attachment theory within clinical supervision: Application of the conceptual to the empirical* (Unpublished doctoral dissertation, University of North Texas).

Yalom, I. D. (2001). *The gift of therapy: An open letter to a new generation of therapists and their patients.* New York: HarperCollins.

17 Supervisor Development

Nadine Pelling and Elisa Agostinelli

Introduction

The practice of clinical supervision has an established history (Bernard & Goodyear, 1997). It was the first educational method in which more experienced colleagues would supervise new and less experienced colleagues to increase their knowledge and competence as practitioners. It was also a way for colleagues to meet and discuss particularly difficult client cases and monitor their own responses to particular issues.

Today the practice of supervision has become more structured and complex. Dealing with supervisee's personal, professional, and ethical issues is not an easy task. It can be difficult to live up to supervisee expectations. Supervision can also be exhausting as, "during the process of supervision, Supervisors make their personality, acquired clinical and theoretical knowledge, and emotional and mental resources available to the learning process" (Yerushalmi, 1999, p. 427).

Recently the idea of supervising supervisors and aiding in their development has emerged in our profession as a possible support for supervisors, but also as a way to control the quality of supervision offered (Ellis, 2006; Emilsson & Johnsson, 2007). It is now widely recognized that supervisors of counsellors can benefit from supervision (Emilsson & Johnsson, 2007; BAC, 1996; BACP, 2007). This recognition fulfils Styczynski's (1980) assertion years ago that as the field of supervision developed, more attention would have to be paid to the training and credentials of supervisors. In other words, if an informed perspective on clinical supervision is to be obtained then an understanding of supervisory development must also be obtained (Watkins, 1997a). This chapter outlines a popular model of supervisor development and then reviews four main influences on supervisory development.

Supervisor development

In most supervisory developmental models, supervisors progress from being vulnerable and anxious about supervising to becoming more autonomous supervisors wherein a supervisory identity takes form (Watkins, 1995a, 1995b, 1995d). At earlier stages of their own development supervisors require more structure and a more secure holding environment, whereas at later stages of development the developing supervisor requires more of a collaborative relationship with their supervisor of supervision (Watkins, 1995a, 1995b, 1995d). Both of these statements are true for the Supervisory Complexity Model as outlined as follows.

DOI: 10.4324/9781003490067-21

Supervisor Complexity Model

The most written about and elaborate model of supervisor development is the Supervisor Complexity Model (SCM). This model was based on the counsellor development models by Hogan (1964) and Stoltenberg (1981), later further developed into the IDM of Stoltenberg, McNeill, and Delworth (1998). According to the SCM (Watkins, 1990a, 1990b, 1993, 1994, 1995a, 1995b, 1995c, 1995d; Hillman, McPherson, Swank, & Watkins, 1998), supervisors progress through four different stages of development in their progression from novice to more competent and expert supervisors. During each of these stages supervisors have specific tasks to accomplish and responsibilities (Watkins, Schneider, Haynes, & Nieberding, 1995). At each stage the supervisor develops greater professional identity, increased acceptance of the supervisee, a less dogmatic approach regarding theory, and an increasing confidence in supervisory skills. Development is viewed as both qualitative and quantitative in nature. Development occurs in the form of an increased sense of professional identity.

Stage One: Role Sock. This stage is encountered by a new supervisor when first entering the supervisor role and is characterized by questions of role boundaries and definitions. Counsellors may feel like imposter supervisors and wonder if they are professionals or students. Supervisors at this stage are also likely to be concrete in their provision of supervision and thus interventions may appear superficial in nature. Supervisors of supervision trainees at this stage of development are best advised to provide a clear and strong holding environment and thus provide a stabilizing and soothing function for supervision trainees. Supervision trainees need to be helped to define the supervision relationship at this stage of development.

Stage Two: Role Recovery and Transition. This stage is characterized by a more realistic perception of one's weaknesses and strengths as a supervisor. Some confidence in one's abilities as a supervisor develops. However, process and transference/countertransference issues are still not well addressed by supervisors at this stage of development. Supervisors of supervision trainees are urged to loosen the hold of their relationship with the supervision trainee at this stage of development and encourage the trainee's development of autonomy.

Stage Three: Role Consolidation. At this stage supervisors have reached a level of increasing consistency in their supervision provision. Supervisors at this level are more realistic about their strengths and weaknesses and can function as a resource for counselling trainees. Supervisors of supervision trainees at this level are more likely to adequately address transference, process, and countertransference issues with their counselling trainees.

Stage Four: Role Mastery. A supervisor at this stage has a sense of mastery about their supervisory competence. Various issues can be addressed competently by supervisors at this level. If supervision is provided for supervisors at this level it is likely to be collaborative, challenging in nature, and on an as-needed basis.

Possible influences on supervisory development

There are four main influences on supervisory competence: personal variables, counselling experience, supervisory training, and supervisory experience.

Personal and relational factors

Looking at fitness to practice, the personal characteristics of the counsellor trainee "invariably affect the supervisory and treatment process" (Haber, 1996, p. 21). According to Bernard and Goodyear (1997), personal growth is part of supervision. It is important to encourage counsellor trainees' personal growth as they learn to encourage parallel growth in their clients (Emerson, 1996). Edwards and Bess (1998) stated, "the development of a therapist's self-awareness must carry at least as much weight in his or her professional education and training as the accumulation of knowledge about theories and methodologies established by the leaders of the profession" (p. 98). R. N. Wendt (Personal communication November 17, 1999) stated that if the therapist measures her self-growth based on her perceived competence as professional, personal development may be impeded. Consequently, counsellor trainees need a training process that integrates personal and technical competencies (Aponte & Winter, 2000).

Systemic theories focus on the person of the therapist in training as a parallel process to the clinical intervention and underline the importance of stimulating therapists in training to critically observe themselves (Andolfi, 2022). Personal issues are seen as potential 'handicaps' and resources at the same time. They are considered 'handicaps' when they prevent the counsellor trainee in establishing a therapeutic relationship with the client and seeing the underlying dynamics between the members of the client-family. They are considered resources when they facilitate the counsellor trainee in making a shift in the affective relationship between members of the client-family (Andolfi,1985). Wendt (1997) suggested that to be able to achieve greater self-awareness and open the boundaries to personal transformation, counsellors and supervisors need to experience vulnerability and failure in their professional life. Through the discussion of personal issues during counselling training, the supervisor may identify counsellor trainees that are hampered in their performance as counsellors because their personal issues are too great to be overcome (Bernard & Goodyear, 1997). This can be a delicate and difficult decision for a supervisor to make and the possibility to discuss the issue with another colleague during the supervision of supervisors could make the process more objective. In addition, to be able to look at the supervisees' personal issues, the supervisors need to constantly look at his or her personal issues and how they affect his work as a supervisor.

Supervisors need to "develop their own capacities for self-observation and to learn more about their own strength and weaknesses" (Whitman & Jacobs, 1998, p. 172). The literature in relational neurobiology has made great strides, the concept of co-regulation in therapy is an essential element that promotes growth and allows changes (Porges, 2007). Specifically, if we are experiencing the conscious or unconscious sympathetic arousal of fear and are unable to recognise and/or regulate it, our ability to judge the situation and create a safe therapeutic environment for our clients will be compromised and consequently the therapeutic relationship impaired (Siegal, 2021). As counsellors, we have to be aware of our reactions and our own limits. We need to be able to recognize that we cannot work with certain kind of clients because of our personal experience or because of specific issues we are going through in a specific time of our life. According to Aponte and Winter (2000), counsellors' effectiveness is not only related to what the counsellor has been able to resolve in his or her life, but also to what the counsellor has learned to recognize and work with in his or her self. "By resolving individual issues, or by learning to work with unchangeable or unresolved issues, a clinician attains greater freedom and ability in the use of self with clients" (Aponte & Winter, 2000, p. 148).

If we think about a therapy session, "ultimately, our single most important instrument is the person we are" (Corey, 2001, p. 38). Competent counsellors are counsellors that are able to recognize their own limitations and refer the client to someone else. As supervisor we have to do the same. Professionally and personally, we cannot be fit to interact with every supervisee. We have to be able to recognize that some of our personal issues in specific times of our life can interfere with our supervisory work with specific supervisees. In this case we need to be able to recognize the problem and refer the supervisee to another supervisor. "Supervisors should be aware that they are participants in the supervisory process, and that their style, inner conflicts, or enactments may directly affect the supervisory relationship and patient treatment" (Whitman & Jacobs, 1998, p. 172). However, at times supervisors may not be able to recognize the effect of their personal issues on the supervisory relationship. Therefore, it is essential for supervisor to have supervision so they can be helped to recognize the reasons for possible impasse in the supervisory relationship and assure a quality services to the counsellor and a safe and effective treatment to the client.

Discussion of personal issues during counselling training reduces the prospect of burnout and increases successful therapeutic outcome (Aponte & Winter, 2000). Similarly, the discussion of personal issues can help the burnout of supervisors. Fear and Woolfe (1999) found that counsellors need to "integrate the epistemological beliefs of their chosen orientation with personal philosophy" (p. 254). If this does not occur it may lead to "a loss of optimal functioning, or in the individual suffering a level of intrapsychic conflict which in turn may result in burnout or abandonment of career" (Fear & Woolfe, 1999, p. 256).

According to Gee (1996), part of the supervisory process is the interpretation of the counsellor trainee's countertransference in relation to the client's transference. In doing so, the supervisor has to focus on aspects of counsellor trainees' personal development related to the relationship between the counsellor trainee and the client, and not on other aspects of their personal development. In the psychoanalytic orientation, countertransference refers to the counsellor's personal issues and "knowing that a counsellor reaction emanates from an area of unresolved conflict requires the counsellor to examine his or her own personal issues" (Rosenberger & Hayes, 2002, p. 269). The supervisor should help the counsellor trainee examine personal issues, but only if these issues relate to problems occurring in the therapeutic relationship between counsellor trainee and client. The focus of recent psychodynamic supervision is to examine and explore during the supervisory experience the intrapersonal and interpersonal dynamics that occur between counsellor trainee and client. "Intrapersonal dynamics consist of covert behaviors and sensory processes such as feelings, thoughts, and perceptions" (Bradley, 1989, p. 68). The supervisor has to focus on counsellor trainees' reactions to clients' transference / countertransference issues. He or she has to be aware of transference and countertransference dynamics between and client that could cause an impasse in the therapeutic process (Borders & Leddick, 1987).

Because of the nature of the relationship, it is likely that counsellor trainees' resistance emerges during the supervisory session and the interpretation of this dynamic by the supervisor is a therapeutic necessity (Bradley, 1989). The processes that occur in the relationship between patient and therapist are often reflected in the relationship between therapist and supervisors (please see the chapter on Alliance Supervision to Enhance Client Outcomes for further discussion of this topic). This is called parallel process, and it is the most unique dynamic in supervision. The same dynamic could occur during supervision of supervisors: A beginner supervisor can experience parallel issues from her own supervision session with a beginner counsellor when she has her own supervision of supervision (Stoltenberg & Delworth, 1987). In this case it is essential that a third parson (the supervisor of supervisors) will analyse and interpret the dynamic between supervisee and supervisor.

Where is the line between therapy and supervision relating to personal and relational variables? Aponte (1992) tried to define the line between supervision and therapy, stating that "because the trainers … consistently redirect the focus of personal exploration to clinical practice, they do not become personal therapists" (p. 275). The supervisor points out to the student the problem he or she had during the session, and connects the problem with the student's personal issues and family issues (Aponte, 1992). This should be translated into the supervision of supervisor relationship.

Counselling experience

Many believe that to be a competent supervisor one must be a competent counsellor. Styczynski (1980) reports that therapist skills are important as they can be imparted to the trainee and also because many of the skills successful in therapeutic interventions are also relevant to the supervisory relationship to "optimize change and development of the student" (p. 31). Watson (1997a, 1997b) echoes this sentiment.

Whereas being a competent counsellor may be a necessary component of being a competent supervisor, counselling skills do not sufficiently enable one to work as an effective supervisor (Farrell, 1996; Watkins, 1991; Watkins et al., 1995). Indeed, Stoltenberg, McNeill, and Delworth (1998) indicate that being a counsellor does not sufficiently enable one to supervisor others' work. Thus, training and experience as a supervisor are also viewed as important aspects of developing supervisory competence in conjunction with counsellor development (Stoltenberg & Delworth, 1987; Pelling, 2008, 2021). Research supports the idea that counsellors develop as they gain experience, namely supervised experience. Similarly, supervisors are expected to develop a more balanced view of themselves and their supervisees as they develop (Watkins, 1993).

Supervisory training

Many authors indicate that training in supervision is needed for therapists to develop their supervisory skills (Bernard & Goodyear, 1992; Farrell, 1996; Stoltenberg & Delworth, 1987; Watkins, 1997a, 1997b). Research also supports the need for training by indicating that systematic training is more likely to facilitate counsellor growth than less systematic training (Lambert & Ogles, 1997). Some authors also advocate that continuing education should be sought by those who perform supervision (Davies, 1997). As indicated by Stoltenberg and Delworth (1987, p. 154) "It seems reasonable at this point to believe that higher functioning supervisors are more effective and that, as with counseling skills, training may improve supervisor functioning." However, as Watkins (1991) states there is a paradox in psychotherapy supervision training, namely, while the supervisory role is considered important, training in how to be a supervisor is very limited.

The SCM specifically identifies training as an agent capable of advancing supervisory identity and skill development, as it can aid the acquisition of competencies in interventions and appropriate supervisory tasks and roles. Supervisory training could be especially helpful for supervisors in the first stage of supervisory development, role shock.

Such training can serve as a buffer for supervisors by indicating what the transition from counsellor to supervisor might entail.

Supervisory experience

Experience as a supervisor has long been believed to have a positive influence on one's development as a supervisor (Stoltenberg & Delworth, 1987). Research supports the idea that supervisory experience can aid supervisory development. Stone (1980) as well as Marikis, Russell, and Dell (1985) indicate that more experienced supervisors made more planning statements. However, Watkins (1993) points out that research indicates that supervisors may not develop and become more competent simply because they conduct supervision. Nevertheless, the more supervisory experience a supervisor accumulates the greater opportunity the supervisory will have to confront more developmental challenges and issues and thus prompt supervisory identity development.

It is possible that supervised supervision experience aids one's development as a supervisor more than independent experience due to the greater amount of reflection, support, and feedback provided by the additional supervisory relationship. Supervision of supervision can provide attachment components that allow for safety and exploration of supervisory behaviours.

Conclusion

Supervision has a long history in the therapeutic professions. Recently the importance of developing supervisors and supporting them in their work has become recognised. Supervisors of supervisors and supervisors of clinicians need to address personal and relational variables, be experienced clinicians, engage in professional developmental training in relation to supervision, and can also benefit from supervision of their own supervision. Reflective practice with clients and/or supervisees means continuous and lifelong learning as well as development.

Acknowledgement

The contents of the present chapter have been previously published in part as follows:

Pelling, N. (2008). The relationship of supervisory experience, counselling experience, and training in supervision to supervisory identity development. *International Journal for the Advancement of Counselling*, 30(4), 235–248.
Schofield, M., & Pelling, N. (2002). Supervision of counsellors. In M. McMahon & W. Patton (Eds.), *Supervision in the helping professions: A practical approach* (pp. 211–222). NSW: Prentice Hall.

Educational questions & activities

1. What does the Supervisor Complexity Model have to say about supervisor development?
2. What are the SCM stages?
3. List four influences on supervisory competence.
4. Which of the four variables above do you see as most influential and why?

References

Andolfi, M. (1985). L'hadicap dello studente come strumento di formazione. In M. Andolfi & D. Piccone (Eds.), *La formazione relazionale: Individuo e gruppo nel processo di apprendimento* (pp. 218–238). Rome: I.T. F.

Andolfi, M. (2022). *The Gift of truth: The inner journey of the therapist.* Rome: Academia Press.

Aponte, H. J. (1992). Training the person of the therapist in structural family therapy. *Journal of Marital and Family Therapy*, 19(3), 269–281.

Aponte, H. J., & Winter, J. E. (2000). The person and the practice of the therapist: Treatment and training. In M. Baldwin (Ed.), *The use of self in therapy* (pp. 127–165). New York: The Haworth.

Bernard, J. M., & Goodyear, R. K. (1992). *Fundamentals of clinical supervision.* Boston: Allyn & Bacon.

Bernard, J. M., & Goodyear, R. K. (1997). *Fundamentals of clinical supervision* (2nd ed.). Boston: Allyn & Bacon.

Borders, L., & Leddick, G. R. (1987). *Handbook of counseling supervision.* Alexandria, VA: Association for Counselor Education and Supervision.

Bradley, L. J. (1989). *Counselor supervision: Principles, process, and practice* (2nd ed.). Muncie, IN: Accelerated Development Inc.

British Association for Counselling (BAC). (1996). *Code of ethics and practice for supervisors of counsellors.* Rugby: BAC.

British Association for Counselling and Psychotherapy. (2007). *Ethical framework for good practice in counselling and psychotherapy.* Leicestershire: BACP.

Corey, G. (2001). *Theory and practice of counseling and psychotherapy* (6th ed.). Pacific Grove, CA: Brooks/Cole.

Davies, D. (1997). *Counselling in psychological services.* Buckingham: Open University Press.

Edwards, J. K., & Bess, J. M. (1998). Developing effectiveness in the therapeutic use of self. *Clinical Social Work Journal*, 26, 89–105.

Ellis, M. V. (2006). Critical incidents in clinical supervision and in supervisor supervision: Assessing supervisory issues. *Training and Education in Professional Psychology*, 8(2), 122–132.

Emerson, S. (1996). Creating a safe place for growth in supervision. *Contemporary Family Therapy*, 18, 393–403.

Emilsson, U. M., & Johnsson E. (2007). Supervision of supervisors: On developing supervision in postgraduate education. *Higher Education Research & Development*, 26, 163–179.

Farrell, W. (1996). Training and professional development in the context of counselling psychology. In R. Wolfe & W. Dryden (Eds.), *Handbook of counselling psychology* (pp. 581–604). London: Sage.

Fear, R., & Woolfe, R. (1999). The personal and professional development of counselors: The relationship between personal philosophy and theoretical orientation. *Counselling Psychology Quarterly*, 12, 253–262.

Gee, H. (1996). Developing insight through supervision: Relating, than defining. *Journal of Analytical Psychology*, 41, 529–552.

Haber, R. (1996). *Dimensions of psychotherapy supervision: Maps and means.* New York: W. W. Norton & Company.

Hillman, S. L., McPherson, R. H., Swank, P. R., & Watkins, C. E. J. (1998). Further validation of the Psychotherapy Supervisor Development Scale. *The Clinical Supervisor*, 17(1), 17–32.

Hogan, R. A. (1964). Issues and approach in supervision. *Psychotherapy, Theory, Research, and Practice*, 1, 139–141.

Lambert, M., & Ogles, B. (1997). The effectiveness of psychotherapy supervision. In C. E. Watkins (Ed.), *Handbook of Psychotherapy Supervision* (pp. 421–446). New York: John Wiley & Sons.

Marikis, D. A., Russell, R. K., & Dell, D. M. (1985). Effects of supervisory experience level on planning and in session verbal behavior. *Journal of Counseling Psychology*, 30, 403–412.

Pelling, N. (2008). The relationship of supervisory experience, counselling experience, and training in supervision to supervisory identity development. *International Journal for the Advancement of Counselling*, 30(4), 235–248.

Pelling, N. (2021). Singaporean supervisory identity development and its relationship to supervisory experience, counselling experience, and training in supervision. *Asia Pacific Journal of Counselling and Psychotherapy*, 12(2), 186–204. https://doi.org/10.1080/21507686.2021.1960400

Porges, S. W. (2007). The polyvagal perspective. *Biological Psychology*, 74, 116–143. https://doi.org/10.1016/j.biopsycho.2006.06.009

Rosenberger, E. W., & Hayes, J. A. (2002). Therapists as subject: A review of the empirical countertransference literature. *Journal of Counselling and Development*, 80, 264–270.

Siegel, D. J. (2021) Interpersonal neurobiology from the inside out. In A. N. Schore, D. J. Siegel, & L. J. Cozolino (Eds.), *Interpersonal neurobiology and clinical practice*. New York: WW Norton.Stoltenberg, C., & Delworth, U. (1987). *Supervising counselors and therapists: A developmental approach*. San Francisco: Jossey-Bass.

Stoltenberg, C., McNeill, B., & Delworth, U. (1998). *IDM Supervision: An integrated developmental model for supervising counselors and therapists*. San Francisco: Jossey-Bass.

Stoltenberg, C. D. (1981). Approaching supervision from a developmental perspective: The counselor complexity model. *Journal of Counseling Psychology*, 28, 59–65.

Stone, G. L. (1980). Effects of experience on supervision planning. *Journal of Counseling Psychology*, 27, 84–88.

Styczynski, L. (1980). The transition from supervisee to supervisor. In A. Hell (Ed.), *Psychotherapy supervision: Theory, research & practice* (pp. 29–40). New York: John Wiley & Sons.

Watkins, C. (1990a). Development of the psychotherapy supervisor. *Psychotherapy*, 27(4), 553–560.

Watkins, C. (1990b). The separation-individuation process in psychotherapy supervision. *Psychotherapy*, 27(2), 202–209.

Watkins, C. (1991). Reflections on the preparation of psychotherapy supervision. *Journal of Clinical Psychology*, 47(6), 145–147.

Watkins, C. (1993). Development of the psychotherapy supervisor: Concepts, assumptions, and hypotheses of the supervisor complexity model. *American Journal of Psychotherapy*, 47(1), 58–74.

Watkins, C. (1994). The supervision of psychotherapy supervisor trainees. *American Journal of Psychotherapy*, 48(3), 417–431.

Watkins, C. (1995a). Psychotherapy supervision in the 1990s: Some observations and reflections. *American Journal of Psychotherapy*, 49(4), 568–581.

Watkins, C. (1995b). Psychotherapy supervisor and supervisee: Developmental models and research nine years later. *Clinical Psychology Review*, 17(7), 647–680.

Watkins, C. (1995c). Psychotherapy supervisor development: On musings, models, and metaphor. *The Journal of Psychotherapy Practice and Research*, 4, 150–158.

Watkins, C. (1995d). Researching psychotherapy supervisor development: Four key considerations. *The Clinical Supervisor*, 13(2), 139.

Watkins, C. (1997a). *Handbook of psychotherapy supervision*. New York: John Wiley & Sons.

Watkins, C. (1997b). The ineffective psychotherapy supervisor: Some reflections about bad behaviors, poor process, and offensive outcomes. *The Clinical Supervisor*, 16(1), 163–180.

Watkins, C., Schneider, L., Haynes, J., & Nieberding, R. (1995). Measuring psychotherapy supervisor development: An initial effort at scale development and validation. *The Clinical Supervisor*, 13(1), 77–90.

Wendt, R. N. (1997). Failure, loss, and marginalization: Toward therapist transformation and thera-peutic honesty. Unpublished paper presented at the IX International Family therapy Association World Conference, Jerusalem, March 9–13, 1997.

Whitman, S. M., & Jacobs, E. G. (1998).Responsibilities of the psychotherapy supervisor. *American Journal of Psychotherapy*, 52(2), 166–175.

Yerushalmi, H. (1999). The roles of group supervision of supervision. *Psychoanalytic Psychology*, 16, 426–447.

18 Multicultural Counselling Supervision

Strengthening Learning and Practice Applications

Nancy Arthur

Multicultural counselling: Identities, social location, and social justice

During the past 25 years, multiculturalism gained momentum as the fourth force (Pedersen, 1999), following psychodynamic, behaviourist, and humanist movements. Renewed interest in social justice and advocacy has contributed to the fifth force, expanding approaches to education, training, and supervision in multicultural counselling (Cohen et al., 2021). Frameworks were developed to enhance multicultural counselling competencies in domains of self-awareness, knowledge, and skills (e.g., Arredondo et al., 1996; Sue et al., 1982, 1998) and the integration of those three domains across core competencies (Collins & Arthur, 2010a, 2010b). Another major shift occurred from defining some clients as culturally diverse (Sue & Sue, 1999) to recognising the complexities and intersections of identities, across time and across contexts, for all people (Arthur, 2018a). There has been greater emphasis on the social processes involved in defining cultural identities and how people are positioned in society with more or less privilege or disadvantage (Ratts et al., 2015), commonly referred to as people's social location.

The call for counsellors to be prepared for multicultural counselling has also raised many questions about the best ways to prepare new counsellors and enhance the competency development of experienced counsellors. Supervision is an important learning context for fostering multicultural cultural competencies. Given that the central goal of supervision is to improve the welfare of clients (Bernard & Goodyear, 2019), the goal of multicultural counselling supervision is to increase the responsiveness of counsellors to all clients, regardless of their life contexts and social locations. Multicultural counselling supervision is a key resource for learning about cultural influences through the supervisory relationship, for enhancing the training experiences of supervisees, and supporting more satisfying supervisory relationships (Constantine, 2003; Crockett & Hays, 2015; Pope-Davis et al., 2003).

Counsellors are encouraged to enhance their preparation for multicultural counselling competence and supervisors are invited to examine their level of preparation for multicultural counselling supervision. The purpose of this chapter is to introduce readers to multicultural counselling supervision and ways to enhance the competency development of supervisors and supervisees. First, the discussion focuses on the broader context of multicultural counselling as ethical practice. Second, perspectives on multicultural counselling supervision are reviewed. Third, some of the challenges associated with learning and development in multicultural counselling supervision are noted. Fourth, case vignettes are offered to illustrate some of the complexities involved in supervisory relationships. At the end of the chapter, reflection questions and some suggested resources are offered. Supervisors and supervisees who read this chapter are encouraged to reflect about ways to

DOI: 10.4324/9781003490067-22

positively engage in exploration of cultural identities, social locations, and social justice as key concepts that underpin ethical practices for multicultural counselling and for multicultural counselling supervision.

Multicultural counselling competency frameworks

Multicultural counselling competence is essential for ethical professional practice and to avoid unintentional forms of oppression with clients (Arredondo & Toporek, 2004; Arthur, 2018a; Pettifor et al., 2011). However, competence is not an end point or final point of achievement. Rather it is an aspirational goal associated with continuous learning and professional development. As noted in the introduction, the field of multicultural counselling has grown considerably. New perspectives, tools, and resources are likely to follow, informing professional learning and practices that underpin ethical practices. A brief review of the broader context of multicultural counselling is offered to set the backdrop for examining advances in multicultural counselling supervision.

Competency frameworks for multicultural counselling have been introduced and revised over several decades. Foundational frameworks were developed by members of the Division of Counseling Psychology of the American Psychological Association (APA), specifically Sue and colleagues (1982, 1998) and Arredondo and colleagues (1996). Although the competencies have continued to evolve over time and have been applied in documents, such as the American Psychological Association (APA, 2003) *Guidelines on Multicultural Education, Training, Research, Practice, and Organizational Change for Psychologists*, the basic model has remained relatively stable over time. Three core categories have been identified as essential to the development of multicultural counselling competence: (a) awareness of one's own cultural assumptions, values, and biases; (b) understanding of client worldviews and perspectives; and (c) implementation of interventions strategies and techniques that are appropriate to the cultural context of the client (Sue et al., 1992). The emphasis on multicultural counselling and advocacy led to updates in competency frameworks to include advocacy competencies connect multicultural counselling and social justice advocacy (Arthur, 2018b; Ratts et al., 2016).

Although the seminal competency frameworks represented advances in the field of multicultural counselling at the time they were developed, there has been critique about their utility and scope (Cohen et al., 2021). First, the definition of what constitutes culture and who 'counts' as culturally diverse (Sue & Sue, 1999) has evolved over time with an emphasis on various populations. For example, the emphasis on race and ethnicity in the early frameworks led to debate about which populations are categorised as culturally diverse, for example, when there are visible differences between the counsellor and client, when presumably the counsellor is White and middle-class. This focus fails to take into account the importance of other salient dimensions of cultural identity such as gender, ability, sexual orientation, age, religion, socioeconomic status and their intersections.

Second, in a more inclusive approach to cultural identity, counsellors are encouraged to explore the complexities of people's cultural identities and their social locations.

'Multicultural complexity' is used herein to refer to the intricacies and convolutions represented by the intersections of multiple grounds of identity, privilege, and marginalization, which define social, historical, and political dimensions for different populations and communities.

(Peters, 2017, p. 2)

Counsellors need to be mindful about the ways that identity might shift across contexts and over time, in response to interactions between members of dominant and non-dominant groups in our society. It is not membership in any one cultural group that is the focus, as knowledge about group membership is not a very reliable source of information about any individual's personal experiences and sense of identity (Petersen et al., 2008). Multicultural counselling is complex as clients may hold multiple identities that become more or less salient in different types of social interactions and shift power relations between people. This is not only a result of which aspects of identity individuals present, but also because some aspects of their identities may be emphasised by other people in social interactions (Arthur, 2018a) Exploration of cultural identity needs to be viewed through the lens of what individuals perceive to be relevant for them, and how they have been positioned by other people in their life experiences. Power dynamics in society lead to varying degrees of privilege and/or marginalisation (Ratts et al., 2015). Over time, people's social location can shift along with changing social status and access to resources.

Third, another common criticism is the risk of an overreliance in multicultural counselling on the application of intervention strategies and techniques derived from competency frameworks (Collins & Arthur, 2010a). Yet, the working alliance is one of the most significant predictors of counselling outcomes (Roysircar et al., 2003; Wampold, 2015). It is through the context of the working alliance and client that the identities of counsellors and clients come together, with the potential for exploration and learning that can improve counselling outcomes. The working alliance was emphasised as a core domain in the original model of culture-infused counselling (Collins & Arthur, 2010a, 2010b) and subsequently applied to the supervisory relationship (Arthur & Collins, 2016; 2017).

Fourth, there is little agreement about how multicultural and social justice competencies should be integrated into curriculum (Cohen et al.). This means that the call for multicultural and social justice approaches in counselling needs to be matched by innovation in pedagogy and evaluation of its effectiveness. Research is also needed to document the process and outcomes of competency development, including demonstration of enhanced outcomes for clients.

Multicultural counselling supervision

Although the terms multicultural supervision and cross-cultural supervision have often been used interchangeably in the literature on supervision, they are not the same. The term cross-cultural supervision emphasises variation in approaches to supervision across different contexts, within and across countries. The term multicultural supervision 'alludes to the study and practice of supervision in and for different cultures. Multicultural supervision would involve the study of different cultural patterns of supervision as pertaining to its content, process, and outcomes' (Brown & Landrum-Brown, 1995, p. 264). These important distinctions invite counsellors to learn about the practices of supervision across countries and contexts, while recognising this is a different pursuit than engaging in multicultural counselling supervision.

There are various ways that supervision has been characterised in the multicultural counselling literature. Readers may notice some similarities between the development of models and competencies in the field of multicultural counselling. In early perspectives, the supervision process emphasised the best ways to support clients who present with diverse cultural identities. For example, supervision might entail discussions of client issues, presenting concerns, and ways to enhance the applications of counselling approaches for working across cultural contexts. Supervision might also focus on the counsellor–client dyad in order to enhance an effective therapeutic alliance.

There have been debates about the pros and cons of trying to match counsellors and clients based on their background experiences and some aspects of their experiences, e.g., ethnicity, gender. Matching has been critiqued on the bases that is a superficial, often based on arbitrary assumptions and stereotypes. There is general agreement that counsellor–client matches ignore the intersectionality of people's cultural identities and variation in their lived experience (Ertl et al., 2019). Similarly, it is impossible to completely match supervisors and supervisees based on assumptions about their lived experience or affiliation to particular groups in society. Arguably, there will also be relative similarities and differences in the worldviews and cultural identities held by supervisors and supervisees. Each supervisory relationship supervision is considered to be a cultural encounter as people's background and life experiences are never exactly the same (Falicov, 2014). As general principles, all counselling relationships and all supervisory relationships are multicultural relationships. Here we see another perspective on supervision, as the focus shifts to the cultural dynamics that exist between the counsellor/supervisee and the supervisor. An underlying assumption is that culture is a central force in the interpersonal process of supervision (Chen, 2001). From this perspective, supervision takes place within a multicultural relationship. Due to their personal life experiences, affiliations, and experiences of privilege and/or marginalisation, supervisees and their supervisors inevitably hold different worldviews that have been shaped over their life course.

A third, and more dynamic perspective, takes into account the interplay of cultural forces that shape the professional relationships in the triadic process between clients, counsellors/supervisees, and their supervisors. There will be relative similarities and differences between individuals involved in a client–counsellor–supervisor triad. From this perspective, multicultural counselling supervision incorporates the interactions among all three parties. Returning to an earlier point raised, the central priority in supervision is to ensure the welfare of clients. Presumably, addressing cultural influences in the counsellor/supervisee–supervisor relationship can facilitate a stronger supervisory process and also improve the delivery of multicultural counselling to clients.

In practice, discussions of cultural identities and social locations through the supervisory relationship can be leveraged as a dual process for exploring these concepts with clients. Arguably, exploration of clients' worldviews are essential for designing ethical and effective counselling goals and processes. Through supervision, modelling reflective practice is aimed at helping supervisees to consider multiple understandings of client behavior and appropriate interventions. The parallel process of developing a relationship between supervisors and supervisees sets the foundation for important competency development. Multicultural supervision from this perspective emphasises exploring complexities in the worldviews and expectations held by clients, supervisees, and supervisors (Vasquez, 2014).

Connecting Multicultural Counselling, Advocacy, and Social Justice

There are strong connections between multicultural competence, social justice, and advocacy that need to be integrated into supervision practices (Dollarhike et al., 2021; Fickling et al., 2019). Many presenting issues in counselling have been developed in contexts where forms of oppression, such as racism, sexism, classism, and homophobia, heavily influence people's mental health and well-being. Clients' concerns may be presented as an individual problem, but the roots of the problem are often connected to social and structural inequalities (Arthur, 2018a).

Unfortunately, when counsellors and supervisors hold stereotypes, these are often enacted as microaggressions that may not be intentional but are harmful in professional relationships (Fernandes & Lane, 2020). Counsellors have an ethical prerogative in their roles and responsibilities for identifying social and political influences on their clients' concerns. The actions or inactions of counsellors are not neutral, and have been framed as political actions (Arthur & Collins, 2014), often bounded by organisational constraints and funding mandates of the agencies where they are employed. Unfortunately, counsellors may have limitations on the degree to which they can actively address the sources of distress in people's lives. There are ethical considerations to be made when counsellors exercise their professional power in ways that perpetuate social and political conditions through helping clients to adjust to the conditions that create mental health issues (Kennedy & Arthur, 2014). In contrast, counsellors are expected to use their professional knowledge for engaging in social justice advocacy to address the systems that are pervasive for negative mental health outcomes.

Connections between multicultural and social justice perspectives sparked the development of new models and competency frameworks. For example, the integration of ecological approaches with multicultural counselling led to the articulation of multiple levels of advocacy competencies (Ratts et al., 2016). During the same time period, the original model of culture-infused counselling (Collins & Arthur, 2010a) was expanded to incorporate a domain that focused on socially just and responsive professional practices. The emphasis on social justice advocacy highlights the important roles that counsellors have for designing relevant interventions to address multiple systems of influence on client's presenting issues, integrating cultural context, identities, and social justice (Arthur, 2018c).

With advancements in the conceptualisation of multicultural counselling, the definitions of multicultural supervision have also shifted to incorporate a stronger social justice orientation. For example, Kemer et al. (2021, p. 2) offered and updated perspective:

> Multicultural supervision is defined as the process through which supervisors can support examining attitudes and beliefs, knowledge, skills, and actions regarding how singular and multiplistic privileged and marginalized identities (e.g., race, disability, nationality, affectional orientation), social structures (e.g., laws, politics), and social-ecological systems (e.g., microsystem, macrosystem, chronosystem) influence the counseling and supervisory processes, relationships, and stakeholders (Falender et al., 2013; Peters, 2017).

This definition highlights the major shift that has occurred from positioning culture as a fixed identity in specific populations deemed to be culturally diverse. Contemporary perspectives acknowledge the complexity and intersections of identities, social structures and social ecologies that are relevant for counselling and for supervision processes. In turn, supervisors have responsibilities for helping supervisees bridge their understanding about societal and structural influences on clients' presenting problems (Mackie & Boucher, 2018). Designing relevant interventions requires thinking systemically, not only of the intrapersonal systems of clients, but the multiple external systems that are influential for mental health and well-being (Arthur, 2018d).

Supervision practices that explore multiple systems of influence open up possibilities for supervisees to expand the ways that they frame client concerns and work collaboratively with clients to design relevant interventions. Supervision can support the development of advocacy competencies for addressing systemic change directly with clients, on their behalf, or for advocacy aimed at education or health promotion (Arthur, 2018d). Fickling et al. (2019) offer suggestions for supervision practices to strengthen advocacy competencies and ecological change, based on the multicultural and social justice competency framework (Ratts et al., 2015). Dollarhide et al. (2021) have developed a new model for social justice supervision that demonstrates the integration of multicultural counselling and social justice perspectives, describing supervision activities in four domains of the model. These recent developments are illustrative of the transformation in conceptual approaches to multicultural counselling as the field shifts to a fourth perspective and the articulation of social justice supervision practices.

Challenges in multicultural counselling supervision

One overriding assumption in multicultural counselling supervision is that both the counsellor/supervisee and the supervisor have received prior training about cultural influences in counselling. It is assumed that through exposure to curriculum, both parties enter the supervisory relationship in a state of readiness for exploring more about cultural influences on counselling practices. Yet, some supervisors may not have received formal training in multicultural counselling, supervision, or in multicultural counselling supervision (Falender et al., 2014). There are also disparities in the approaches taken to curriculum within cultural education curriculum and the extent to which counsellors and supervisors feel equipped with skills for practice. Although strides have been made to integrate multicultural counselling curriculum, and many programmes offer specialist courses, counsellor education programmes tend to emphasise the self-awareness and knowledge domains of multicultural competence. Students in counsellor education programmes benefit from supervision to help them translate concepts about multicultural counselling into skills for practice, including direct client contact and practicum site supervision (Brown et al., 2014; Collins et al., 2015). However, the development of multicultural competencies is an ongoing learning process and not something that ends when completing workshops or a counselling degree programme. Rather, continuous learning is embedded in an ethical foundation for multicultural counselling.

Supervisors are called upon to strive for self-awareness as a foundation for culturally competent practice (Falendar & Shafranske, 2004, 2007). In order for supervisors to facilitate supervisees' exploration of their cultural identities, they need to have personally engaged in such exploration (Constantine et al., 2005). A foundational aspect of multicultural supervision is capability of supervisors to engage supervisees in an exploration to increase their self-awareness. Supervisors may choose to share with supervisees the process they used to gain awareness about their cultural identities and some of the growing edges of that experience (Falender et al., 2014).

To a large degree, most barriers in supervision reflect cultural biases and assumptions on the part of either supervisors or supervisees that have not be adequately addressed. Ignoring cultural identities and social locations sends a clear message of disinterest and minimises the importance of attending to salient cultural influences that are important for supervises and for clients (Estrada et al., 2004). To this point, supervisors are cautioned about making assumptions regarding the homogeneity of supervisees. Even though the majority of students in counsellor education programmes are typically white, middle-class and female, the demographics are changing, with more diversity in the life experiences of supervisees that could be integrated into supervision discussions (Davis, 2014). Assumptions about supervisees may lead to greater defensiveness, misunderstandings, and invisible and unspoken barriers of power differences in supervisory relationships.

For supervision to be maximally effective, both supervisors and counsellors/supervisees need to be willing to explore the potential influences of their cultural identities and social locations for the supervisory relationship. Discussion of dimensions of personal identity such as race, ethnicity, gender, sexual orientation, age, religion, and socio-economic status have been implicated for the strength of the supervisory working alliance and the supervisee's satisfaction with supervision (Constantine, 2003; Davis, 2014; Gatmon et al., 2001). When supervisors have not considered their experiences of privilege, it may make it more difficult for them to self-assess power differentials and appreciate the experiences of supervisees or clients who have not held similar levels of social advantage. In turn, supervisees who have enjoyed privilege associated with their cultural identities may feel stretched to relate to a supervisor whose life experiences have included experiences of oppression. However, supervisors can take the onus to introduce how life experiences of privilege and/or oppression is relevant for multicultural counselling (Lowe & Davis, 2010; Wong et al., 2013). It is important to offer a cautionary note that assumptions should not be made about the backgrounds of either supervisees or supervisors, and it is the exploration of cultural identities and social locations that leads to greater understanding for multicultural counselling (Davis, 2014; Wong et al., 2013).

However, it should not be assumed that either member of the supervision dyad necessarily embraces multiculturalism as a positive or desirable direction in their professional practice. Some counsellors/supervisees have higher levels of interest and expertise in examining cultural influences in supervision than their supervisors, or vice versa (Falender et al., 2014). As a former instructor and supervisor of students in practicum placements, I have noticed varying degrees of interest by students and their site supervisors to incorporate multicultural and social justice competencies into supervision. Even if there is a willingness on behalf of supervisors to explore cultural influences through supervision, disparate levels of competency can be problematic for counsellors/trainees. There is a risk of exploitation when supervisors depend upon their supervisees, often students, as the main source of education about culture or about the multicultural counselling process (Estrada et al., 2004).

The personal cultural biases and assumptions made by supervisors may surface in ways that are challenging, but might have consequences for evaluating the performance of counselling supervisees. For example, supervisees may be inappropriately judged according to the supervisor's worldview and the viewpoints of the supervisee may be minimised or discounted. In this instance, supervisees may feel compelled to work as if in agreement with supervisors. Miscommunication or cultural misunderstandings may also surface as barriers to effective supervisor–supervisee interactions. This includes lack of understanding about the verbal or nonverbal communication patterns used by the counsellor/supervisee. Such misinterpretations may be channelled into evaluations about the competence level of the counsellor/supervisee when rigid standards for communication skills are upheld (Hird et al., 2001). Supervisees may question the clinical judgement of the supervisor (Brown et al., 2014) but intentionally withhold disclosing their concerns, which poses risks for their work with clients.

Inherent power differences in supervision roles make it difficult for counsellors/supervisees to feel comfortable and confident about challenging their supervisor's views of multicultural counselling. Power differences between supervisors and supervisees can easily spill over into case conceptualisation and impact whose views are considered to be more expert and legitimate. The imposition of power differences may be unintentional; supervisors who have not explored their roles in multicultural counselling supervision may be unaware and inadvertently dominate supervisees (Hird et al., 2001; Wong et al., 2013). Supervisors are encouraged to take the lead and introduce dialogue about cultural identities and social location, while openly acknowledging the power differentials in the supervisor relationship (Toporek et al., 2004).

Strengthening the working alliance in multicultural supervision

Trainees' perceptions about the multicultural competence of their supervisors is a key factor for supporting an effective supervisory working alliance and has also been implicated in research on perceived supervision satisfaction (Crockett & Hayes, 2015; Inman, 2006). A consistent finding in the literature on supervisory relationships is that trust in supervisory working alliance is an essential prerequisite for supervisees to engage in discussion about cultural influences on their own lives and on the lives of their clients. A trusting relationship is the departure point for examining complex client concerns and an examination of challenging cultural influences that permeate the client-supervisee-supervisor triad. Conversely, a lack of trust or serious rupture in trust may result in either supervisors or supervisees going into a protective or defensive stance. Caution about risk-taking or exposing vulnerabilities may lead to silence about important multicultural counselling issues in supervision and/or in the dynamics between supervisees and their clients. The common challenges introduced in this chapter may prompt reflection about how supervisors can build trusting and respectful relationships with supervisees. It is proposed that the open discussion about cultural identities and social locations in the supervisory relationship is a learning process that can strengthen multicultural counselling. The suggestions below are framed as enhancing supervision practices through collaboration and cultural humility.

The extent to which counsellors/supervisees view their supervisors as culturally aware and receptive to alternate points of view can strengthen or detract from a satisfactory supervisory relationship (Constantine, 2003). There are a number of positive ways that supervisors and counsellors/trainees can work together to enhance multicultural counselling supervision. For example, supervisors can initiate and facilitate shared learning, taking an empowerment approach through feedback about supervisees' existing strengths and discussing areas for continued learning (Wiley et al., 2021), Negotiating a stance of co-discovery promotes greater levels of collaboration and mutuality between supervisees and supervisors in their respective roles.

Both supervisors and their counsellors/supervisees need to examine their expectations about expertise in the supervisory relationship. Historically, supervision unfolded in a top-down fashion in which the supervisor maintained control of knowledge in an expert role (Bernard & Goodyear, 2019). This placed the supervisor in a position of authority in which expertise is imparted to a supervisee, who serves in a type of apprenticeship to the profession. The sharing of multicultural expertise is presumably a major goal, yet supervisors may lack models from which to feel confident and competent for shifting from an expert stance to collaboration and sharing of power and expertise with supervisees (Cary & Marques, 2007).

When counsellors/supervisees possess more knowledge and experience about multicultural counselling, a renegotiation of the expectations for supervision seems warranted. This is not an unusual situation in cases where supervisees are exposed to new curriculum through professional education. Regardless, there are many possibilities for collaborative learning, if expectations for the supervisory relationship can be openly discussed For example, the supervisor might be better positioned to offer more knowledge about the therapeutic process and the process of supervision and be willing to engage counsellors/supervisees in sharing their culture-specific expertise. It is the active negotiation that is characteristic of building a strong working alliance in supervisory relationships.

It is also possible that, by virtue of life experience, some supervisors or supervisees may be more attuned to issues of privilege and disadvantage, or the ways that social inequities influence mental health and well-being. The results of research on multicultural counselling supervision has suggested that supervisors from non-dominant racial/ethnic groups spend significant more time discussing cultural issues in supervision than their White counterparts (Hird et al., 2005). It has also been proposed that supervisees who have experienced oppression and disadvantage in their social locations may have acquired life experience that supports increased self-awareness. The dynamics of supervision can be enhanced through exchanges about relative experiences of privilege and/or oppression in their lives, including the implications for relating to the lives of their clients (Davis, 2014).

Toporek and colleagues (2004) noted that 'the relationship may be a pivotal component of multicultural supervision that moderates how all other experiences are perceived' (p. 80). Within the supervisory relationship, trust must be established but cultural expectations influence how trust and expertise are shared within the context of a supervisory relationship. For example, it should not be assumed that all counsellors/supervisees want to initially engage in a collaborative and mutually negotiated relationship. Some supervisees may hold expectations (implicit or explicit) about the supervisor's role as expert and the formal evaluative nature of the relationship. For example, supervisors who adopt a nondirective approach may be matched with supervisees who have been culturally socialised to listen to persons in authority and who wait to receive specific direction. Supervisees may be reluctant to bring up issues that challenge the expertise of the supervisor due to cultural upbringing about relationships of authority or fears about the evaluative components of supervision.

The sharing of personal reflections by supervisors with supervisees may facilitate the imparting of multicultural counselling competencies. It has been suggested that self-disclosure about struggles and uncertainties experienced with multicultural counselling may be comforting to supervisees and help them to address their own issues as they attempt to integrate multicultural perspectives into counselling (Hird et al., 2001). Through discussing their personal experiences, supervisors model the ongoing process of reflective practice and multicultural development. In this way, supervisors reveal themselves as lifelong learners interested in improving their understanding about the influences of culture in professional practice. For examples of personal reflections, readers are referred to the contributions of chapter authors and their applications to culture-infused counselling in Arthur (2018d).

The willingness of supervisors to demonstrate cultural humility has been emphasised in the counsellor–client relationship and has been extended to the supervisor–supervisee relationship (Hook et al., 2013, 2016), Cultural humility is defined as the 'ability to maintain an interpersonal stance that is other-oriented (or open to the other) in relation to aspects of cultural identity that are most important to the client [or supervisee]' (Hook et al., 2013, p. 354). The demonstration of cultural humility may set the stage for building trust and supporting supervisees to move beyond intentional non-disclosure of personal and performance vulnerabilities (Cook et al., 2020; Hook et al., 2016).

Essentially, the onus is on supervisors to initiate discussions about difficult and uncomfortable topics that surface in multicultural counselling (Constantine, 2003), such as ethical dilemmas, experiences of relative privilege or marginalisation, and unintentional racism (Collins & Arthur, 2018). There are many benefits from supervisors taking the lead and positioning discussions about cultural influences as central to the agenda for supervision. Through regularly scheduled meeting, supervisees can be supported to gain more confidence and competence for multicultural counselling and to take more of a lead role in bringing forward challenging issues to discuss in a trusted supervisory relationship.

Supervision scenarios

The following supervision scenarios were developed by the author to illustrate how cultural beliefs interface with expectations about supervision. Versions of the first five scenarios were published in earlier publications on supervision (Arthur & Collins, 2016, 2017) based on the original model of culture-infused counselling (Collins & Arthur, 2010a, 2010b). Two new supervision scenarios were developed by the author for this chapter to encourage readers to reflect about social justice and advocacy competencies, as described in the revised model (Arthur, 2018c).

Scenario 1

Janet was a graduate student who was increasingly frustrated at her practicum site as she was disappointed by the quality of supervision. She chose the setting due to the reputation of the supervisor for excellent clinical practice. Yet, she was discouraged as the supervisor rarely offered his opinion and always asked her what she thought. Janet was also very interested in discussing multicultural counselling. As the supervisor never brought up the topic, she did not believe it was an area of interest for the supervisor.

This scenario expands our consideration of mismatches when cultural influences and expectations in supervision are not discussed openly. The sense of frustration felt by the supervisee in this vignette may have been avoided through active negotiation of roles and expectations early in the supervisory relationship. In fact, to do so at the interview and selection stage may prevent mismatches in supervision preferences from occurring. Some supervisors or supervisees may self-select out of working together. However, such negotiation is more likely to open the door to working more effectively together.

Scenario 2

Michelle was very impressed with the clinical work of her supervisor but dreaded their supervision sessions. Like many new supervisees, Michelle was reluctant to bring up any concerns or show areas of weakness for fear of being judged as incompetent. Yet, when Michelle asked for help, the supervisor gave her ideas that she always found to be useful. When invited to discuss what was 'missing' in the supervisory relationship, Michelle noted that she would like to have more informal discussion and have the supervisor show more interest in her as a person, rather than immediately launching into case consultation. The supervisee wondered if her experience might be different working with a female supervisor.

In this second vignette, a different kind of mismatch in supervisory relationship expectations is highlighted. Two of the key dimensions in counsellor supervision can be characterised as content needs (focus on case conceptualisation and intervention planning) and relational needs (developing a trusting working relationship between the supervisor and the supervisee). If we think about these dimensions on a continuum, Michelle's supervision needs at this time might be characterised as higher on relational needs, whereas the supervisor appeared to be basing supervision strongly on content to improve counselling competencies. In reality, these two dimensions are not mutually exclusive. For supervisees whose worldview emphasises relationships as a primary component of learning, an immediate focus on the *business* of supervision will be unsettling. Supervisors may need to consider how to create a basis of comfort and ways of establishing rapport, prior to structuring supervision time around case conceptualisation). It is also possible that gender issues may emerge as salient in negotiating the nature of the supervisory relationship.

Scenario 3

Quan believed that there has been a high level of conflict with his supervisor, to the point that he feared a negative evaluation. Quan was concerned with the amount of supervision time taken on non-essential matters and a lot of time seemed to be wasted, when he really needed help with strategies for working with clients. Quan felt a lot of pressure to disclose about himself and this was not something he felt comfortable doing in a relationship that he considered to be a work environment. He attempted to discuss his cultural values with his supervisor, but this only seemed to make a temporary difference in how supervision was approached. Quan was concerned that unless he showed more evidence of personal reflection, he would be penalised. His beliefs about the cultural appropriateness of personal disclosure resulted in a lot of anxiety about supervision and what he might need to do to meet the supervisor's expectations, despite his personal convictions.

The third scenario describes the experiences of a supervisee who felt that his cultural boundaries around privacy were violated through supervision. There is general agreement in the multicultural counselling literature on the importance of self-awareness and counsellors are encouraged to be continually reflective about the influence of their personal culture (Davis, 2014; Torres-Rivera et al., 2001). Supervision approaches based on models of personal development also emphasise personal reflection and awareness as foundational to the development of higher-level counselling skills. This can be a particularly sensitive area in multicultural supervision, as trainees are encouraged to engage in personal reflection and disclosure with their supervisor about areas of potential vulnerability.

Underlying the process of gaining self-awareness are cultural norms about sharing personal information in public contexts. Depending upon the cultural backgrounds of either the counsellor/supervisee or the supervisor, mismatches can occur in expectations about the degree of disclosure expected and how that disclosure is managed. Without attention to expectations and the personal cultural identities of both the supervisor and the counsellor/supervisee, there is a risk that conflicting expectations will be detrimental to the supervisory relationship. In this scenario, the female supervisor who was trained in Western perspectives was inadvertently challenging the gender role beliefs of a male who was socialised in a collectivist, patriarchal Eastern culture. Rather than insisting on a high level of verbal disclosure, the supervisor may have expanded her methods for ascertaining this supervisee's level of reflective practice. For example, allowing the supervisee the option of writing personal reflections and selecting which content to bring forward to supervision may be more compatible than the supervisee's perception that he was pressured into disclosure upon demand by the supervisor.

Scenario 4

*Nick was an experienced counsellor, and he was very keen to enhance his multicultural coun-
selling competencies through his graduate practicum. The instructor who coordinated his practicum placement encouraged him to discuss his interests with his site supervisor to see if it
would be possible to place a greater emphasis on cultural influences on his work with clients.
The supervisor was really interested in this idea, and they negotiated agreement that either
of them could raise issues about culture in their supervision sessions. This openness motivated
Nick to pay more close attention to the ways that he was approaching multicultural counselling and how his personal socialisation was potentially influential in the way that he worked
with clients. Discussions with his supervisor included aspects of Nick's cultural identity that
were considerably different than the cultural identity of his supervisor. Through more open
sharing of their worldviews, their supervisory relationship was also strengthened.*

The fourth scenario depicts a counsellor/supervisee who has high levels of multicultural competencies and who was proactive about pursuing his learning needs related to
culture-infused supervision. A major contributing factor to Nick's positive experience of
supervision was the openness of the supervisor to explore Nick's expressed learning needs.
In this vignette, the receptivity of the supervisor to engage in a discussion of cultural
identities provided an indication of support and acceptance. The supervisor also felt that
the supervision discussions were highly rewarding as they offered new perspectives and
learning.

Scenario 5

*Angie was a supervisee who was really worried about finding a suitable supervision placement
in her graduate programme. She took the initiative to call a supervisor known for multicultural counselling competency. During the initial phone contact, Angie offered several times
to come and meet the supervisor and, in fact, insisted on an appointment. The supervisor
reflected at the time that the student seemed very keen but also seemed 'pushy.' Their relationship began with Angie frequently asking for the supervisor's opinion and the supervisor
noted that Angie most often paraphrased content but did not offer her own opinion. After
two months of working together, the supervisor had concerns about the level of growth that
was needed in Angie's counselling skills. Angie had the courage to tell the supervisor that she
felt she was not trusted to take on more independence in working with clients. The supervisor
agreed, with some caution, to let Angie work more independently. Angie's descriptions of her
clients and her counselling sessions led the supervisor to believe that everything was going well.
However, within the next week, there were two complaints levied by clients and requests to
be transferred to another counsellor. The supervisor interviewed the clients and determined
that Angie would need more structured supervision and more time co-counselling before she
would be allowed to counsel clients independently. Angie was very angry with the supervisor
for making this decision.*

The fifth scenario depicts a supervisory relationship where expectations between the
supervisor and supervisee were misaligned. There were cues about potential cultural
misunderstandings early in their relationship. Angie was focused on pleasing the supervisor, as a person of authority, and her continued stance of agreement was a sign of respect.
At the same time, she expected the supervisor to recognise her loyalty and offer her more
opportunities to demonstrate her skills. The supervisor seemed to feel conflicted about
the supervisory relationship from the first point of contact. A serious rupture occurred in

the supervisory relationship when the supervisor intervened and restricted Angie's level of contact with clients. From Angie's point of view, she felt betrayed that the supervisor did not recognise her skill development. From the supervisor's point of view, matters of ethical practice were paramount. Both parties were left to question the multicultural competence held by the other person and held by themselves. From this scenario, readers are invited to consider the potentially confounding issues between *what is cultural* and *what is competence*, and the potential for supervisee's skills to be over- or under-rated by their supervisors.

Scenario 6

Melinda sent her practicum course instructor an email to say that she was enjoying her practicum setting and the experiences that she was gaining through working with a range of clients and their presenting issues. She commented that she was working with one client who was experiencing multiple barriers and was having difficulties committing to counselling. Melinda commented that she might have framed this a lack of motivation on the behalf the client but then realised the toll that dealing with daily life demands on a limited budget was taking on the client's time and energy to make longer-term changes. Melinda said she was very excited about her work to connect the client to two other community agencies that would help with food security and finding suitable accommodation. She noted it took a lot of time to set up those arrangements, but it was worth it when the client expressed relief about sharing the burden of finding resources. Melinda also wrote to the practicum course instructor to ask for advice about what her practicum site supervisor said when she shared her advocacy actions and the outcomes. The question, 'How many clients did you see today?' seemed to discount her advocacy.

Melinda reaching out to consult about the place of advocacy offered the possibility to discuss the roles and responsibilities that counsellors have for helping clients to overcome barriers that are linked to their presenting issues. What Melinda seemed to be facing was an example of the constraints found in many public agencies where counselling occurs, when funding mandates are based on seeing high numbers of clients with limited time. The problem with such organisational constraints is that counsellors may feel they are not supported for advocacy work, even though it would likely address more complex social and structural systems. In this case, the course instructor encouraged Melinda to engage her practicum site supervisor in a conversation about expectations for seeing clients and to seek her advice about how time for advocacy could be built into her practicum placement.

Scenario 7

Miguel was a novice counsellor who worked in a university counselling setting. After working there for a year, he noticed that many of the international students he was seeing presented with common concerns related to their adjustment to new norms in their academic programme and for interacting with people in the local community. Although Miguel recognised that there were unique cultural influences for each international student, he felt that their issues might be addressed through different modalities. Miguel discussed his ideas with his supervisor, and they were able to make a plan for expanding his role and giving him more time for outreach and education with international students. As a result, Miguel was able to work more closely with the staff who coordinated international student services for the purpose of referral and consultation. Miguel was invited to present a workshop to new international students to educate them about campus resources, including peer-support and counselling. Miguel was also successful in securing funding from the university to develop some new resources for international students, including videos and online material on topics relevant to mental health and well-being.

In this scenario, the counsellor identified that providing alternate ways of service-delivery might enhance education and health promotion, while also improving access to counselling services. The support of his supervisor was pivotal for encouraging outreach and advocacy. Making contact with other professionals on the student services team allowed him to have a higher profile for referral and consultation about international students. Miguel was able to use this professional knowledge and connections to grow resources available to international students. Through tracking the number of times that the online resources were used, he was able to include the information on an evaluation report. Miguel was able to share his learning and increase awareness of other counsellors about the contexts and identities of international students and how to provide culturally appropriate services.

Scenario learnings

The previous supervision scenarios illustrate some of the ways that the expectations and behaviours of both supervisors and supervisees come together in unique ways. Five positions are embedded in the main themes of the scenarios: (a) supervisors avoid addressing cultural issues with supervisees, either intentionally or unintentionally; (b) supervisors wait for supervisees to bring up cultural issues and address them if they come up in the process of supervision; (c) supervisors proactively engage in supervision discussions about cultural influences; (d) supervisors have to carefully navigate issues of power and competence; and (e) conditions in the sites where supervision occurs may be discouraging or empowering for enacting social justice advocacy. It is inevitable that some cultural (mis)understandings will surface in supervisory relationships but the willingness of supervisors and supervisees to seek clarification and negotiate understanding afford critical learning that can transfer to the counsellor–client dyad. Supervisees can also be supported to integrate multicultural and social justice competencies into their roles and responsibilities for ethical practices.

Tools for reflective practice

During the past decade, new resources have emerged to support the development of multicultural competence in supervision (e.g., Falender et al., 2014; Inman & Ladany, 2014). Supervisors are encouraged to select one or more of the multicultural competency frameworks introduced in this chapter as tools for setting learning goals and as a reference for reviewing competency development of supervisees. Along with new and revised multicultural counselling models and competency frameworks, there are additional resources and guidelines for supervision. For example, questionnaires designed for assessing multicultural supervision competencies have been developed (e.g., Sangganjanavanich et al., 2019). Supervisors and supervisees can reflect about cultural identities and social locations in supervision through focusing on questionnaire items, and select topics to target for professional learning and development. Another practical tool involves both supervisors and supervisees creating cultural genograms as a foundation for discussing their personal cultural identities and improving supervision and counselling relationships (Estrada et al., 2004). Mitchell and Butler (2021) have offered a developmental framework with multicultural elements that supervisors can use to structure supervision and guide supervisees. Peters (2017) has suggested action plans for supervisors and supervisees to explore the intersectionality of people's identities and social locations.

Any of these tools can be used to enhance multicultural counselling supervision with the dual purpose of enhancing competencies for working with clients. The tools offer stimulus for engaging in deeper conversations and targeted learning through supervision. Moving from informal discussions to structured and targeted learning goals, supervisors and supervisees can collaborate in designing practical steps for growth and development. This process has been described as cultural auditing (Arthur & Collins, 2017) to inform and revise learning plans in supervision, tailored to meet the current and emerging learning needs of supervisees.

Summary and conclusion

Counselling students, graduates, more experienced counsellors, and those who hold supervisory roles need to consider how culture is infused into their professional roles and relationships. Culture impacts the reciprocal relationships between counsellors/ supervisees, supervisors, and clients. Supervision practices can support cultural learning during counsellor education programmes or through ongoing professional practice in the workplace. Supervisors are encouraged to become familiar with resources on the multicultural supervision literature in general (e.g., Bernard & Goodyear, 2019; Falender et al., 2014; Inman & Ladany, 2014). The multicultural and social justice competency frameworks overviewed in this chapter can be used by supervisors to help them identify their personal strengths and areas for continued professional development. In conjunction with supervisees, these frameworks can be used to guide exploration of multicultural counselling competencies and identify specific ideas for learning and development.

The shift to social justice and advocacy competencies needs to be integrated into multicultural counselling supervision. To date, there has been more written about the necessity of social justice perspectives in supervision practices than scholarship to inform supervision approaches (Kemer et al., 2021). However, this appears to be symptomatic of a field in transition and there is inevitably a lag time for conceptual and competency frameworks to be developed and tested through research. At the same time, there are opportunities to capture best of practices and encourage supervisors and supervisees to share their approaches and strategies for strengthening social justice supervision.

In summary, the multicultural counselling supervision literature has shifted from a focus on the cultural diversity of clients to the intersections of supervisor–counsellor–client identities and social locations. The supervisory relationship has the potential to be a rich learning platform from which counsellors can improve their multicultural counselling competencies for designing interventions to support clients directly and to address systemic and structural inequalities. Collaboration in supervisory relationships is a foundation for exploring the intersections of cultural identities, social locations, and social justice. Ultimately, supervision offers both supervisors and supervisees a professional relationship through which they strengthen their personal learning for ethical practice.

Acknowledgement

An earlier version of this chapter was published as Arthur, N. & Collins, S. (2017). Culture-infused counsellor supervision. In N. Pelling & P. Armstrong (Eds.), *The practice of counselling and clinical supervision* (pp. 267–295). Bowen Hills, QLD: Australian Academic Press.

Educational questions & activities

1. Individual and Small Group Reflection Exercise The following reflection questions are intended to promote discussion about culture-infused supervision. Reflect about the way that you currently supervise students, or, if you are a student/supervisee, the way that you are supervised during your practicum or field placement.

   a. How do you incorporate discussions about clients' cultural contents as an ongoing aspect of supervision?

   b. How do introduce supervisor and supervisee cultural identities into supervision discussions?

   c. What cultural influences in the relationship between supervisors and supervisees have you experienced?

   d. What are some topics related to cultural contexts, cultural identities, and/or social justice that you would like to discuss with your supervisor/supervisee?

   e. What barriers have you experienced in multicultural counselling supervision? How have you overcome those barriers?

   f. What has helped you to build a strong working alliance with your supervisee/ supervisor in which you discussed ideas about cultural contexts, cultural identities and/or social justice advocacy?

2. What does social justice advocacy mean to you? Give some examples of how counsellors can integrate advocacy roles into their practices.

3. Describe how you might approach intervention planning when a client's presenting issue is connected to a structural or social barrier?

4. What does the phrase, 'the professional is political' mean to you?

Selected references for further reading

Selected internet resources

American Psychological Association (2017). Multicultural Guidelines: An Ecological Approach to Context, Identity, and Intersectionality. www.apa.org/about/policy/ multicultural-guidelines.pdf

- These guidelines were developed to provide an updated approach and ecological framework to enhance knowledge about a person's context, identity, and intersectionality as foundational for intervention planning.

Home page of the Association for Counselor Education and Supervision, a division of the American Counseling Association. www.acesonline.net

The Association for Counselor Education and Supervision (ACES) emphasises the need for quality education and supervision of counsellors in all work settings. *Counselor Education and Supervision* is the official journal of the Association for Counselor Education and Supervision. http://onlinelibrary.wiley.com/journal/10.1002/ (ISSN)1556-6978/issues

The Clinical Supervisor is a journal devoted exclusively to articles on the art and science of clinical supervision. An interdisciplinary, refereed publication, the journal facilitates the communication of ideas, experiences, skills, techniques, concerns, and needs of supervisors in psychotherapy and mental health. https://www.tandfonline.com/journ als/wcsu20

The Journal of Multicultural Counseling and Development publishes research and conceptual articles related to multicultural counselling and social justice competencies. Articles on multicultural supervision are also published in this journal. https://onlinelibrary. wiley.com/journal/21611912

References

American Psychological Association (APA) (2003). Guidelines on multicultural education, training, research, practice, and organizational change for Psychologists. *American Psychologist, 58*(5), 377–402. https://doi.org/10.1037/0003-066X.58.5.377

Arredondo, P., & Toporek, R. (2004). Multicultural counseling competencies = ethical practice. *Journal of Mental Health Counseling, 26*(1), 44–55. https://doi.org/10.17744/mehc.26.1.hw2enjqve2p2tj6q

Arredondo, P., Toporek, R., Brown, S., Sanchez, J., Locke, D. C., Sanchez, J., & Stadler, H. (1996). Operationalization of the multicultural counseling competencies. *Journal of Multicultural Counseling & Development, 24*(1), 42–78. https://doi.org/10.1002/j.2161-1912.1996. tb00288.x

Arthur, N. (2018a). Infusing culture and social justice in ethical practices with all clients. In N. Arthur (Ed.), *Counseling in cultural contexts – identities and social justice* (pp. 3–28). New York, NY: Springer.

Arthur, N. (2018b). Culture-Infused Counselling: Context, identities, and social justice. In N. Arthur (Ed.), *Counseling in cultural contexts – identities and social justice* (pp. 29–62). New York, NY: Springer.Arthur, N. (2018c). Culture-infused counselling: Applied activism and advocacy. In N. Arthur (Ed.), *Counseling in cultural contexts – Identities and social justice* (pp. 383–406). New York, NY: Springer.

Arthur, N. (2018d). *Counseling in cultural contexts – identities and social justice*. Cham: Springer.

Arthur, N., & Collins, S. (2014). Counsellors, counselling, and social justice: The professional is political. *Canadian Journal of Counselling and Psychotherapy, 48*(3), 171–185. http://cjc-rcc.ucalg ary.ca/cjc/index.php/rcc/article/view/2764/2532

Arthur, N., & Collins, S. (2016). Culture-infused counselling supervision: Applying concepts in clinical supervision practices. In B. Shepard, L. Martin, & B. Robinson (Eds.), *Clinical supervision of the Canadian counselling and psychotherapy profession* (pp. 353–378). Ottawa: Canadian Counselling and Psychotherapy Association.

Arthur, N., & Collins, S. (2017). Culture-infused counsellor supervision. In N. Pelling, A. Moir-Bussy, & P. Armstrong (Eds.), *The practice of counselling and clinical supervision* (pp. 267–295). Bowen Hills, QLD: Australian Academic Press.

Bernard, J. M., & Goodyear, R. K. (2019). *Fundamentals of clinical supervision* (6th ed.). Boston, MA: Pearson.

Brown, C., Collins, S., & Arthur, N. (2014). Fostering multicultural and social justice competence through counsellor education pedagogy. *Canadian Journal of Counselling and Psychotherapy, 48*(3), 300–320. http://cjc-rcc.ucalgary.ca/cjc/index.php/rcc/article/view/2730

Brown, M. T., & Landrum-Brown, J. (1995). Counselor supervision: Cross-cultural perspectives. In J. G. Ponterotto, J. M. Casas, L. A. Suzuki, & C. M. Alexander (Eds.), *Handbook of multicultural counselling* (pp. 263–286). Thousand Oaks, CA: Sage.

Cary, D., & Marques, P. (2007). From expert to collaborator: Developing cultural competency in clinical supervision. *The Clinical Supervisor, 26*(1–2), 141–157. https://doi.org/10.1300/J001v26n01_10

Chen, E. C. (2001). Multicultural counselling supervision: An interactional approach. In J. G. Ponterotto, J. M. Casas, L. A. Suzuki, & C. M. Alexander (Eds.), *Handbook of multicultural counselling* (2nd ed., pp. 801–824). Thousand Oaks, CA: Sage.

Cohen, J., Kassan, A., Wada, K., Arthur, N., & Goopy, S. (2021). Enhancing multicultural and social justice competencies in Canadian counselling psychology training. *Canadian Psychology*, online, 1–15.

Collins, S., & Arthur, N. (2010a). Culture-infused counselling: A fresh look at a classic framework of multicultural counselling competencies. *Counseling Psychology Quarterly, 23*(2), 203–216. https://doi.org/10.1080/09515071003798204

Collins, S., & Arthur, N. (2010b). Culture-infused counseling: A model for developing cultural competence. *Counseling Psychology Quarterly, 23*(2), 217–233. https://doi:10.1080/095150 71003798212

Collins, S., & Arthur, N. (2018). Challenging conversations: Deepening personal and professional commitment to culture-infused and socially-just counseling practices. In D. Pare & C. Oudette (Eds.), *Social justice and counseling: Discourse in practice* (pp. 29–42). New York, NY: Routledge.

Collins, S., Arthur, N., Brown, C., & Kennedy, B. (2015). Student perspectives: Graduate education facilitation of multicultural and social justice competency. *Training and Education in Professional Psychology, 19*(2), 153–160. https://doi:10.1037/tep0000070

Constantine, M. (2003). Multicultural competence in supervision. In D. B. Pope-Davis, H. L. K. Coleman, W. M. Liu, & R. Torporek (Eds.), *Handbook of multicultural competencies in counseling and psychology* (pp. 383–391). Thousand Oaks, CA: Sage.

Constantine, M., Warren, A. K., & Milville, M. L. (2005). White racial identity dyadic interactions in supervision: Implications for supervisee's multicultural counseling competence. *Journal of Counseling Psychology, 52*(4), 490–496. https://doi:10.1037/0022-0167.52.4.490490

Cook, R. M., Jones, C. T., & Welfare, L. E. (2020). Supervisor cultural humility predicts intentional nondisclosure by post-master's counselors. *Counselor Education and Supervision, 59*, 160–167. https://doi.org/10.1002/ceas.12173

Crockett, S., & Hays, D. G. (2015). The influence of supervisor multicultural competency on the supervisory working alliance, supervisee counseling self-efficacy, and supervisee satisfaction with supervision: A mediation model. *Counselor Education and Supervision, 54*(4), 258–273. https://doi:10.1002/ceas.12025

Davis, D. (2014). Complexity overlooked: Enhancing cultural competency in the White lesbian counseling trainee through education and supervision. *Journal of Lesbian Studies, 18*(2), 192–201. https://doi:10.1080/10894160.2014.849166

Dollarhide, C. T., Hale, S. C., & Stone-Sabali, S. (2021). A new model for social justice supervision. *Journal of Counseling & Development, 99*(1), 104–113. https://doi.org/10.1002/jcad.12358

Ertl, M., Mann-Saumier, M., Martin, R., Graves, D., & Altarriba, J. (2019). The impossibility of client–therapist "match": Implications and future directions for multicultural competency. *Journal of Mental Health Counseling, 41*, 312–326. https://doi.org/10.17744/mehc.41.4.03

Estrada, D., Frame, M. W., & Williams, C. B. (2004). Cross-cultural supervision: Guiding the conversation toward race and ethnicity. *Multicultural Counseling and Development, 32*, 307–319. www.wyomingcounselingassociation.com/wp-content/uploads/Estrada-et-al-2004-Cross-Sultu ral-Supervision.pdf

Falender, C. A., Burnes, T. R., & Ellis, M. V. (2013). Multicultural clinical supervision and benchmarks: Empirical support informing practice and supervisor training. *The Counseling Psychologist, 41*(1), 8–27. https://doi.org/10.1177/0011000012438417

Falender, C. A., & Shafranske, E. P. (2004). *Clinical supervision: A competency-based approach.* Washington, DC: American Psychological Association.

Falender, C. A., & Shafranske, E. P. (2007). Competence in competency-based supervision practice: Construct and application. *Professional Psychology: Research and Practice, 38*(3), 232–240. https://doi:10.1037/0735-7028.38.3.232

Falender, C. A., Shafranske, E. P., & Falicov, C. J. (2014). Diversity and multiculturalism in supervision. In C. Falender, E. Shafranske, & C. Falicov (Eds.), *Multiculturalism and diversity in clinical supervision: A competency-based approach* (pp. 3–28). Washington, DC: American Psychological Association.

Falicov, C. (2014). Psychotherapy and supervision as cultural encounters: The multidimensional ecological comparative approach framework. In C. Falender, E. Shafranske, & C. Falicov (Eds.), *Multiculturalism and diversity in clinical supervision: A competency-based approach* (pp. 29–58). Washington, DC: American Psychological Association.

Fernandes, C., & Lane, D. (2020). Best practices in multicultural supervision in counseling. *Journal of Counseling Research and Practice, 6.* https://egrove.olemiss.edu/jcrp/vol6/iss1/4

Fickling, M., Tangen, J., Graden, M., & Grays, D. (2019). Multicultural and social justice competence in clinical supervision. *Counselor Education and Supervision, 58,* 309–316. https://doi.org/10.1002/ceas.12159

Gatmon, D., Jackson, D., Koshkarian, L., Martos-Perry, N., Molina, A., Patel, N., & Rodolfa, E. (2001). Exploring ethnic, gender, and sexual orientation variables in supervision: Do they really matter? *Journal of Multicultural Counseling and Development, 29,* 102–113. https://doi.org/10.1002/j.2161-1912.2001.tb00508.x

Hird, J. S., Cavalieri, C. E., Dulko, J. P., Felice, A. A, & Ho, T. A. (2001). Visions and realities: Supervisee perspectives of multicultural supervision. *Journal of Multicultural Counseling and Development, 29*(2), 114–130. https://doi:10.1002/j.2161-1912.2001.tb00509.x

Hird, J. S., Tao, K. W., & Gloria, A. M. (2005). Examining supervisors' multicultural competence in racially similar and different supervision dyads. *The Clinical Supervisor, 23*(2), 107–122. https://doi:10.1300/j001v23n02_07

Hook, J. N., Davis, D. E., Owen, J., Worthington, E. L., Jr., & Utsey, S. O. (2013). Cultural humility: Measuring openness to culturally diverse clients. *Journal of Counseling Psychology, 60,* 353–366. https://doi.org/10.1037/a0032595

Hook, J. N., Watkins, C. E. Jr., Davis, D. E., Owen J., Van Tongeren, D. R., & Ramos, M. J. (2016). Cultural humility in psychotherapy supervision. *American Journal of Psychotherapy, 70,* 149–66. https://doi: 10.1176/appi.psychotherapy.2016.70.2.149. PMID: 27329404.

Inman, A. G. (2006). Supervisor multicultural competence and its relation to supervisory process and outcome. *Journal of Marital and Family Therapy, 32,* 73–85. https://doi.org/10.1111/j.1752-0606.2006.tb01589.x

Inman, A. G., & Ladany, N. (2014). *Multicultural competencies in psychotherapy supervision.* Washington, DC: American Psychological Association.

Kemer, G., Li, C., Attia, M., Chan, C. D., Chung, M., Li, D., Neuer Colburn, A., Peters, H. C., Ramaswamy, A., & Sunal, Z. (2021). Multicultural supervision in counseling: A content analysis of peer-reviewed literature. *Counselor Education and Supervision,* 1–13. https://doi.org/10.1002/ceas.12220

Kennedy, B., & Arthur, N. (2014). Social justice and counselling psychology: Recommitment through action. *Canadian Journal of Counselling and Psychotherapy, 48,* 186–205. https://cjc-rcc.ucalgary.ca/article/view/61013

Lowe, S. M., & Davis, C. (2010). Sharing wisdom: Ethnic minority supervisor perspectives. *Training and Education in Professional Psychology, 4*(1), 1–2. https://doi:10.1037/a0018560

Mackie, K., & Boucher, M. (2018). Just supervision: Thinking about clinical supervision that moves toward social justice. In C. Audet & D. Paré (Eds.), *Social justice and counseling: Discourse in practice* (pp. 57–68). New York: Routledge.

Mitchell, M. D. and Butler, S. K. (2021). Acknowledging intersectional identity in supervision: The Multicultural Integrated Supervision Model. *Journal of Multicultural Counseling and Development, 49,* 101–115. https://doi.org/10.1002/jmcd.12209

Pedersen, P. (Ed.) (1999). *Multiculturalism as a fourth force.* Philadelphia: Brunner/Mazel.

Peters, H. C. (2017). Multicultural complexity: An intersectional lens for clinical supervision. *International Journal for the Advancement of Counselling, 39,* 176–187. https://doi.org/10.1007/s10447-017-9290-2

Pettifor, J., McCarron, M. E., Schoepp, G., Stark, C., & Stewart, D. (2011). Ethical supervision in teaching, research, practice, and administration. *Canadian Psychology, 52*(3), 198–205. https://doi.org/10.1037/a0024549

Pope-Davis, D. B., Toporek, R. L., & Ortega-Villalobos, L. (2003). Assessing supervisors' and supervisees' perceptions of multicultural competence in supervision using the Multicultural Supervision Inventory. In D. B. Pope-Davis, H. L. K. Coleman, W. M. Liu, & R. Torporek (Eds.), *Handbook of multicultural competencies in counseling and psychology* (pp. 211–224). Thousand Oaks: Sage.

Ratts, M. J., Singh, A. A., Nassar-McMillan, S., Butler, S. K., & McCullough, J. R. (2015). *Multicultural and social justice counseling competencies.* www.counseling.org/docs/default-source/competencies/multicultural-and-social-justice-counseling-competencies.pdf

Ratts, M. J., Singh, A. A., Nassar-McMillan, S., Butler, S. K., & McCullough, J. R. (2016). Multicultural and social justice competencies: Guidelines for the counseling profession. *Journal of Multicultural Counseling & Development, 44*, 28–48. https://doi.org/10.1002/jmcd.12035

Roysircar, G., Hubbell, R., & Gard, G. (2003). Multicultural research on counselor and client variables. In D.B. Pope-Davis, H.L.K. Coleman, W.M. Lui, & R.L. Toporek (Eds.), *Handbook of multicultural counseling and psychology* (pp. 247–266). Thousand Oaks, CA: Sage.

Sangganjanavanich, V., Dang, Y., & Liang, X. (2019). The validation of the Multicultural Supervision Scale. *The Journal of Counselor Preparation and Supervision, 12*(4). https://repository.wcsu.edu/jcps/vol12/iss4/8

Sue, D. W., Arredondo, P., & McDavis, R. J. (1992). Multicultural counseling competencies and standards: a call to the profession. *Journal of Counseling and Development, 70*, 477–483. https://doi.org/10.1002/j.1556-6676.1992.tb01642.x

Sue, D. W., Bernier, J. B., Durran, M., Feinberg, L., Pedersen, P., Smith, E., . . . Vasquez-Nuttall, E. (1982).Cross-cultural counseling competencies. *The Counseling Psychologist, 10*, 45–52. https://doi:10.1177/0011000082102008

Sue, D. W., Carter, R. T., Casas, J. M., Fouad, N. A., Ivey, A. E., Jensen, M., … Vasquez- Nuttall, E. (1998). *Multicultural counseling competencies: Individual and organizational development.* Thousand Oaks: Sage.

Sue, D.W., & Sue, D. (1999). *Counseling the culturally different: Theory and practice* (3rd ed.). New York: Wiley.

Toporek, R. L., Ortega-Villalobos, L., & Pope-Davis, D. B. (2004). Critical incidents in multicultural supervision: Exploring supervisees' and supervisors' experiences. *Journal of Multicultural Counseling and Development, 32*(2), 66–83. https://doi:10.1002/j.2161-1912.2004.tb00362.x

Torres-Rivera, E., Phan, L.T., Maddux, C., Wilbur, M. P., & Garrett, M. T. (2001). Process versus content: Integrating personal awareness and counselling skills to meet the multicultural challenge of the twenty-first century. *Counselor Education & Supervision, 41*, 28–40. https://doi.org/10.1002/j.1556-6978.2001.tb01266.x

Vasquez, M. (2014). Foreward. In C. Falender, E. Shafranske, & C. Falicov (Eds.), *Multiculturalism and diversity in clinical supervision: A competency-based approach* (pp. xi–xv). Washington, DC: American Psychological Association.

Wampold, B. E. (2015). How important are the common factors in psychotherapy? An update. *World Psychiatry, 14*, 270–277. https://doi: 10.1002/wps.20238

Wiley, E. D., Phillips, J. C., & Palladino Schultheiss, D. E. (2021). Supervisors' perceptions of their integration of strength-based and multicultural approaches to supervision. *The Counseling Psychologist, 49*, 1038–1069. https://doi.org/10.1177/00110000211024595

Wong, L., Wong, P., & Ishiyama, I. (2013). What helps and what hinders in cross-cultural supervision: A critical incidents study. *The Counseling Psychologist, 41*(1), 66–85. https://doi:10.1177/0011000012442652

Part 5

Evaluation

Part 5, **Evaluation**, is a word often dreaded by supervisees and supervisors alike. It can be unnerving to be evaluated and also to complete evaluations. This section contains three chapters and provides both general and specific information about evaluation. For instance, Chapter 19 explores supervision as gatekeeping into the counselling profession. Chapter 20 explores the various ways of defining and assessing competence in counselling. And in Chapter 21 the specifics of supervising a clinical placement are explored.

Chapter overview

Chapter 19, **Supervision as Gatekeeping: Managing professional competency problems in student supervisees**, by Brian Sullivan and Elisa Agostinelli, discusses the often-feared aspect of evaluation relating to student professional competency problems. In a gentle manner they review the three main domains of counselling competence – cognitive, affective, and relational – as well as overall performance assessment and argue for the use of clear and shared terminology regarding competency problems. The use of supervision in decisions to remediate or dismiss students is reviewed.

Chapter themes

In this chapter you will explore the following themes:

- Professional training standards
- Beginning with the end in sight
- The 'self' of the counsellor
- The three dimensions of counselling mastery
  - Cognitive
  - Affective domain
  - Relational domain
- Student performance concerns
- Clear, shared, and consistent terminology
- Our critical role as gatekeepers
- Remediation
- Dismissal
- Recommendations
- Conclusions

DOI: 10.4324/9781003490067-23

Chapter **20**, **Counsellor Competence**, by Nadine Pelling, is a literature analysis regarding how the counselling and psychology professions struggle to define what makes therapists competent in their applied work. Additionally, the controversy over for whom and for what purpose competency is defined and how it is measured is presented. This is a broad introduction to the issues of assessment and therapist competence.

Chapter themes

In this chapter you will explore the following themes:

- Defining competence
- Assessment of competence
- Purpose of assessment
- Who will assess competence?
- Training/supervisor assessment
- Manager assessment
- External judge assessment
- Self-assessment
- Peer assessment
- Client assessment
- How do we measure competence?
- Questionnaires/rating scales
- Journals
- Exams
- Identifying a minimum level of counsellor competence
- Enforcing minimum levels of counsellor competence
- Can/does licensure and certification ensure counsellor competence?

Chapter **21**, **Supervising Clinical Placement**, by John Barletta and Jason Dixon, brings this section to a close by exploring the crucial role of internship and practicum experiences in the development of trainees. It is in these contexts that students are happily inducted into the profession and supervisors perform the potentially burdensome role of gate-keeper. This chapter educates the novice as to the possible supervisory approaches they will be exposed to, while providing a useful template on how to provide a client history to a supervisor, group, or peer. Table 21.1, which highlights the development of the therapist, will be an invaluable resource to normalise and validate the feelings and steps of trainees on their professional journey.

Chapter themes

In this chapter you will explore the following themes:

- Definition and purpose
- What to expect from the supervision experience
- Approaches a supervisor may employ
- Live supervision and supervision with pre-recorded work
- Characteristics of effective supervisors
- Case conceptualisation, critical thinking and note taking

- Client history intake form
- Therapist development
- The journey of professional therapists
- Critical incidents and case studies
- Case presentations
- Circumstances requiring immediate action to prevent imminent harm
- Sample suicide contract

19 Supervision as Gatekeeping

Managing Professional Competency Problems in Student Supervisees

Brian Sullivan and Elisa Agostinelli

Introduction

Supervision is a mandatory requirement for professional counsellors and for any accountable and accredited counselling programme (ACA, 2020). Supervision covers multiple roles, including oversite of student skill and competency development, ensuring the standards of the profession are upheld, and protecting clients by ensuring that counsellor-trainees undertake and maintain safe and ethical practice (PACFA, 2022). The key characteristics of a profession are to: 'screen and select new members; to educate, train, and socialize those who are selected; and to articulate standards of ethical practice' (Forrest, Elman, Gizara, & Vacha-Haase, 1999, p. 628). Yet while the counselling literature acknowledges this critical role of counsellor education programmes, there is little substantive direction for faculty in directing that process (Wilkerson, 2006). This chapter is about the broad concept of supervision in regards to counsellor trainees, the students in our counsellor education programmes. In this specific context, supervision includes the tri-partite work of counsellor educators in facilitating training in traditional course work (theoretical and skills-based), personal development, and supervised practice with programme-based and on-site supervisors and trainers (Rønnestad & Skovholt, 2001). In particular, this chapter is about how we as counsellor educators, trainers, and supervisors, manage students who are manifesting problematic performance in the programme, be that academic difficulties, skills deficits, personal limitations, interpersonal problems, mental health issues, ethical concerns or any combination of these, as they may overlap (Forrest et al., 1999; Ladany, Friedlander, & Nelson, 2005).

The two most critical tasks of counsellor educators are the selection screening and ongoing evaluation of student counsellors (Enochs & Etzbach, 2004; Forest et al., 1999). If we do not attend prudently to these twin tasks, we run the risk of graduating students who may not be appropriate candidates to be professional counsellors, and ultimately this is potentially harmful to the public who use counselling services. Not only is there the potential of harm to clients and future clients, but also to the reputation of the training programme and faculty, the counselling profession itself, and of course the negative consequences of career unsuitability on the individual graduate. These supervisory tasks involve not only academic and attitudinal considerations, but ethical and legal implications as well (Enochs & Etzbach, 2004; Ladany et al., 2005).

As counsellor educators, we need to begin with the end in sight. We need to have specific key performance indicators, clearly articulated to our students, so that there are no surprises, no catches, and no hidden agenda in our counselling programmes (Bhat, 2005; Kaslow, Rubin, Forrest et al., 2007). What should a graduate from our programmes be

DOI: 10.4324/9781003490067-24

able to do? What kind of person (cognitively, ethically, attitudinally, and behaviourally) should our candidates and graduates be? Ensuring that students who graduate from our programmes are likely to be professionally competent is a basic objective of counsellor trainers and supervisors. This is a foundational principle of ethical and accountable counsellor education programmes (Kaslow et al., 2007).

Professional training standards

The Psychotherapy and Counselling Federation of Australia (PACFA) in its 2022 Professional Training Standards stated that 'Prospective students need to demonstrate the presence of a set of human capacities as a pre-requisite for acceptance into counselling, psychotherapy or Aboriginal and Torres Strait Islander Indigenous Healing Practice programs' (p. 8). The capacities so important for selection of suitable candidates may be demonstrated for those who are doing the selection via live interviews, observing student's participation in experiential workshops, referees reports, among other means. Whatever means a training programme chooses to select candidates for admission, prospective students:

- need to have demonstrated self-awareness and a relational capacity, including the capacity to relate in a facilitative way with others and to reflect on and examine the impact of these actions;
- need to demonstrate a capacity to understand and practice ethical behaviour in accordance with the PACFA (or other professional association) Code of Ethics;
- [need] a certain level of mature life experience on the part of the applicant as shown by the capacity to reflect on and learn from experience, including being open to positive and challenging feedback (PACFA, 2022, p. 8).

Professional Standards typically enunciate student requirements of self-awareness, maturity, and ethical behaviour (McCaughan & Hill, 2015).

While these standards provide counsellor educators and supervisors guidelines for the selection of suitable candidates and an example of means to undertake that selection process, they do not elucidate gatekeepers on the specifics of the management of those who are accepted onto the programme and then show diminished functioning in any of the relational skills, self-awareness, maturity, and/or ethical behaviour aspects of student development.

Beginning with the end in sight

As professional counsellors, our noble vocation (Skovholt & Jennings, 2005) is:

> to understand; to help; to speak the truth; to make a meaningful connection with our clients that fosters their sense of agency, their capacity for enjoyment and mastery, and their ability to tolerate grief and limitation, whether or not their behaviour is unconventional and inconvenient according to ordinary cultural norms.
>
> (McWilliams, 2005, p. 140)

Obviously, this work is *not* for everyone. So counsellor educators and those responsible for the supervision of trainees need to ensure that it *is* for those who have been selected and have embarked on their training to become professional counsellors. Supervisors need to work with their supervisees to ensure that those who are in training are being true to and growing in that vocation. This of course is for the good of our clients, both present and future. It is also for the good of our trainees; for the good of our training institutions and supervisory faculty; and ultimately it is for the good of the counselling profession.

Good counsellors are both born and bred. However, our natural proclivities and personal qualities should be nurtured in and through the quality of our training and supervision. It is not an either/or situation. Our training and what we bring to that training are both vital for our development as counsellors (Sullivan, 2008; Wheeler, 2002). Wheeler (2002) has employed a culinary analogy that captures this synthesis of trainer, trainee, and training:

> the way the pudding is stirred and baked has much to answer for, but without handpicked, good-quality ingredients, the result may be less than satisfactory. So it is with counsellor training: the outcome depends not only on the programme delivered but also on the suitability of the participants.
>
> (Wheeler, 2002, p. 427)

For the best end product, we need good programmes of training, with highly effective trainers and supervisors, and we need good quality candidates. Good training and supervision provides structured learning experiences and professional direction for those with innate personal qualities. Good training and supervision will enhance and deepen those innate personal qualities (Sullivan, 2008; Wheeler & Richards, 2007).

The 'self' of the counsellor

In counselling, we typically work with those who have been 'bruised by life' to varying degrees, both with 'the walking wounded' and 'the worried well' (Aveline, 2005, p. 157). There is much at stake for our clients when they access our services. However, we must not lose sight of the fact that as human beings and as trainees, or counsellors, we too are 'wounded' albeit aspiring to be 'wounded healers' (Wheeler, 2002, p. 435). As counsellors we are not somehow outside of, immune to, or exempt from the human condition, the struggles and pain of human living and relating. We wrestle with the questions, issues, and challenges that concern most people. They are concerns about the meaning of our lives, about the ways of achieving and living good and happy lives, about how to be healthy both physically and mentally, and being in good and happy relationships (Sullivan, 2008). With that in mind then, let us briefly consider the qualities and characteristics of good counsellors that have been shown to be effective with clients. It is critical for us as trainers and supervisors to consider these qualities and characteristics, especially when selecting trainees for our programmes, and when dealing with trainees who may be exhibiting cognitive difficulties, problematic behaviours, and ethical deficiencies? There is much at stake for us when we select, accept, and commit to train students to become professional counsellors. We should remember too that there is much at stake for students who embark on this journey to become professional counsellors.

The three dimensions of counselling mastery

The research of Skovholt, Jennings, and colleagues (Jennings & Skovholt, 1999; Rønnestad & Skovholt, 2003; Skovholt, 2005; Sullivan, Skovholt, & Jennings, 2005; Skovholt &

Jennings, 2005; Jennings, Goh, Skovholt, Hanson, & Banerjee-Stevens, 2003) has largely sought to find answers to the question of 'What are the personal characteristics of expert counsellors?'

Three dimensions or domains have been identified that belong to the highly effective counsellor (Jennings & Skovholt, 1999; Skovholt, 2005). These domains, the cognitive, emotional, and relational, are integral areas of functioning for the effective counsellor. Master therapists blend these three domains and have the three domains available to them in their work with clients. In their qualitative research with 'master therapists,' Jennings and Skovholt (1999) identified that within each of these three domains there were three categories:

Cognitive domain

1. Master therapists are voracious learners.
2. Accumulated experiences have become a major resource.
3. Master therapists value cognitive complexity and the ambiguity of the human condition.

Affective domain

1. Master therapists are self-aware, reflective, non-defensive, and open to feedback.
2. Master therapists are congruent, mentally healthy, and mature individuals who attend to their own emotional well-being.
3. Master therapists are aware of how their emotional health affects the quality to their work; they are willing to work on their own emotional health.

Relational domain

1. Master therapists possess strong relational skills, such as warmth, respect, caring, and a genuine interest in people.
2. Master therapists believe that the foundation for therapeutic change is a strong working alliance.
3. Master therapists are experts at using their exceptional relationship skills in therapy. They provide safety and support for their clients and also are not afraid to challenge them. They are not afraid of strong emotion and, having the courage to deal with their own painful areas, can be present with their clients' pain.

When considering the types of students we admit to our counselling programmes, these characteristics and qualities of master counsellors could be a reliable guide in the selection and screening of candidates. While not expecting trainees to be instant experts or immediate master counsellors, counsellor educators and supervisors are looking for trainees and supervisees who are open to growth, receptive of feedback, and capable of achieving a developmental trajectory in that direction. And for our trainees to graduate, we are as supervisors and educators saying to the public and to the profession, that at this stage of their development, these graduates are professionally competent, personally sound, and ethically appropriate in their practice. They are 'good enough' to practice as professional counsellors.

In balancing the needs of potential counsellor trainees and other stakeholders (e.g., the profession, the public, and the counsellor education programme), Russell and her colleagues (2007) posed three questions that counsellor educators and supervisors might ask themselves. These questions are: 1) would I be comfortable hiring this person? 2) Would I be willing to supervise this person as my employee? 3) Would I refer a family member to this counsellor? (cf., p. 239). If as educators and supervisors of counsellors we honestly discussed our responses to these questions about our students with the counselling faculty, we may in fact save ourselves (and others) much grief and anxiety later in the programme.

Student performance concerns

As educators and supervisors in graduate programmes we are also aware of some students about whom we have serious professional concerns, in regards to their clinical competency, personal soundness, and/or ethically appropriateness. These concerns may arise through our direct observation, observation of other faculty, practicum supervisor reports, other student feedback, or indeed from information that the trainee gives to us directly (Forest et al., 1999). The American Counseling Association has used the term 'personal limitations' of supervisees that are likely to negatively affect professional competence (Code of Ethics and Standards of Practice F.3., 1995). The rates of problematic students in programmes, at least from American research run at about 5% (Forrest et al., 1999; Rapisarda & Britton, 2007). If this statistic was similar in our Australian counselling programmes, it would mean that out of forty students over a two-year full-time equivalent programme, there would be two students who are presenting with professional problems. At any rate, the literature suggests that most graduate programmes have at least one trainee who is not meeting a satisfactory standard of professional performance (Elman & Forrest, 2007). These students demand an inordinate amount of the faculty's time, energy, and resources. How we manage them, and what we in fact do with them and for them, is critical for all stakeholders.

Forrest and her colleagues (1999) summarised the ethical mandates incumbent upon trainers, educators, and supervisors, in managing problematic student performance. These include: a) attending to the possibility that their trainees' personal problems might lead to harm of others; b) making sure that trainees are not harming clients or others under their care; c) attending to the possibility that trainees may misuse their influence; d) evaluate whether trainees are performing responsibly, competently, and ethically; e) articulating a clear set of professional standards; and f) evaluating trainees based on these relevant and established requirements (cf., p. 636).

Clearly, being aware of potential harm, articulating performance criteria and standards, and evaluating student performance are essential aspects of ethical counsellor education and supervision. The faculty of responsible and ethical counsellor education programmes needs to respond to the following questions:

1. How do we identify and respond to the trainee who is showing serious limitations in any or all of the domains: cognitive; relational; or affective?
2. How do we understand the difference and overlap between impaired, incompetent, and unethical behaviours in our trainees (Forest et al., 1999)?
3. Are these problems, with appropriate intervention, always surmountable?
4. Or do they indicate that a trainee may in fact be unsuitable for the profession and should be counselled off or even dismissed from the programme?
5. What, if in our supervisory evaluation and with faculty consultation, a trainee is deemed not professionally 'good enough' and so unsuitable for the profession?

6. When is dismissal warranted and necessary for the protection of clients, the trainee, and the profession?
7. What is the threshold for dismissal on our programme?
8. What are our professional, ethical, and legal responsibilities as trainers and supervisors to this trainee, to the public, to the profession, and to our training institutes?

Certainly it has been my experience in discussing these questions with colleagues that as a profession, counsellor educators and supervisors are struggling to fully comprehend and implement their role and responsibilities as gatekeepers for professional counselling quality control (Forest et al., 1999). As educators and supervisors, we are accountable to and for our programmes, to our trainees, to the profession, and ultimately to future clients. How we operationalize our accountability is crucial to our role as gatekeepers to and for the profession. There is a tension between our need to support and nurture students and facilitate their growth as professionals, and our evaluative role as gatekeepers. It may be that there is a tension between university requirements to maintain full occupancy in academic programmes for economic viability (the 'innkeeper' role) and our professional roles to screen and evaluate. This means that not everyone who begins the programme is necessarily fit for graduation as a competent and ethical professional counsellor. Counselling certain students out of the programme or even their dismissal are real options.

Clear, shared, and consistent terminology

Over the past twenty years or so, there has been much conjecture and controversy over which terminology we as counsellor educators and supervisors use when referring to students who are not 'measuring up' to programme and professional expectations. When looking at the problem emotions, behaviours, and attitudes that students can manifest, it is obvious that these problems are on a continuum, ranging 'from interpersonal skill deficits to major psychopathology' (Ladany et al., 2005, p. 183). These problems have been referred to as: a) *impairment*, where students have shown prior professional competency, but are experiencing diminished functioning due to some external stressors; *incompetence* (where students have never shown a level of competent professional functioning); *unethical behaviour*, where students have shown they are not performing in accord with the counselling profession's code of ethics. Impairment, incompetence, and unethical behaviour are not mutually exclusive and may of course overlap (Forrest et al., 1999). Other terminology that has been used includes: *undesirable, unsuitable, emotionally troubled*, and *personality problems* (Elman & Forrest, 2007). The problem with these terms is that they lack specificity and precision, blur behaviour and personality, and mix-up cause and consequences. These terms can be seen as labels that are detrimental to the career future of the student, not only in the counselling profession. (see Elman & Forrest 2007 for a complete discussion on this). Elman and Forrest have proposed and argued for a more behaviourally precise term, *professional competence problems*. This term may cover the breadth and depth of the problems and concerns that counsellor educators and supervisors encounter in students who are not, for whatever reason, meeting professional standards of practice. Because it is behaviourally focused, the term may lead to more attentive monitoring and evaluation of students, which will in turn lead 'improved identification, remediation, and effective outcomes' (Elman & Forrest, 2007, p. 508).

Our role as gatekeepers

Let us now discuss our gatekeeper role, which for many of us may be fraught with difficulties. The American Counseling Association (2014) defined 'gatekeeping as "the initial and ongoing academic, skill, and dispositional assessment of students" competency for professional practice, including remediation and termination as appropriate' (p. 20) Gatekeeping is challenging and complicated. It is also defined as the process of intervening with counselling students such that only those who are competent and ethical graduate and enter the profession of counselling (Foster et al., 2014). Within the metaphor of the 'gatekeeping' role are three contributing components worth noting. Firstly, there is the 'gate' or the expectations, obligations, and standards of professional and ethical practice which are evaluated via a set of criteria within the structured programme of counsellor education and professional bodies. Secondly, there is the one trying to access and progress through the gate, that is the student who is being evaluated and assessed, and is attempting to meet professional competency and ethical standards. Thirdly, there is the 'gatekeeper' who is the evaluator, the trainer, or supervisor who is responsible for professional quality control in the form of evaluation. Ultimately the purpose of the process of gatekeeping is twofold: to protect the profession for which training is being provided and to protect the public who will access the profession.

Brear, Dorrian, and Luscri (2008) have identified the twofold challenge for gatekeepers: 'to develop a set of relevant and explicit criteria against which students can be measured, and to develop a fair and valid framework within which the gatekeeping mechanism can operate' (p. 94). They go on to summarise the seven functions of effective gatekeeping for the counselling profession as:

1. promoting student equity
2. fulfilling the educational and ethical responsibilities of the educator
3. guarding the integrity of training programmes
4. ensuring the quality of graduates
5. enhancing the quality of the profession
6. maintaining societal sanction
7. protecting the interests of the community, particularly consumers of counselling services, i.e., our clients and future clients

Bemak, Epp, and Keys (1999) designed a five-step model of gatekeeping, with the goal being ongoing evaluation of students. The five steps are: a) before the application process begins, potential applicants have programme expectations clearly clarified and communicated to them, where unacceptable or inappropriate behaviours, attitudes, and outlooks that could lead to dismissal are explicitly stated; b) contractual agreement, signed by the student, indicating comprehension of and agreement to the above; c) early identification of problematic concerns, where prompt review with the student and faculty staff is undertaken; d) remediation recommendations in the form of a plan are designed with the student and counsellor educators and supervisors; and, e) ongoing monitoring and evaluation of progress and outcomes, where this student is informed of this. At this stage is satisfactory progress is not made, then dismissal becomes a real possibility. Ziomek-Daigle & Christensen (2010) in their emergent theory of gatekeeping posited four phases of gatekeeping practices: preadmission; postadmission; remediation plan; and remediation outcome. Potential students and students need to be informed of these phases of gatekeeping, prior to acceptance and during the course of their studies. Staff need to be upskilled in the programme's gatekeeping philosophy, policies, and practice, to ensure as far as possible, competent and ethical graduates for the profession.

Christine Suniti Bhat's (2005) idea of designing performance appraisals for student counsellors has much merit. They are used for evaluating employees and could in fact be a useful tool for us as gatekeepers of the profession, as they are defined in terms of behavioural and measurable objectives. A performance appraisal process encapsulates much of the Bemak, Epp, and Keys five-step model.

Remediation

Counsellor educators and supervisors need to know when to initiate remediation assistance for students who are manifesting professional competence problems – the earlier the better (Bhat, 2005). While there is some literature that refers to remediation in terms of 'sanctioned' or 'mandated' supervision (Cobia & Pipes, 2002; Rapisarda & Britton, 2007), it may be better to use the term *required performance or clinical monitoring,* which in reality is an increased and focused level of supervision (cf., Rapisarda & Britton, 2007). 'Sanctioned' and 'mandated' suggest a sense of being involuntary, punitive, and coercive. And as such may indicate the student lacks motivation and commitment to the process. While this may be the case for some students presenting with performance problems, it is not necessarily the case for all. If the student's performance and functioning has diminished, he or she may welcome remediation steps to regain or achieve satisfactory performance standards, and so be able to continue successfully to graduation.

In summarising the remediation literature, Forrest and her colleagues (1999) suggested that remediation plans should:

1. identify and describe deficiencies that are directly tied to the programme's evaluation criteria,
2. identify specific goals or changes that need to be made by the trainee,
3. identify possible methods for meeting those goals,
4. establish criteria for judging whether remediation has been successful, and
5. determine a timeline for re-evaluation.

The remediation plans generally include increased mentoring and advising, intensified and focused supervision, additional field experience, remedial or repeating coursework or practicum, and personal counselling is often encouraged. Forrest and her team believe that while remediation plans are discussed in the literature, there has not been the data gathering or research to support how we should design, implement, and monitor remediation plans designed to manage and address students' performance problems (Forrest et al., 1999).

Dismissal

When remediation plans do not achieve positive outcomes for students, we need to face the fact that these students need to be counselled off the programme, or even dismissed from the programme as being unsuitable for the profession, in that they never had or have not been able to achieve an adequate level of professional competence. If such students are known to the faculty and to other students, and are permitted to continue to graduation, then the Training Institute, University, and programme faculty (as well as the graduate) may be held legally liable for malpractice, for any harm done to clients in the future (Enochs & Etzbach, 2004). Obviously due process needs to be followed according to the policies of the University or Training Institute, where students have been duly informed of professional competencies, standards, and expectations, remedial plans that have not achieved sufficient change in the student's professional competency levels are recorded, and extensive and detailed documentation is completed and placed in the student's file (Wilkerson, 2006).

Some of the reasons for dismissal include continued poor academic performance, poor clinical performance, failed competency tests, ethical violations, psychopathology, emotional instability, personality disorder, unprofessional demeanour, poor interpersonal skills, sexual misconduct, and substance abuse (Forrest et al., 1999). Obviously, these are serious issues and are going to affect a student's ability to meet successfully professional competency standards, and lead to potential harm done to clients, the profession, and the programme itself. Ultimately, we do no favour to a student who is professionally incompetent if we permit him or her to graduate.

Recommendations

The following recommendations are a compilation of recommendations from some of the relevant literature. If implemented these could contribute positively to the selection, review, remediation, and retention policies and practices in our programmes (Bhat, 2005; Bemak, Epp, & Keys, 1999; Enochs & Etzbach, 2004; Foster et al., 2014; Freeman et al., 2020; Russell et al., 2007). They include:

- Screening and selection procedures are clearly outlined and defined, including required professional and personal characteristics, students' openness to feedback, and willingness to undertake personal counselling.
- A programme's gatekeeping policies and procedures should be clearly articulated during admission procedures, upon entrance into the programme, in formal and informal meetings with advisors and supervisors, and regularly throughout the programme. These standards, once promulgated, should be implemented consistently and justly.
- Screening and selection should not be an isolated process at the programme's beginning, but the evaluation and review process needs to be ongoing. Just because a student wins initial selection onto the programme should not ensure certain graduation. He or she may exhibit such behaviour on the programme that means the individual is not appropriate to continue in the programme.
- Counsellor educators and supervisors should establish clear performance-based contracts with students early in training, where learning objectives and professional competencies are unequivocally articulated, performance reviews and competency interviews regularly undertaken. Students are informed of the gatekeeping role of the faculty and onsite supervisors. Students are also alerted to the expectations of professional codes of conduct and standards of practice.
- Counsellor educators and supervisors require regular and ongoing opportunities to consult together about students' dispositions and progress.
- The gatekeeping role of counsellor educators and supervisors is an ethical obligation so as to take appropriate action to protect clients and future clients form harm. Therefore, the faculty need to be professionally developed and trained in the gatekeeping role.

The role needs to be defined in a systematic and structured way, with clear policies and procedures.

• Universities need to have 'clear and precise procedures for dismissing students who are inappropriate for the program' (Enochs & Etzbach, 2004, p. 399) because of continued professional competency problems.

These recommendations are intended to strengthen our role as gatekeepers and lessen the stressful effects of not dealing early enough or adequately with students' professional competency problems.

Conclusions

The review of supervision literature (mainly examining studies undertaken with trainees) by Wheeler and Richards indicated that supervision has positive effects on the supervisee where the growth and development is enhanced. Supervisees' self-efficacy and skills are improved via supervision. 'Supervision does seem to offer opportunities for supervisees to improve practice and gain in confidence' (Wheeler & Richards, 2007, p. 63). This is evidence that: we as supervisors of trainees need to take this role seriously; we need to consider the recommendations from the literature for our programmes; we need to professionally develop ourselves as gatekeepers; we need to articulate professional performance standards, requirements, and programme expectation; and finally we need to communicate clearly, strongly and early to our students that this is one of our key roles in the programme. Gatekeeping within training programmes is a 'global imperative' that should be implemented by counsellors, supervisors, and counsellor educators locally and internationally (Mccaughan & Hill, 2015, p. 39). Gatekeeping is a process of protecting the profession, protecting the public, and importantly protecting counsellor-supervisees themselves.

Educational questions & activities

1. If the three domains of counselling mastery are the cognitive, the affective, and the relational (Jennings & Skovholt, 1999), how can we best evaluate if our programme applicants are likely to be effective in these areas? In what ways can counsellor educators and supervisors assist potential students fairly in demonstrating their capacities to be worthy candidates for a postgraduate counselling programme?
2. Forrest and her colleagues (1999) summarised the ethical mandates incumbent upon trainers, educators and supervisors, in managing problematic student performance. These include:
   • Attending to the possibility that their trainees' personal problems might lead to harm of others
   • Making sure that trainees are not harming clients or others under their care
   • Attending to the possibility that trainees may misuse their influence
   • Evaluating whether trainees are performing responsibly, competently, and ethically
   • Articulating a clear set of professional standards
   • Evaluating trainees based on these relevant and established requirements (cf., p. 636).

Discuss how your programme attends to these mandates effectively?

3. Discuss the significance of the language we use in defining and labelling certain behaviours and/or individuals who are problematic. What are the benefits and dangers in using the following terminology in regards to students? a) 'Incompetence'; b) 'impairment'; c) 'personal limitations'; d) 'inappropriateness'; e) 'unsuitability'; f) 'unfit to practice'; professional competence problems?

4. Discuss how you can design, implement, and monitor remediation plans shaped to manage and address individual student's performance problems. Who should take responsibility for these plans in your programme? Should the three tasks of design, implementation and monitoring be undertaken by different individuals on the faculty?

5. Discuss with your colleagues what behaviours, attitudes, and contexts demand the dismissal of a student from your programme. What are our professional, ethical, and legal responsibilities as trainers and supervisors to this trainee, to the public, to the profession, and to our training institutes?

References

American Counseling Association (ACA) Code of Ethics (2014). Retrieved on 3 January 2024 from ACA 2014 Code of Ethics (counseling.org).

Australian Counselling Association (ACA) Inc. 2nd ed. (2020). Scope of Practice for Counsellors. Newmarket, Queensland: Philip Armstrong, retrieved on 3 January 2024 from Scope_of_Practice_2nd_Edition.pdf (theaca.net.au).

Aveline, M. (2005). The person of the therapist. *Psychotherapy Research*, 15(3), 155–164.

Bemak, F., Epp, L.R., & Keys, S.G. (1999). Impaired graduate students: A process model of graduate program monitoring and intervention. *International Journal for the Advancement of Counseling*, 21, 19–30.

Bhat, C.S. (2005). Enhancing counseling gatekeeping with performance appraisal protocols. *International Journal for the Advancement of Counselling*, 27(3), 399–411.

Brear, P., Dorrian, J., & Luscri, G. (2008). Preparing our future counselling professionals: Gatekeeping and the implications for research. *Counselling and Psychotherapy Research*, 8(2), 93–101.

Cobia, Debra, & Pipes, Randolph. (2002). Mandated supervision: An intervention for disciplined professionals. *Journal of Counseling & Development*. 80(2). 10.1002/j.1556-6678.2002.tb00176.x.

Elman, N.S. & Forrest, L. (2007). From *trainee impairment* to *professional competence problems*: Seeking new terminology that facilitates effective action. *Professional Psychology: Research and Practice*, 38(5), 501–509.

Enochs, W.K. & Etzbach, C.A. (2004). Impaired student counselors: Ethical and legal considerations for the family. *The Family Journal: Counseling and Therapy for Couples and Families*, 12(4), 396–400.

Forrest, L., Elman, N., Gizara, S., & Vacha-Haase, T. (1999). Trainee impairment: A review of identification, remediation, dismissal, and legal issues. *The Counseling Psychologist*, 27, 627–686.

Foster, J.M., Leppma, M., & Hutchinson, T.S. (2014). Students' perspectives on gatekeeping in counselor education: A case study. *Counselor Education and Supervision*, 53(3), 190–203. https://doi.org/10.1002/j.1556-6978.2014.00057.x

Freeman, B., Woodliff, T., & Martinez, M. (2020). Teaching gatekeeping to doctoral students: A qualitative study of a developmental experiential approach. *The Professional Counselor, Suppl. Special Issue: Doctoral Counselor Education*, 10(4), 562–580. https://doi.org/10.15241/bf.10.4.562

Jennings, L., Goh, M., Skovholt, T.M., Hanson, M., & Banerjee-Stevens, D. (2003). Multiple factors in the development of the expert counselor and therapist. *Journal of Career Development*, *30*(1), 59–72.

Jennings, L., & Skovholt, T.M. (1999). The cognitive, emotional and relational characteristics of master therapists. *Journal of Counseling Psychology*, *46*(1), 3–11.

Kaslow, N.J., Rubin, N.J., Forrest, L., et al. (2007). Recognizing, assessing, and intervening with problems of professional competence. *Professional Psychology: Research and Practice*, *38*(5), 479–492.

Ladany, N., Friedlander, M.L., & Nelson, M.L. (2005). Addressing problematic emotions, attitudes, and behaviours: Counseling in versus counseling out, pp. 183–210. *Critical Events in Psychotherapy Supervision: An Interpersonal Approach*. Washington, DC: APA.

Mccaughan, A.M., & Hill, N.R. (2015). The gatekeeping imperative in counselor education admission protocols: The criticality of personal qualities. *International Journal for the Advancement of Counselling*, *37*(1), 28–40. https://doi.org/10.1007/s10447-014-9223-2

McWilliams, N. (2005). Preserving our humanity as therapists. *Psychotherapy: Theory, Research, Practice, Training*, *42*(2), 139–151.

Psychotherapy and Counselling Federation of Australia (PACFA) Training Standards (2022). Retrieved from the PACFA website www.pacfa.com.au on 3 January 2022.

Rapisarda, C.A., & Britton, P.J. (2007). Sanctioned supervision: Voices from the experts. *Journal of Mental Health Counseling*, *29*(1), 81–92.

Rønnestad, M.H., & Skoholt, T.M. (2001). Learning arenas for professional development: Retrospective accounts of senior therapists. *Professional Psychology: Research and Practice*, *32*, 181–187.

Rønnestad, M.H., & Skovholt, T.M. (2003). The journey of the counselor and therapist: Research findings and perspectives on professional development. *Journal of Career Development*, *30*(1), 5–44.

Russell, C.S., Beggs, M.A., Peterson, C.M. & Anderson, M.P. (2007). Responding to remediation and gatekeeping challenges in supervision. *Journal of Marital and Family Therapy*, *33*(2), 227–244.

Skovholt, T., & Jennings, L. (2005). Mastery and expertise in counseling. *Journal of Mental Health Counseling*, *27*(1), 13–18.

Skovholt, T.M. (2005). The cycle of caring: A model of expertise in the helping professions. *Journal of Mental Health Counseling*, *27*(1), 82–93.

Sullivan, B.F. (2008). *Counsellors and Counselling: A New Conversation*. French's Forest, NSW: Pearson Education.

Wheeler, S. (2002). Nature or nurture: Are therapists born or trained? *Psychodynamic Practice*, *8*(4), 427–441.

Wheeler, S., & Richards, K. (2007). The impact of clinical supervision on counsellors and therapists, their practice and their clients. A systematic review of the literature. *Counselling and Psychotherapy Research*, *7*(1), 54–65.

Wilkerson, K. (2006). Impaired students: Applying the therapeutic process model to graduate training programs. *Counselor Education and Supervision*, *45*(3), 207–217.

Ziomek-Daigle, J., & Christensen, T.M. (2010). An emergent theory of gatekeeping practices in counselor education. *Journal of Counseling and Development*, *88*(4), 407–415. https://doi.org/10.1002/j.1556-6678.2010.tb00040.x

20 Counsellor Competence

Nadine Pelling

Introduction

The topic of counselling competence has increased in importance in recent years along with a growing demand for high-quality counselling, an increase in credentialing efforts, and a focus on the professionalisation of counselling. There are many ways of defining and assessing counsellor competence. This chapter describes some of the main issues relating to the definition and assessment of counsellor competence including who is assessing competence and for what purpose.

The importance and complexity of counsellor competence

The topic of counsellor competence became very important in the 1990s in the United States of America (USA) (McLeod, 1992). In fact, a plethora of professional ethical codes regarding counsellor competence, a synopsis of which can be found in Corey, Corey, and Callanan (1992), developed. Anderson says that this was due to five discernible forces influencing the counselling profession in the USA:

> (a) a growing demand for quality mental health counseling; (b) an increasing public awareness of specific issues in mental health care and general health care consumerism; (c) increasing demands for quality assurance, accountability, and containment of mental health care cost; (d) a progressive state-by-state wave of credentialism and licensure; and (e) increasing national emphasis on counselor professionalism.
>
> (Anderson, 1992, p. 22)

As a result, counsellor licensure and certification have long been viewed as a validation of qualifications needed for effective and competent counselling in the USA (McLeod, 1992). Counsellor licensure and certification have become expected in the USA. The goal of counsellor licensure and certification is to increase counsellor professionalism and protect consumers from incompetent practitioners.

A similar focus on counselling competency is currently developing in Australia. This is evident in the two main generalist counselling associations' recent focus on educational standards and credentialing efforts. These two associations are often seen as competitors due to their overlapping and similar functions as well as, at times, different philosophies regarding the credentialing of counselling. It is sufficient to say that different counselling associations in Australia are defining competence or readiness for counselling differently. This is not surprising given that counsellor competence is so difficult to define

DOI: 10.4324/9781003490067-25

and measure. Add this to indecisiveness regarding who will measure counsellor competence and the complexity of assessing competent counselling services in Australia becomes clear (Armstrong, 2006; Pelling, 2003; Pelling, 2006; Pelling & Sullivan, 2006; Pelling & Whetham, 2006; Pelling, Brear, & Lau, 2006; Schofield, Grant, Holmes, & Barletta, 2006; Sullivan, 2003).

Defining competence

How does one define counsellor competence? The literature on counsellor competence centres on the idea of skill (Egan, 1990; Ivey & Authier, 1978). Thus, a competent counsellor would be one who has mastered a set of counselling skills. The National Counsellor Examination's testing of professional knowledge on basic counselling information and skills in eight basic areas of counselling practice seems to subscribe to this view of competence as skill (Corey, Corey, & Callanan, 1992).

However, there are those who believe that competence cannot be reduced to the level of skill. These people argue that counselling is not simply the accumulation of a set of skills. As stated by McLeod (1992, p. 360) "the person of the counselor, including her values and philosophy, is a key factor in the counseling relationship, and that this factor is not readily observable within discrete, 'micro' interactions."

Thus, although the literature on competence focuses on the idea of skill it also seems agreed upon that competence subsumes skill and refers (McLeod, 1992, p. 360) "to any qualities or abilities of the person which contribute to effective performance of a role or task." As stated by McLeod (1992, p. 359) "Counseling is an activity in which, almost uniquely, the quality of work and the outcome of effort is largely hidden form external scrutiny and affirmation." This sentiment is echoed by Gross and Robinson (1987, p. 7) who view counsellor competence as containing five basic aspects, the fourth issue being most closely associated with competence as skill, which are an "(1) accurate representation of professional qualifications; (2) professional growth through involvement in continuing education; (3) provision of only those services for which one is qualified; (4) maintenance of accurate knowledge and expertise in specialized areas; and (5) assistance in solving personal issues which impede effectiveness."

As stated by McLeod (1992, p. 367) "Within the thousands of counseling and psychotherapy trainers, tutors and supervisors there certainly must exist a deep well of experience and knowledge about how best to assess the competence of counselors. Very little of this knowledge is written down, however, and even less of it has been subject to systematic research." Thus, obviously, defining counsellor competence is difficult and one's definition clearly depends on many factors, including the purpose of one's definition. Capturing the essence of and what is meant by competence is elusive (Goh, 2005). Nevertheless, this difficulty has not prevented many efforts at measuring counsellor competence.

The assessment of competence

The measurement of counsellor competence is complicated by its very nature. First, there is no precise definition of competence. Second, the purpose of competence measurement will affect the definition of competence and thus the assessment technique used. Third, the measurement of competence will also be influenced by who is measuring competence.

Purpose of assessment

The measurement of counsellor competence takes two forms, formative and summative, depending on what function the assessment is to serve. Summative assessment's purpose is to evaluate the competence of a person and formative assessment's purpose is to generate information concerning the developmental needs of the counsellor. Summative assessment would therefore most likely be used in evaluating a counsellor's competence to perform a particular job or whether the person should receive a professional certification or license. In contrast, formative assessments are designed to generate information about the developmental needs of the counsellor that could be used to define learning objectives in work settings or in continuing education programs (McLeod, 1992).

Who will assess competence?

Counsellor competence can be assessed by counsellor trainers, managers, supervisors, external judges, themselves, peers, and clients. These different assessors usually differ in their purpose, their corresponding definition of competence, and their measurement techniques. Some general statement concerning the advantages and disadvantages of each of the before mentioned competence evaluators are as follows (McLeod, 1992).

Trainer/Supervisor Assessment. Competence assessment is a necessity when one is in a training program. Unfortunately, the validity and reliability of assessment by a trainer or supervisor may be negatively impacted by many factors. For example, trainers may not have equal exposure to all their trainees and the contact they do have may be coloured by 'impression management' on the trainees part who want to be evaluated favourably. Moreover, supervision is said to involve aspects of assessment, training, support, and personal therapy which can complicate the assessment process (McLeod, 1992; Corey, Corey, & Callanan, 1992).

Manager Assessment. Some managers are not members of the counselling profession and thus their assessment of counsellor competence might be resisted due to the belief that only counsellors should judge counsellor competence. Such managers might consider a counsellor effective if they work well with other staff members, engage in professional development, and if clients return to see the counsellor in question.

External Judge Assessment. Judgments made by an external judge are less likely to be biased. However, the counselling work they are exposed to is likely to be limited and thus may not be representative of the counsellor's overall competence.

Self-Assessment. The main argument against counsellor self-assessment of competence is that incompetent counsellors are not likely to know how to make accurate judgement of their own competence (McLeod, 1992). In contrast, Gross and Robinson (1987) purport that an internal frame of reference is best used to ensure competence, although the necessity for some level of external enforcement is conceded. Gross and Robinson (1987) believes that each counsellor should take full responsibility for their own conduct and their adherence to the rules and regulations of their profession. Self-assessment, of course, depends on the honesty of the assessor or counsellor. In Australia counsellors themselves are likely the most common assessors of competence as counselling is currently a legally unregulated activity. Thus, in Australia competence assessments are not specifically required for counselling practice.

Peer Assessment. This type of assessment is less impacted by the 'impression management,' which can impact supervisory assessment. However, if peer assessment is to be utilised an appropriate culture regarding the giving and receiving of feedback must be created and maintained.

Client Assessment. As stated by McLeod (1992, p. 363) "The ultimate criterion of counselor competence must be that of client benefit." In other words, did the client benefit from his or her counselling experience? Unfortunately, research in this area is limited and can be very expensive.

How do we measure competence?

The measurement of competence is very complicated, depends on the definition of competence utilized, and can be accomplished in a number of ways. Moreover, the multifarious measurement of competence is even further complicated by the general exclusion of validity and reliability data on counsellor competence measurements (McLeod, 1992). In general, the measurement of counsellor competence is best assessed in a safe and open environment, when assessment techniques are based in research, target competencies are specific, and multitudes of measurement techniques are used. The main techniques used for the measurement of counsellor competence are as follows: questionnaires and rating scales, video/audio tapes, role-play exercises/simulations, journals, and exams (McLeod, 1992).

Questionnaires/Rating Scales. There are two types of questionnaires/rating scales; those with an evaluative component and those designed to estimate how often a counsellor does something (i.e., reflect the client's feelings), whose results would then be interpreted in relation to the theory the counsellor is using. Both Carkhuff (1969) as well as Ivey and Authier (1978) have developed rating scales that assess various counselling skills. Similarly, specific scales have been devised and used to measure different types of counselling competence, such as multicultural competence (Holcomb-McCoy, 2005). In contrast, Sachs (1983) has developed a rating scale designed to measure the absence of competence via its focus on therapist errors. It seems that those using questionnaires and rating scales are supervising counsellors set cut-off levels between acceptable and unacceptable levels of competence. The counselling behaviour assessed can be live, on video/audiotape, or role-play/simulation situations.

Journals. Learning journals and diaries containing the participant's subjective record of their development and learning can also be used to assess counsellor competence. Competence is assessed by examining the amount of insight the counsellor has into his or her actions and interventions.

Exams. Formal examinations are widely accepted as able to assess dimensions of cognitive skill and knowledge rather than interpersonal skills that is required for working with clients. This technique assumes that counsellor competence is largely due to one's ability to learn difficult theoretical material. However, empirical testing of this assumption has not been flattering and many sources believe that (McLeod, 1992, p. 366; Chevron & Rounsaville, 1983) "too high an emphasis on theoretical knowledge may distract the counselor from her primary task, that of establishing a therapeutic relationship with her client." In fact, Chevron and Rounsaville (1983) found, in their study of psychotherapy evaluating techniques, that only supervisor's ratings were correlated with patient outcome.

In Australia, the Psychology Board of Australia has instituted a National Psychology Exam that most wishing to become registered psychologists will have to pass to qualify for general registration. Pelling (2017) discusses the use of exams in counselling and psychology in a Pelling and Burton (2017) study guide for the exam.

Identifying a minimum level of counsellor competence

To summarise, there is a lack of information regarding the reliability and validity of assessments of counsellor competence. The research findings of Chevron and Rounsaville (1983) suggest that competence assessments and client outcome lack a relationship. Thus, developing counsellor competence and designating a minimum level of counsellor competence to be measured does not at this time seem realistic. It seems more logical to focus on the gradations of competence rather than on identifying various absolute levels of competence when skill and direct work with clients is concerned. It is easier to judge whether a counsellor is grossly incompetent versus designating competence. This is the reasoning behind Sachs' (1983) study of negative factors in psychotherapy. Nevertheless, there are authors that have proposed minimum standards of competence for counsellors, one example is Anderson (1992) who has proposed eight minimum standards.

Enforcing minimum levels of counsellor competence

How does one ensure counsellor competence given the lack of consensus regarding a definition of competence and the multitude of assessors as well as assessment techniques? It seems that the most efficient and common method of ensuring counsellor competence is the counsellors' self and peer assessment; if an open, safe, and honest environment can be maintained. This is important to ensure that a 'police state' does not result in the counselling profession. Yes, we want to ensure that only competent counsellors are practicing counselling but a professional emphasis in assessment must be on formative versus summative assessment aimed at continuously increasing counsellor competence if the counselling profession is to be an inclusive occupation and not exclusive in Australia. This is the approach taken by Nagy (1989) who has proposed nine guidelines for counsellors to avoid practicing beyond their limits of competence, including skills areas and personal problem management.

Can/does licensure and certification ensure counsellor competence?

Unfortunately, legal regulation and certification cannot ensure counsellor competence. They may serve to create very general minimum standards of competence but they certainly cannot (Corey, Corey, & Callanan, 1992) confer overall competence. As pointed out by Nagy (1989) counsellor competence can be exceeded both on purpose as well as accidentally and steps must be taken by the counsellor him/herself to ensure that one does not work outside their boundaries of competence. Evidently we must patrol ourselves to ensure that our peers and we learn how to stay within our boundaries of competence when working with clients. We must understand and believe that this is in our and our clients' best interests.

Within the profession 'incompetence' is generally recognisable by both the counsellor him/herself and also his/her peers. Differing levels of competence are less definable due to the: subjective nature of defining competence, differing reasons for competence measurement, and the plethora of people who may be in charge of competence assessment. Given all this subjectivity it seems impossible to decisively measure competence with purely objective measures and thus designate a minimum level of competence as well as objective gradations of competence. Counsellors subjectively know what competence and incompetence are and how to evaluate them ... an objective measurement and testing of this is less likely and some would argue not desired. A starting point for competence assessment is clearly stating our definition of competence and who and for what purpose competence is to be assessed while keeping in mind the difficulty in assessing such a concept.

Acknowledgement

The contents of the present chapter have been previously published as follows:

Pelling, N. (2006). Counsellor competence: A survey of Australian counsellor self perceived competence, *Counselling Australia*, 6(1), 3–14.
Pelling, N. (2007). Counsellor competence (Chapter 2). In N. Pelling, R. Bowers, & P. Armstrong (Eds.), *The practice of counselling* (pp. 36–45). Melbourne, Australia: Thomson.

Educational questions & activities

1. Discuss how you define competence.
2. List two forms of assessment.
3. Who are some stakeholders who can assess competence?

References

Anderson, D. (1992). A case for standards of counselling practice. *Journal of Counselling & Development*, 71, 22–26.
Armstrong, P. (2006). The Australian Counselling Association: Meeting the needs of Australian counsellors. *International Journal of Psychology*, 41(3), 156–162.
Carkhuff, R. (1969). *Helping and Human Relations* (2nd ed.). New York: Holdt.
Chevron, E., & Rounsaville, B. (1983). Evaluating the clinical skills of psychotherapists. *Archives of General Psychiatry*, 40, 1129–1132.
Corey, G., Corey, M., & Callanan, P. (1992). *Issues and Ethics in the Helping Professions* (4th ed.). California: Brooks/Cole.
Egan, G. (1990). *The Skilled Helper* (4th ed.). San Francisco: Brooks/Cole.
Goh, M. (2005). Cultural competence and master therapists: An inextricable relationship. *Journal of Mental Health Counseling*, 27(1), 71–82.
Gross, D.R., & Robinson, S.E. (1987). Ethics in counseling: A multiple role perspective. *TACD Journal*, 15(1), 5–15.
Holcomb-McCoy, C. (2005). Investigating school counselors' perceived multicultural competence. *Professional School Counseling*, 8(5), 414–424.
Ivey, A., & Authier, A. (1978). *Microcounselling: Innovations in Interviewing, Counselling, Psychotherapy and Psychoeducation* (2nd ed.). Illinois: Thomas.
McLeod, J. (1992). What do we know about how best to assess counsellor competence? *Counselling Psychology Quarterly*, 5(4), 359–372.
Nagy, T. (1989). Boundaries of Competence: Training and Therapist Impairment. Annual Meeting of the California State Psychological Association, San Francisco, 25–28 February.

Pelling, J. (2017). Preface: Rationale for an elements book. In N.J. Pelling, & L.J. Burton (Eds.), *The elements of applied psychological practice in Australia*. London: Taylor and Francis.

Pelling, N. (2003). Counselling in Australia Comment. *Counselling Today*, 45(7), 4 & 30.

Pelling, N. (2006). Introduction to the special issue on counselling in Australia. *International Journal of Psychology*, 41(3), 153–155.

Pelling, N., Brear, P., & Lau, M. (2006). A survey of advertised Australian counsellors. *International Journal of Psychology*, 41(3), 204–215.

Pelling, N., & Sullivan, B. (2006). The credentialing of counselling in Australia. *International Journal of Psychology*, 41(3), 194–203.

Pelling, N., & Whetham, P. (2006). The professional preparation of Australian counsellors. *International Journal of Psychology*, 41(3), 189–193.

Pelling, N.J., & Burton, L.J. (Eds.). (2017). *The elements of applied psychological practice in Australia*. London: Taylor and Francis.

Sachs, J. (1983). Negative factors in brief psychotherapy: An empirical assessment. *Journal of Consulting and Clinical Psychology*, 51, 557–564.

Sullivan, B. (2003). Counselling in Australia Comment. *Counselling Today*, 45(7), 30.

21 Supervising Clinical Placement

John Barletta and Jason Dixon

Introduction to internship and practicum

Internship and practicum are the pinnacle of the therapist training experience. During these fieldwork experiences trainees are challenged to apply what they have learnt in coursework and research to the clinical workplace. Internship is where the rigorous science of the profession and the creative art of the practice intersect, and trainees begin to develop competence and clinical wisdom. The trainee therapist, being prepared for their responsibilities, and having a successful relationship with their supervisor, can optimise the gains from this integrated experience. In this chapter, an introduction to supervised internship and practicum encounters is provided with the trainee therapist and future supervisor firmly in mind.

Definition and purpose

Supervision is critical to clients and to the trainee. In the simplest of terms supervision is a service provided directly to trainees with an effect on the clinical outcomes for clients. Understanding the nature of supervision and internship or practicum will prepare trainees to effectively engage and benefit from these experiences.

There are several definitions of supervision used in the helping professions. Some of these definitions solely emphasise the relationship between the supervisor and the supervisee (e.g., Gilbert & Evans, 2000), while others focus only on the client's experience. The task of supervision maybe as narrow as only administrative responsibilities or as broad as encompassing all aspects relating to work as a therapist (Loganbill, Hardy, & Delworth, 1982). Bernard and Goodyear's (2018) definition of supervision is usefully comprehensive as it relates to provision of therapy in that supervision is defined as a relationship between the supervisor and supervisee that is evaluative, extends over time, enhances supervisee functioning, monitors the quality of professional services, and serves as gate-keeping to the profession.

In the United Kingdom, the literature of Proctor and Kadushin is very influential in the field of supervision. They outline three functions of supervision being normative (administrative), formative (educational), and restorative (supportive) and these are common across the professions of social work, nursing, medicine, educational psychology, and teaching (Kilminster & Jolly, 2000). In the United States of America, Bernard and Goodyear (2018) are arguably the most influential authors in the field of supervision and state that the fundamental purpose of supervision is to foster supervisee professional development and ensure client welfare. What we know is that individual clinical supervision not only functions to improve the development of a clinician and reduce risks to clients, but that attending professional conferences is also an aspect of supervision in a broad sense. As

DOI: 10.4324/9781003490067-26

trainees experience supervision they discover areas of proficiency and shortcomings that they will need to explore through professional development.

What to expect from the supervision experience

The fieldwork experience should be organised so that it is not so effortless that it becomes tedious and not too challenging that it is overwhelming. Thankfully, in the experience of internship and practicum, trainees are likely to have more than one supervisor who monitors progress. This will probably be someone from the academic institution where trainees are studying, and a field supervisor who will oversee tasks in the clinical setting. This section focuses on the collaboration trainees undertake with the field supervisor.

Approaches of a supervisor

In general, the field supervisor may employ at least three broad approaches to working with trainees. Supervisors may assist through teaching, counselling, and/or consultation (Barletta, 2007). In the case of teaching, trainees will have the already familiar learning role. However, unlike the classroom experience where a general syllabus is provided to outline the learning objectives, teaching in the supervisory setting will be designed to the trainee's specific needs, strengths, and weaknesses (Bernard & Goodyear, 2018). Without the structure of a syllabus, the learning trainees will do in supervision is andragogic (i.e., adult learning), which means that trainees develop the way they learn and to some extent what they learn, from and beyond supervision (Granello & Hazler, 1998; Marshak, 1983). This allows for greater control over learning experiences and helps develop an insight into managing professional development above and beyond supervision and internship.

Trainees' clients will personally change them in different ways. Depending on trainees' experiences, a supervisor may use a counselling approach with them. Most of trainees' encounters in helping clients will lead to a deep sense of occupational satisfaction and encouragement. However, sometimes clients will have a negative personal impact on trainees. This goes with the territory in all the helping professions. Well-documented is the clinician's experience of vicarious or secondary trauma of those working with people with posttraumatic stress disorder (Zimmering, Munroe, & Gulliver, 2003). Sometimes even less dramatic experiences can also effect therapists negatively. One of the authors of this chapter had a supervisee who was shocked at a teenage client who was questioning his sexuality and presented her with pornographic drawings. In this case the author used counselling interventions to assist the supervisee to work through their shock and integrate this situation into her understanding of the client's case, and thus improve her effectiveness in helping the teenager. However it is important to remember that a supervisor is not the trainee's therapist per se and has an ethical responsibility to refer trainees to another professional should they present with issues with an aetiology independent from client work (Ladany, Lehrman-Waterman, Molinaro, & Wolgast, 1999)

Especially in the Australian context, the trainees a supervisor works with may or may not be from the same profession. This will depend on which profession the trainee is pursuing. When a supervisor is from a different profession, for example, the supervisor is a psychologist and the trainee is a counsellor, the supervisor may employ more of a consultation approach. Consultation is often used when the supervisee is an experienced clinician and has the purpose of handling difficult and complicated cases or for the need to retrieve objectivity. It is also suggested that consultation is useful for experienced clinicians moving into a new area of clinical practice. It should be remembered that if trainees are experiencing hurdles during internship, and the field supervisory relationship only allows for consultation, trainees should consider seeking advice from the supervisor at the academic institution.

Live supervision and supervision with pre-recorded work. The practice of live supervision has decades of history in the helping professions. Live supervision is a training component used across a wide range of helping professions, including counselling, social work, and psychology (Champe & Kleist, 2003). Live supervision along with recordings reviewed by a supervisor are ways of addressing possible conscious and unconscious distortion in the reporting of clinical work by the supervisee (Noelle, 2002).

Live supervision is delivered in different ways. Supervisors can view trainees' work from behind a two-way mirror in a clinical or training facility (Hunt & Sharpe, 2008) and give instructions via a 'bug in the ear.' The supervisor may not be on site and trainees receive guidance via teleconferencing, or the supervisor can co-counsel with the trainee who is given a model of practice to emulate. Live supervision works best when it is collaborative and supportive in nature.

Interpersonal Process Recall (IPR) (Kagan, 1975) is an approach that has been applied to supervision and training. In this technique the trainee and the supervisor review a recorded therapy session. Either the trainee or supervisor stops the recording at any time to explore matters relating to the therapeutic process. The supervisor will establish the space to recall and examine the trainee's experiences as they relate to the therapeutic process. Results from an empirical study of counsellor trainees was used to draw conclusions that the IPR method of training was best suited for trainee counsellors who had mastered advanced counselling skills and are ready to personalise diverse theoretical concepts to client helping practices. Thus, this approach is well-suited to those who are entering the practicum and internship phases of their therapist training.

Characteristics of effective supervisors

When considering the role of the trainee as a supervisee, one might wonder how they know if the supervision being received is effective. One of the most important core conditions for the therapeutic environment is interpersonal trust (Hazler & Barwick, 2001). One way to gauge the effectiveness of supervision experience is to consider if the supervisor is able to develop and maintain trust and a successful working alliance. This is similar to counselling and other intimate relationships. Also, the supervisor should be providing trainees with clear and practical feedback. Supervisees need to feel that, in a professional capacity, they are receiving appropriate support and care. In a study of Educational Psychologists in the UK, the most important requirements for effective supervision were problem solving, appropriate guidance and support accommodating supervisees' needs and effective communication (Atkinson & Woods, 2007). Maintaining trust and an effective working alliance is, as in any effective relationship, a task that requires commitment and dedication from both parties involved.

Case conceptualisation, critical thinking, and note taking

The way trainees think about a case and the notes they take are related to the way they conceptualise the client's experience and the paradigm and worldview from which they operate. By collaborating with the supervisor, the trainee will develop the skills to accurately articulate in clinical language the client's status. The dialogue with the supervisor will assist the trainee in discovering unexplored areas of the client's experience and further the depth and spectrum of the way they conceptualise the case.

In a study of trainee counsellors, Ladany, Marotta, and Muse-Burke (2001) found that the more client and supervision sessions a counsellor experiences, the more integrated and complex etiologic and treatment conceptualisations are made. This means that the way a trainee sees the client's issues will develop in depth and sophistication through the process of supervision.

Note taking is an integral requirement of clinical practice and is an art that will improve as the internship progresses. Note taking is a central part of the clinical interview and an ongoing task of professional work.

In the practical sense note taking serves the functions of:

- A description of the presenting problem closely reflecting the language used by the client.
- A description of how the presenting problem impairs the client's life (e.g., social, occupational, affective, cognitive, physical).
- A history of the presenting problem (i.e., predisposing, precipitating, and perpetuating factors).
- A record of the primary support network, which includes family and close social relationships and the strengths and stressors of these relationships.
- A record of cultural, religious, and ethnic background.
- A description of any medical condition and medications.
- A record of information pertaining to the client's presenting problems in relation to the approaches of the profession (e.g., psychologists may incorporate more information on symptomatology, and social workers may include more details about psychosocial aspects).
- An outline of treatment recommendations.
- Record of client and therapist goals (clinical outcomes), process (specific interventions), prognosis (prediction), and progress (actual client change toward the goals).

Once a trainee understands the basic functions of note taking, there may appear to be a tremendous amount of work involved in this task. Much of this work can be part of, but not limited to, the first clinical interview and is an opportunity to 'start establishing the therapeutic relationship between (therapist) and client, which conveys a sense of client worth and worthiness for treatment' (Faiver, Eisengart, & Colona, 2000, p. 46). Building trust and rapport with the client should take precedence over taking notes, yet both tasks need to be accomplished. As trainees spend more time with clients, notes will be added to create a comprehensive clinical picture. Depending on the trainee's unique way of interacting with people, they may wish to take notes during each session and/or at the conclusion of each session. Creating clinical notes (written) and the presentation of client material in supervision (verbal) are both ways to practice and improve how to conceptualise and articulate the client's world. Refer to Figure 21.1 for an example of a client intake form.

Therapist development

Supervision seen as a developmental process has a long history in the counselling literature, and is useful as developmental models are not tied to any particular system of therapy

Client: _____   DOB: _____

Agency: _____   Phone: _____

Identifying Information:

Referral Source:

Presenting Concern/Goals:

Previous Treatment:

Mental Status:

Family History:

Siblings:

Education:

Employment History:

Social Development and Connections:

Marital and Dating History:

Medical Information and Medication:

Lifestyle Issues:

Personality Style:

Religious Affiliation:

Strengths and Supports:

Diagnostic Impressions:

Summary:

Treatment Plans and Recommendations:

_____   _____
        Therapist   Date

Figure 21.1 Client intake form

(Bernard & Goodyear, 2018). Developmental models give an insight into the development as a therapist for internship and practical training and into a career as a successful and competent professional. Stoltenberg and Delworth's (1987) and Stoltenberg, McNeill, and Delworth's (2009) Integrated Developmental Model of supervision is a popular approach to understanding the supervision experience.

According to this model, in the journey as a helping professional, trainees experience issues around anxiety-dependence. Simply put, they might be motivated but experience the need to check and monitor their work as a therapist. At this stage the supervisor can provide the structure and feedback needed. As the trainee continues to develop they will experience a dependency-autonomy conflict where they need less supervisory structure and more emotional encouragement from the supervisor. Following this the trainee will

Table 21.1 The journey of professional therapists

The Person (The Role)	Awareness and Skill (Affect)	Phases of Professional Development (Ronnestad & Skovholt)	Focus of Approach	Consideration and Attention (Virtues)
1 HUMAN (Accidental Helper) Observe	Unconscious Incompetence (Ignorance)	Conventional	Instinct & Experience	SELF (Hope & Will)
2 THERAPY STUDENT (Apprentice) Discover	Conscious Incompetence (Confusion)	Transition	Theory	OTHERS (Self-discipline & Responsibility)
3 EMERGING THERAPIST (Novice) Hypothesise	Conscious Competence (Confidence)	Imitation of Experts	Skills	RELATIONSHIP (Competence & Fidelity)
4 THERAPIST (Practitioner) Verify	Conscious Competence (Certainty)	Conditional Autonomy and Exploration	Values	THERAPEUTIC FRAME (Humility & Care)
5 SENIOR THERAPIST (Expert) Communicate	Unconscious Competence (Satisfaction)	Integration Individuation Integrity	Being	CONTEXT & CULTURE (Wisdom & Love)

start to experience collegial supervision where they have confidence, insight and competence and the supervisor will start interacting with them more like what seems like a professional peer. Finally, the trainee will find themselves at the integrated level where they experience autonomy, self and other awareness, security, and the ability to self-confront. This self-confrontation or self-challenging is the beginning of the ability to engage in a form of 'self-supervision' (Lowe, 2002), developing a reliable 'internal supervisor' (Gilbert & Kenneth, 2000) or autonomous professional development. Barletta's table (Table 21.1) outlines a developmental model that integrates a range of concepts that can be explored to describe the growth of a helping professional. It highlights the changing role, levels of awareness and skill, focus of clinical attention and associated virtues. See Table 21.1 for an overview of therapist development.

Critical incidents and case studies

The study of critical incidents grew out of the practice of industrial and organisational psychology in the USA military during World War II (Butterfield, Borgen, Amundson, & Maglio, 2005). Critical incidents in clinical supervision for counselling have been defined as an incident, milestone, or turning point that results in a change in the supervisee's perception of their effectiveness as a counsellor (Heppner & Roehlke, 1984). Critical incidents can be perceived as both positive and/or negative. For example, a trainee might help a client who gives them positive feedback on the work they did, or the trainee might experience a difficult client who seems unresponsive to their efforts. Both types of these incidents are useful for the development as a counsellor. Positive incidents reinforce confidence in competence as a therapist, while negative incidents can be an indication of what areas need further development. Heppner and Roehlke (1984) found that critical incidents can be classified in terms of counsellor development. They can be incidents related to self-awareness, professional development, competency and personal issues affecting therapy. Whether the incidents are positive the field supervisor can help the trainee work with these experiences to gain the most benefit from them.

As trainees review the literature of their particular helping profession, they will routinely come across examples of case studies. Case studies are an excellent way to present, in detail, a client and the complexities that surround them (Page, Stritzke, & McLean, 2008). We learn from the narrative, that is, the stories. Client cases used in supervision can function in a similar way to Interpersonal Process Recall (IPR) that is used to recall in an experiential manner the therapeutic process by viewing a recorded therapy session. Producing case studies functions in a similar way to IPR in that the therapist recalls and articulates in writing their knowledge about a case and the therapeutic process. Critical incidents can be incorporated into the writing-up of case studies and can be presented during supervision sessions. Trainees should take the initiative to write up a case study for experience, and provided here is a simple guide to facilitating the process:

- Describe the background to the case including the presenting problem and historical information.
- What was happening for you when working with this client?
- What do you feel was happening for the client?
- Describe what approaches were or were not effective?
- Was there anything of a personal nature on your part hindering or promoting therapeutic change?

As in the IPR approach, trainees need to recall how they felt, what they might have liked to have done, their thoughts about what happened, and any imagery they had or have about the experience.

Case presentations

Case presentations are useful if trainees are participating in group supervision, particularly if it is multidisciplinary, or peer consultation. The content presented will be similar to what one would include in writing up a case study except it is presented for feedback and discussion amongst professional peers. The supervisor and/or group will have in place a format and procedure for trainees to follow. They may use specific technologies such as presentation software or audio/visual records of client sessions to assist in communicating to peers. Case presentations in a group setting can be very useful as trainees will benefit from several people thinking about and working with them on a particular issue. In spite of the initial anxiety associated with presenting in front of others, greater understandings and new ideas will invariably be the outcome.

Cases requiring immediate action

Included in the incidents described above, trainees need to be prepared for circumstances where their immediate action is necessary to prevent imminent harm to the client or someone else.

The most obvious circumstance of imminent harm is potential suicide. Suicide can be understood as a continuum of behaviour which includes fleeting thoughts of suicide, suicidal ideation, suicide planning and means, suicidal attempts and completed suicide (Kanel, 2003). The way to gain an indication of where the client is relative to suicide is to ask within the context of the therapeutic relationship. More detailed methods to explore this clinical issue exist in a plethora of literature on the topic of suicide.

While there is still no universally accepted assessment instrument for suicidal risk or prediction, the Suicide Assessment Scale (SUAS) has some reliability and validity (Nimeus, Alsen, & Traskman-Bendz, 2000). The SUAS has also been modified to an interview version and has high reliability and predictive validity (for manual and scale, see Nimeus, Stahlfors, Sunnqvist, Stanley, & Traskman-Bendz, 2006). Trainees can discuss the use of such assessments and instruments with their field supervisor.

In any event, at the first indication of potential suicidal behaviour the trainee may put into place a suicide contract. While the internship site may already have a preferred document for contracting, Figure 21.2 is an example of a contract that can be modified. Keep in mind that there is some controversy regarding the use of suicide contracts. Indeed, one of the editors of this book prefers the use of coping planning over the use of a suicide contract and notes they would not normally implement such a contract when working with clients/supervisees (Pelling, personal communication, 25 June 2022; Stallman, 2019).

Although less prevalent than suicide, some clients will disclose their intention to harm others or property. As with client suicide, a client who threatens the safety of others presents a dilemma in the duty of care to protect the client's rights to privacy and the trainee's responsibility to protect society from harm. It is here that informed consent is the greatest ally as it protects the trainee's position and informs the client of professional responsibilities. For these and other legal and ethical responsibilities, it is important that trainees review the code of ethics relevant to their profession. Below is a brief procedure of an ethical decision-making model that can be applied to ethical dilemmas (adapted from Miller & Davis, 2006). It is good practice to keep a record of the details of this process as it relates to a specific client in the clinical notes. Please note that the field and academic supervisor must be informed of any ethical dilemmas a trainee might have during their internship and will be ready to assist them in the decision-making process.

1. Identify the problem.
2. Apply the relevant Code of Ethics.
3. Determine the nature and dimensions of the dilemma.
4. Generate potential courses of action.
5. Consider the potential consequences of all options; choose an action.
6. Evaluate the selected course of action.
7. Implement the course of action.

Pelling (2019) provides an overview of ethical principles and ethical dilemma examination that is relevant to counselling, although focused on applied Australian psychological practice, for interested readers.

Concluding statement

Clinical fieldwork in the training context is a critical component of the formation of the therapist. It gives the trainee, academic institution, and professional community a sense

I, _____, (client), hereby agree that I will take the following actions if I feel suicidal.

1. I will not suicide.

2. I will phone _____ at _____.

3. If the above person can not be reached, I will contact the following services in the order below:

Name/Agency	Phone
_____	_____
_____	_____
_____	_____

4. I will also seek social support from any or all of the following people:

Name	Phone
_____	_____
_____	_____
_____	_____

5. If none of these actions are helpful or available, I will present at the Emergency Department at one of the following:

Hospital	Address	Phone
_____	_____	_____
_____	_____	_____
_____	_____	_____

6. If I am not able in any way to undertake the above-mentioned actions, I will phone Emergency Services on _____ if I feel I am in immediate danger of harming myself.

7. I agree to discuss any crisis leading to suicidal thoughts or planning to _____ (therapist's name) at our next session.

Client's signature: _____

Therapist's signature: _____   Date: __/__/____

Figure 21.2 Example suicide contract

of the potential for the novice. As trainees are challenged and supported to apply what they have learnt in the classroom and research to the workplace, they are exploring how the science of the profession becomes the art of clinical practice. This chapter provided an overview of the key elements to the supervision of placement experiences to facilitate the development of clinical competence in the trainee, via a quality relationship and thoughtful structured supervisory experiences.

Educational questions & activities

1. Activity: Note-taking, Simulation, Self-Appraisal, Specific and General Discussion. Provide each student with a copy of the intake form (Figure 21.1) in this chapter. Prepare a comprehensive description of a complex clinical case.

   Step 1. Read the case to the class while students fill in the information on the intake form.

   Step 2. Allow students to ask you questions and ask you to repeat information they may have missed. (This allows students to be active and intentional in thinking about information they need from a client)

   Step 3. In pairs, have students compare and contrast their notes, while adding information to make this record more comprehensive.

   Step 4. Engage in an open-ended class discussion including the content of their record, what other information should be gathered initially, what could be gathered in later client sessions, and student reactions to the note-taking process.

2. Use Barletta's developmental model (Table 21.1) to discuss the concept of the growth of a helping professional, with particular attention to the student's current phase, individual plans to facilitate additional progress, and expectations of what the future phases might be like.

Selected references for further reading

Carrington, G. (2004). Supervision as a reciprocal learning process. *Educational Psychology Practice*, *20*(1), 31–42.

Carroll, M., & Gilbert, M.C. (2006). *On being a supervisee: Creating learning partnerships*. Kew, Victoria: PsychOz.

Skovholt, T.M., & Ronnestad, M.H. (1995). *The evolving professional self: Stages and themes in therapist and counselor development*. New York: John Wiley.

Van Exan, J. (2004). The legal and ethical issues surrounding the duty to warn in the practice of psychology. *Windsor Review of Legal and Social Issues*, *18*, 123–126.

Zimering, R., Munroe, J., & Gulliver, S. B. (2003). Secondary traumatization in mental health providers. *Psychiatric Times*, *20*(4), 43.

References

Atkinson, Cathy, & Woods, Kevin. (2007). A model of effective fieldwork supervision for trainee educational psychologists. *Educational Psychology in Practice*, *23*, 299–316. 10.1080/02667360701660902.

Barletta, J. (2007). Clinical supervision. In N. Pelling, R. Bowers, & P. Armstrong (Eds.), *The practice of counselling* (pp. 118–135). Melbourne, Australia: Thomson.

Bernard, J.M., & Goodyear, R.K. (2018). *Fundamentals of clinical supervision* (6th ed.). Upper Saddle River, NJ: Pearson.

Butterfield, Lee, Borgen, William, Amundson, Norman, & Maglio, Asa-Sophia. (2005). Fifty years of the critical incident technique: 1954–2004 and beyond. *Qualitative Research, 5*, 475–497.

Champe, J., & Kleist, D.M. (2003). Live supervision: A review of the research. *The Family Journal, 11*, 268–275.

Faiver, C., Eisengart, S., & Colona, R. (2000). *The counselor intern's handbook* (2nd ed.). Belmont, CA: Wadsworth/Thomson.

Gilbert, M.C., & Evans, K. (2000). *Psychotherapy supervision: An integrative relational approach to psychotherapy supervision.* Philadelphia, PA: Open University.

Granello, D., & Hazler, R. (1998). A developmental rationale for curriculum order and teaching styles in counselor education programs. *Counselor Education and Supervision, 38*(2), 89.

Hazler, R.J., & Barwick, N. (2001). *The therapeutic environment.* Philadelphia, PA: Open University.

Heppner, P.P., & Roehlke, H.J. (1984). Differences among supervisees at different levels of training: Implications for a developmental model of supervision. *Journal of Counseling Psychology, 31*(1), 76–90.

Hunt, C., & Sharpe, L. (2008). Within-session supervision communication in the training of clinical psychologists. *Australian Psychologist, 43*(2), 121–126.

Kagan, N. (1975). Influencing human interaction: Eleven years with IPR. *Canadian Counsellor, 9*(2), 74–97.

Kanel, K. (2003). When crisis is a danger. In Kim Svetich-Will (Ed.), *A guide to crisis intervention* (2nd ed., pp. 74–90). Pacific Grove, CA: Brooks-Cole.

Kilminster, S.M., & Jolly, B.C. (2000). Effective supervision in clinical practice settings: A literature review. *Medical Education, 34*, 827–840.

Ladany, N., Lehrman-Waterman, D., Molinaro, M., & Wolgast, B. (1999). Psychotherapy supervisor ethical practices: Adherence to guidelines, the supervisory working alliance, and supervisee satisfaction. *The Counseling Psychologist, 27*(3), 443–475.

Ladany, N., Marotta, S., & Muse-Burke, J.L. (2001). Counselor experience related to complexity of case conceptualization and supervision preference. *Counselor Education and Supervision, 40*, 203–219.

Loganbill, C., Hardy, E., & Delworth, U. (1982). Supervision: A conceptual model. *The Counseling Psychologist, 10*(1), 3–42.

Lowe, R. (2002). Self-supervision: From developmental goal to systemic practice. In M. McMahon & W. Patton (Eds.), *Supervision in the helping professions: A practical approach* (pp. 67–78). Frenchs Forest, NSW: Pearson.

Marshak, R.J. (1983). What's between pedagogy and andragogy? *Training and Development Journal, 30*(10), 80–81.

Miller, H.F., & Davis, T. (2006). *A practitioner's guide to ethical decision making.* Alexandria, VA: American Counseling Association.

Nimeus, A., Alsen, M., & Traskman-Bendz, L. (2000). The Suicide Assessment Scale: An instrument assessing suicide risk of suicide attempters. *European Psychiatry, 15*, 416–423.

Nimeus, A., Stahlfors, F.H., Sunnqvist, C., Stanley, B., & Traskman-Bendz, L. (2006). Evaluation of a modified interview version of a self-rating version of the Suicide Assessment Scale. *European Psychiatry, 21*, 471–477.

Noelle, M. (2002). Self-report in supervision: Positive and negative slants. *Clinical Supervisor, 21*, 125–134.

Page, A., Stritzke, G., & McLean, N. (2008). Toward science-informed supervision of clinical case formulation: A training model and supervision method. *Australian Psychologist, 43*(2), 88–95.

Pelling, N.J. (2019). Overview of ethics in Australian psychology. In N. Pelling & L. Burton (Eds.), *The elements of ethical pracice: Applied psychology ethics in Australia* (pp. 12–38). Abingdon, Oxon: Routledge.

Stallman, H. M. (2019). An ethical response to disclosures of suicidal ideation or behaviour. In N. Pelling, & L. Burton (Eds.), *The elements of ethical practice: Applied psychology ethics in Australia* (pp. 155–166). Abingdon, Oxon: Routledge.

Stoltenberg, C.D., & Delworth, U. (1987). *Supervising counselors and therapists: A developmental approach*. San Francisco, CA: Jossey-Bass.

Stoltenberg, C.D., McNeill, B.W., & Delworth, U. (2009). *IDM Supervision: An integrated developmental model for supervising counselors and therapists*. New York, NY: Routledge.

Part 6

Research

Part 6, **Research**, presents supervision relevant research and scholarship information. Chapter 22 presents the nature of recent scholarship in supervision and provides recommendations as to where research and scholarly activities should be directed. This chapter serves as a timely reminder that supervision is not only an applied speciality but also a research and scholarly focus. Chapter 23 specifically provides an overview of psychotherapy research in Asia. Evidence based therapies in Asian countries are then presented in Chapter 24.

Chapter overview

Chapter 22, **The State of Supervision Scholarship in the Twenty-First Century**, by Nadine Pelling, Deah Abbott, and Caleb Lack asserts that supervision is not just an applied specialty area but also one that can be the focus of research and scholarly efforts. Supporting the scientist-practitioner model of training and practice, the authors review the results of literature searches of standard counselling and psychological library databases.

Chapter themes

In this chapter you will explore the following themes:

- Clinical supervision: An applied activity and research focus
- Method
- Scholarly Review Results
- Discussion
- Concluding statements and recommended future directions

Chapter overview

Chapter 23, **An Overview of Psychotherapy Research in Asia**, by Deah Abbott and Caleb Lack provides information on Asia-specific research.

DOI: 10.4324/9781003490067-27

Chapter themes

In this chapter you will explore the following themes:

- Regionally-specific research on psychotherapy and counselling
- Method
- Results
- Discussion

Chapter overview

Chapter 24, **Research on Evidence-Based Therapies in Asian Countries,** by Kyle Haws, Yasmin Shiralli, and Caleb Lack, outlines information on evidence-based therapies being applied and explored in Asian countries.

Chapter themes

In this chapter you will explore the following themes:

- Method
- Results
- Discussion

22 The State of Supervision Scholarship in the Twenty-First Century

Nadine Pelling, Deah Abbott, and Caleb W. Lack

Clinical supervision: An applied activity and research focus

Clinical supervision is a huge part of one's training in the applied areas of psychology, counselling, social work, and nursing. Supervisors use skills to provide feedback and help support and develop novice practitioners in a manner that increases their competence when working with clients. Indeed, the majority of this book outlines the ethics, methods, models, and interventions one can use in applied supervisory interactions. However, there is another aspect to clinical supervision that is less often reviewed and even neglected in many discussions: research.

The typical model of training used in psychology and related fields in many countries is that of the scientist-practitioner (Pelling, 2004). According to this model clinicians are expected to be both competent basic researchers (both in conducting their own research as well as evaluating the research of others) and competent practitioners. This balance allows clinicians to apply the latest scholarly knowledge to their work in order to both benefit clients and allow for constant self-reflection and examination. By continuously examining their actions and their results with clients, clinicians will continue to grow in their skills sets and abilities throughout their career, rather than stagnate.

Unfortunately, as many have noted, there are divides in the realm of scholarship regarding clinical supervision, both between scientists and clinicians and among researchers who use qualitative versus quantitative methodologies (Pelling, 2000). Many clinicians are not actively engaged in the production or ingestion of research. Indeed, clinicians have been known to remark that published research tends to not apply to their work and, in essence, gives them metaphoric indigestion.

Given its massive importance in training and continued professional development, plus the divisions that are seen, the focus of this chapter is to outline the current state of supervision scholarship. We will be examining what is being published in articles on supervision, where the scholarship is originating, and what methods are being used in supervision scholarship. In doing so we are updating a previously published book chapter (Pelling, 2009) by seeing whether and how the literature has evolved in the past several years. To answer these questions a series of literature searches were conducted to provide an overview of the current supervision scholarship. Please note that the following is not meant to be and is not an annotative bibliography on the scholarship in supervision, but instead a brief content analysis of the scholarship on supervision during the first 16 years of the twenty-first century.

DOI: 10.4324/9781003490067-28

Method

Two brief literature searches were conducted in order to examine the current state of supervision scholarship. First, a search was conducted in May 2008 covering all published articles (not books or book chapters or book reviews) from the start of 2000 onward. Second, in May 2016 a final search from June 2008 onward was conducted. Key search words included *supervision*, *clinical* or *counselling/ counseling*. All searches were computer based and used standard databases in the counselling and psychological fields including ERIC, PsychLit, and PsychInfo.

Relevant publications were then printed on paper or saved electronically, and the abstracts and/or articles collected were examined for author country of origin, basic methodology employed, or whether the paper was a review/editorial, and general supervision research subtopic including psychology, counselling, and medicine.

Results

Article publications were found in a diversity of journals. For instance, *Professional Psychology: Research & Practice, Computers in Human Behavior, The Clinical Supervisor,* and *Australian Psychiatry* were all represented. Additionally, solo, joint, and teams of authors consisting of eight or more authors contributed to the groups of published manuscripts obtained in the conducted searches. While a few publications originated from Scandinavia, Israel, South Korea, and elsewhere, these are not represented on the following tables for simplicity's sake as the majority of publications came from Australia, New Zealand, Hong Kong, the United States of America (USA), Canada, and the United Kingdom (UK).

Table 22.1 shows scholarship type and general topic by country published from January 2000 to May 2008. Table 21.2 shows scholarship type and general topic by country published since June 2008 to May 2016.

It is clear from both of these tables that for the first 16 years of the twenty-first-century discussion or review papers have been the most popular type of scholarship in clinical supervision (39% and 34%, respectively). Generally such publications include models for the use of supervision or the outlining of various topics in supervision. For instance, Aten, Strain, and Gillespie (2008) outline the transtheoretical model of supervision. Quantitative research articles were increasingly popular, accounting for 25 per cent of the literature in the first eight years and 32 per cent in the second eight years. Examples of this type of published research included Riva and Erickson Cornish's (2008) examination of group supervision practices as psychology predoctoral internship programs and Britt and Gleave's (2011) examination of clinical psychology doctoral students' satisfaction with their supervision.

Researchers in the USA published the majority of articles on supervision in both time periods, accounting for 27 per cent in the first eight years and increasing to 66 per cent of the literature in the second eight years. Australia published the second most of articles in the first eight years (25%), but in the second eight years was surpassed by the United Kingdom at 14 per cent (as opposed to Australia's diminished 8%). These publications included an article on the perspectives of wise supervisors when working with conflict in clinical supervision from an article by a Wisconsin group of authors (Nelson, Barnes, Evans, & Triggiano, 2008), Gonsalvez and McLeod's (2008) on a science-informed practice of clinical supervision in the Australian context, and an article on supervision for the

Table 22.1 Clinical supervision scholarship type and general topic by country published from January 2000 to May 2008

		Country						
		Australia	New Zealand	Hong Kong	USA	Canada	UK	TOTAL
Scholarship Type	Quantitative	5	1	2	1		2	11
	Qualitative	1	1		2	1		5
	Discussion or Review Paper	2	4	1	8		2	17
	Unable to Determine from Abstract	3	1	5	1			10
	TOTAL	11	7	8	12	1	4	43
Scholarship Topic	Psychology	1		3	9		3	16
	Counselling	5	4	4	2		1	16
	Medical (psychiatry, nursing, medical practitioner training)	5	3	1				10
	Other (psychotherapy, group, school psychology, music therapy)				1	1		2
	Totals	11	7	8	12	1	4	44

Note: Categories are not necessarily mutually exclusive (i.e., some mixed method research exists and is counted in both quantitative and qualitative sections).

treatment of depression by a group of British authors (Simpson-Southward, Waller, & Hardy, 2016).

For the first 16 years of the twenty-first century, psychology and counselling has increasingly dominated the literature in this area, with first 36 per cent and then 45 per cent relating to psychology and 37 per cent then 39 per cent relating to counselling. Other areas of supervision were also included, such as nursing supervision and music therapy supervision, but to a lesser extent.

Discussion

The topic of clinical supervision in psychotherapy has garnered an increased amount of scientific interest in the twenty-first century thus far. The literature review that covered the first eight years consisted of less than 50 total publications. The second eight-year period resulted in more than six times that number of articles, with more than 300 new articles on the subject.

In regards to scholarship type, it is no surprise that a largely applied area such as clinical supervision would engender a large amount of scholarship that is applied (model-based/ review material) in nature versus research-based scholarship. However, if supervisory practices are to be grounded in research, then more quantitative, qualitative, and mixed model research (versus commentary) is in order. Similarly, more quantitative versus

Table 22.2 Clinical supervision scholarship type and general topic by country published from June 2008 to May 2016

		Country						
		Australia	New Zealand	China (Including Hong Kong)	USA	Canada	UK	TOTAL
Scholarship Type	Quantitative	7	3	5	76	3	9	103
	Qualitative	9	1	6	42	3	16	77
	Discussion or Review Paper	10	2		68	10	19	109
	Unable to Determine from Abstract			1	25	2	1	29
	TOTAL	26	6	12	211	18	45	318
Scholarship Topic	Psychology	11	2	4	113	11	33	174
	Counselling	6	3	9	108	9	16	151
	Medical (psychiatry, nursing, medical practitioner training)	7	1		16		4	28
	Other (psychotherapy, group, school psychology, music therapy)	3		3	21	2	4	33
	Totals	27	6	16	258	22	57	386

Note: Categories are not necessarily mutually exclusive (i.e., some mixed method research exists and is counted in both quantitative and qualitative sections).

qualitative or case studies of supervision, were published. It is possible that the supervisory arena could benefit from an increase in a diversity of methodology that may be more relevant to practitioners (i.e., qualitative and case study presentations).

It was also not a revelation that the majority of publications were based on research conducted in the USA, given the large population of that country and high number of active researchers. Also because of the high number of researchers it was not surprising that the UK published a significant portion of the articles in the second literature review. However, the large number of publications from Australia in the first literature review was unexpected. However, the fact that the *Australian Psychologist* published a special section on clinical supervision in May of 2008 (Gonsalvez, 2008) may in part explain this finding.

Given that the databases searched were generally psychological, education, and counselling related it is not surprising that counselling and psychology were highly represented topics relating to clinical supervision. As a result, it is possible that if specifically medical or legal databases were searched that different results regarding applied/clinical supervision would result.

This brief overview of recent supervision scholarship has its limits in that it is simply meant as a concise overview, a snapshot in time which is likely to change as academic knowledge and training continues to move forward. Additionally, electronic database searches do have their limits. Firstly, there are some delays as to when certain articles are published and then available on the databases. Secondly, not all journals are indexed by all databases. For instance, a quantitative examination of supervisory development published by one of the current authors before the May 2008 literature review was not available at that time via some databases due to a time-lag between publishing and indexing (Pelling, 2008).

Concluding statement

A few general recommendations can be made based on this recent supervision scholarship snapshot. Firstly, that more research and less editorialising is needed and that research should include quantitative and qualitative methodologies and case studies. Secondly, that those mental health professionals in countries where little supervision research is being conducted should be sought out by American, Australian, and British researchers for collaborative efforts. It would be great to see some additional cross cultural/international research on clinical supervision being published which can help broaden the researchers' and readers' perspectives. Similar collaborations could be made with those in non-psychology or counselling-related fields involved with supervision such as medicine and nursing. Finally, we must remember that as scientist-practitioners we not only supervise applied work via clinical supervision but also produce research via research supervision. The research supervision field appears wide open to many research possibilities relating to the relationship, process, and productivity variables.

Educational questions & activities

1. What is the typical model used in psychology training?
2. Why do some believe that clinicians should also be competent basic researchers?
3. What divide has historically existed among researchers?
4. What is the most popular type of scholarship in clinical supervision?
5. What country accounts for most of the publications found in the searches conducted?
6. What does the author recommend regarding supervision scholarship?

Selected references for further reading

Selected reference

Falender, C.A., & Shafranske, E.P. (2008). *Casebook for clinical supervision: A competency-based approach*. Washington, DC: American Psychological Association.

Selected internet resources

The website for the *Journal Counselor Education and Counseling Supervision* https://onlinelibrary.wiley.com/journal/15566978

- Houses one of the main supervision-related journals in counselling.

The website for the Association for Counselor Education and Supervision
www.acesonline.net/

- Lists information on conferences and current news regarding supervision in the USA.

References

Aten, J., Strain, J., & Gillespie, R. (2008). A transtheoretical model of clinical supervision. *Training and Education in Professional Psychology*, *2*(1), 1–9. doi:10.1037/1931-3918.2.1.1

Britt, E., & Gleaves, D.H. (2011). Measurement and prediction of clinical psychology students' satisfaction with clinical supervision. *The Clinical Supervisor*, *30*(2), 172–182. doi:10.1080/07325223.2011.604274

Gonsalvez, C. (2008). Introduction to the special section on clinical supervision. *Australian Psychologist*, *42*(2), 76–78. doi:10.1080/00050060802068547

Gonsalvez, C., & McLeod, H. (2008). Toward the science-0informed practice of clinical supervision: The Australian context. *Australian Psychologist*, *43*(2), 79–87. doi:10.1080/00050060802054869

Nelson, M., Barnes, K., Evans, A., & Triggiano, P. (2008). Working with conflict in clinical supervision: Wise supervisors' perspectives. *Journal of Counseling Psychology*, *55*(2), 172–184. doi:10.1037/0022-0167.55.2.172

Pelling, N. (2000). Scientists versus practitioners: A growing dichotomy in need of integration. *Counselling Psychology Review*, *15*(4), 3–7.

Pelling, N. (2004). Counselling psychology: Diversity and commonalities across the western world. *Counselling Psychology Quarterly*, *17*(3), 239–245. doi:10.1080/09515070412331317611

Pelling, N. (2008). The relationship of supervisory experience, counseling experience, and training in supervision to supervisory identity development. *International Journal for the Advancement of Counselling*, *30*(4), 235–248. doi:10.1007/s10447-008-9060-2

Pelling, N. (2009). Recent supervision scholarship. In N. Pelling, J. Barletta, & P. Armstrong (Eds.), *The Practice of Clinical Supervision*, pp. 81–86. Bowen Hills, Queensland: Australian Academic Press.

Riva, M., & Erickson Cornish, J. (2008). Group supervision practices at psychology predoctoral internship programs: 15 years later. *Training and Education in Professional Psychology*, *2*(1), 18–25. doi:10.1037/1931-3918.2.1.18

Simpson-Southward, C., Waller, G., & Hardy, G.E. (2016). Supervision for treatment of depression: An experimental study of the role of therapist gender and anxiety. *Behaviour Research and Therapy*, *77*, 17–22. doi:10.1016/j.brat.2015.11.013

23 An Overview of Psychotherapy Research in Asia

Deah Abbott and Caleb W. Lack

Regionally-specific research on psychotherapy and counselling

The majority of the prominent counselling and psychotherapeutic treatments currently in widespread use were developed by European or American psychologists and psychiatrists. Given their geographic placement, psychotherapy research has also been historically centred on those populations. There has thus historically been much more research about the efficacy of such treatments on those populations than on Asian populations. However, the prevalence of psychological treatment in East and Southeast Asian countries has increased considerably over the past two decades, leading to a massive increase in research on psychotherapy and counselling.

The people living in the geographical regions of East Asia (including China, Japan, South Korea, and Taiwan) and Southeast Asia (including Singapore, the Philippines, Malaysia, Thailand, and Vietnam) constitute approximately one-fourth of the world's population. It is imperative that research be conducted in this region, whether that is to assess the efficacy of treatments of western origin on those living in this area of the world, to validate newer treatments of originating from this region, or to assess the prevalence and popularity of various treatments currently being administered in this region.

The purpose of this chapter is to examine recent research trends. To do this we examined the available research on psychotherapy and counselling practices and their efficacy over the most time period of 2011 through 2015. We examined the literature for relevant peer-reviewed articles from eight different countries: China, Japan, South Korea, the Philippines, Thailand, Vietnam, Malaysia, and Singapore. We then categorized all pertinent articles to provide a picture of what is being researched, how it is being researched, and where it is being researched. From this broad-scope perspective we have also made suggestions for areas of future research.

Method

A literature search examining the current state of counselling in South East Asia was conducted. Key search words included *counselling/counseling, psychotherapy, therapy, Asia, Japan, Korea, the Philippines, Thailand, Vietnam, Malaysia, China, Hong Kong, Taiwan,* and *Singapore*. All searches were computer-based and used standard databases in the counselling and psychological fields including PsychARTICLES, PsychINFO, and PubMED.

Relevant publications were then electronically saved and reviewed with the most pertinent information in the articles being categorized by participants' country, researcher's university location, scholarship type, participant population, problem of focus, and

DOI: 10.4324/9781003490067-29

theoretical orientation of treatment. It was also noted if the articles focused on local legal or ethical concerns related to counselling.

Results

The literature review produced 222 articles that were included in final analysis from the pool of more than 43,000 articles produced using the related search terms. The articles were published in a variety of journals including the *International Journal for the Advancement of Counselling*, *Chinese Journal of Clinical Psychology*, *Asia Pacific Journal of Counselling and Psychotherapy*, and *The Counseling Psychologist*. The majority of researchers publishing articles on counselling in this region were at universities in East or Southeast Asia. Less than 30 per cent of the articles had one or more author from a European, North American, South American, African, or Australian university. Of those articles, the majority had a primary investigator from an Asian country.

Table 23.1 depicts scholarship type and population type of the published research on psychotherapy and counselling in East and Southeast Asia by country from 2011 to 2015. Quantitative research was by far the most prevalent, accounting for 45 per cent of the total research on the topic. The second most prevalent were discussion and review articles which accounted for an additional 24 per cent. Qualitative and case study articles were far less prevalent, only accounting for 15 per cent and 11 per cent respectively.

As Table 23.1 depicts, the largest percentage (39%) of articles focused on treatment for adults. The next largest proportion did not specify the population of focus. An approximately equal amount of articles focused on family, child, and adolescent populations, averaging around 10 per cent for each. Very few articles, less than 5 per cent, addressed treatment for the elder population.

The vast majority of the research was focused on the Chinese population, accounting for 60 per cent of the articles. This category included articles which focused on counselling in mainland China, Taiwan, and Hong Kong. The next highest percentage, approximately 16 per cent, was about counselling in Japan. Articles that addressed Korean counselling accounted for approximately 10 per cent of the research. Articles about the five other countries, Singapore, Thailand, Malaysia, the Philippines, and Vietnam, accounted for the remaining 18 per cent of research, with the research for each country's population accounting for less than 5 per cent of the total research.

Table 23.2 shows the treatment types by problem of focus from 2011 to 2015. Nearly half of the articles (46%) did not specify what the problem of focus was for counselling. Of these, many were discussion or review articles. These addressed the available research about a region, the history and status of a particular treatment type in one of the countries of interest, or ethical and legal concerns of counselling in a specific area. Examples of these include Tuason, Fernandez, Catipon, Trivino-Dey, and Arellano-Carandang's (2012) discussion of the history, current state, and future directions of counselling in the Philippines, Ono et al.'s (2011) review of the literature on cognitive-behavioral therapy in Japan, and Zhao et al.'s (2011) article on the ethical practices of Chinese psychotherapists. Additionally, a few of the articles in this category focused on the person of the counsellor, their training, and orientation within a given region, such as Pelling's (2013) article "Advertised psychologists and counsellors in Hong Kong and Singapore."

Of the articles that did discuss the problem of focus for treatment, the largest number of them were about treating depressive disorder. This accounted for 18 per cent of the

Table 23.1 East and Southeast Asian psychotherapy scholarship type and population by country from 2011 to 2015

		Country								
		China	Japan	South Korea	Philippines	Thailand	Vietnam	Malaysia	Singapore	TOTAL
Scholarship Type	Quantitative	61	19	14	2	5	1	4	4	110
	Qualitative	22	3	2	4	0	1	3	2	37
	Discussion or Review	43	8	5	1	3	3	2	3	68
	Case Study	12	7	3	0	2	1	2	0	27
	TOTAL	138	37	24	7	10	6	11	9	242
Population Type	Unspecified	48	7	3	2	3	1	1	1	66
	Family	16	0	2	3	0	1	0	3	25
	Child	13	4	2	1	0	1	1	3	25
	Adolescent	7	5	3	2	3	1	0	2	23
	Adult	54	18	11	2	3	1	6	3	98
	Elder	6	3	2	1	0	0	0	0	12
	TOTAL	144	37	23	11	9	5	8	12	249

Note: Categories are not necessarily mutually exclusive (i.e., a study that included adult and adolescent participants would count in both the Child and Adolescent sections).

Table 23.2 Treatment type for East and Southeast Asian psychotherapy by problem of focus from 2011 to 2015

Treatment Type	Problem of Focus										
	Unknown/ Unspecified	Psychotic Disorders	Depressive Disorders	Anxiety Disorders	Trauma- and Stressor-Related Issues	Somatoform Disorders	Disruptive Behavior Disorders	Substance Use Disorders	Neuro-cognitive Disorders	Other	TOTAL
Unspecified/Non-Specific	50	1	10	5	6	1	2	3	0	2	80
Family Therapy	17	0	1	0	0	0	2	0	0	1	21
Cognitive Behavioral Therapy	7	4	17	6	2	2	3	2	2	4	49
Interpersonal Therapy	0	0	6	2	0	0	0	0	0	0	8
Mindfulness-Focused Therapy	1	1	1	1	0	0	1	0	0	0	5
Existential Therapy	2	0	0	0	0	0	0	0	0	0	2
Psychodynamic/Psychoanalytic	5	0	0	0	0	0	0	0	0	0	5
Expressive/Experiential therapy	3	0	3	6	9	1	2	3	1	1	29
Adlerian Therapy	5	0	0	0	0	0	0	0	0	0	5
Solution Focused Therapy	2	0	0	0	0	0	0	0	0	0	2
Religious/Spiritual Therapy	9	0	1	0	1	0	0	0	0	0	11
Narrative Therapy	2	0	1	0	1	0	0	1	0	0	5
Other	10	0	5	5	4	0	0	0	1	1	26
TOTAL	113	6	45	25	23	4	10	9	4	9	248

Note: Categories are not necessarily mutually exclusive (i.e., a treatment type may include a Buddhist component in psychoanalysis and would count in both Psychodynamic/ Psychoanalytic and Religious/Spiritual Therapy sections).

total articles. An example of this is Chung, Tsu, Kua, Lin, and Chang's (2014) article on the efficacy of group interpersonal therapy on Taiwanese patients with depressive disorder.

The second most prevalent group of disorders in the literature were anxiety disorders, which accounted for 10 per cent of the research. An example of this is Shirotsuki, Kodama, and Nomura's (2014) study on cognitive-behavioral therapy for social anxiety disorder in Japan. Trauma- and stressor-related issues followed close behind anxiety disorders and accounted for 9 per cent of the research. Ho's (2015) article on dance therapy for Chinese survivors of childhood sexual abuse provides an example of the research on this topic.

Just as many of the articles did not specify the reason for treatments, many of them did not specify the type of treatment that was administered (32%). Many of the discussion and reviews mentioned above were included in this category. The most popular treatment specifically mentioned in the literature was cognitive-behavioral therapy, which accounted for 20 per cent of the articles.

The second most researched treatment type were the expressive and experiential therapies. These accounted for 12 per cent of the total articles. These articles included a variety of interventions such as art therapy, music therapy, dance therapy, and adventure therapy. Notably, some of these articles, like Kim's (2015) study on music therapy for Korean children exposed to abuse and poverty, found no statistically significant results from the treatment.

Family therapy was the third most prevalent in the literature. This type of treatment accounted for 8 per cent of the articles. Most of these articles, such as Deng, Lin, Lan, and Fang's (2013) article in *Contemporary Family Therapy: An International Journal*, focused on counselling in China. Each remaining treatment type accounted for less than 5 per cent of the total research.

Discussion

While there is certainly enough published research on counselling in East and Southeast Asia to provide a broad picture of what may be popular or effective in the region, it is in some ways surprising that there was so little research on the subject. That there were only slightly more than 200 articles published across a five year time span from a region that constitutes around 25 per cent of the world's population should be a wake-up call to researchers in these countries and elsewhere.

As one would expect due to population size and the number of research universities, the majority of the research concentrated on counselling in China. For the same reasons, it is not surprising that the second most researched country was Japan. There was relatively little research on each of the remaining countries during this five year time frame.

It is not surprising that the largest segment of the articles focused on adult participants. It is somewhat surprising, though, how few studies researched the elderly, given the emphasis many of these cultures place on respecting and caring for this segment of the population.

It is also reasonable that cognitive-behavioral therapy was the type of therapy on which most of the articles focused, because in the West this therapy is considered a gold standard and evidence-based practice for many disorders and other issues. It is also not surprising that there was so much research on family therapy. Most cultures in these countries value community and collectivism more than most Eurocentric countries. It makes sense that therapy involving many members of the family may be more popular in these regions than in the West.

It was somewhat surprising that the second most common category of therapy researched was that of the expressive and experiential therapies. Admittedly, this may have in part been because this category grouped together many different types of therapy, from music therapy to dance therapy to art therapy and beyond. But this still does not explain why this form of therapy has nearly four times the number of articles as Interpersonal Therapy, a practice solidly considered as evidence-based in the West for depression (in both adult and adolescent populations), the most common disorder found in the literature. It also does not explain why research on expressive therapy would be nearly six times as prevalent as mindfulness-based therapy, which draws its principles from and has cultural and historical roots in this region.

This chapter is only intended as a broad overview of the available research on this region and as such there are several limitations to this overview. Neither of the researchers spoke the native languages of the countries of focus, and as such only articles and abstracts written or translated into English could be utilized in this chapter. This review also has a fairly narrow scope as it only includes research from a five year time period (2011–2015). Additionally, in order to ensure that all related articles would be catalogued and accessible by psychology databases, the most recently published research (from January 2016 forward) was not included in analysis. For instance, Pelling's (2021) research on Singaporean supervisory development is not included. While this ensures the most complete and accurate image of the available research, it also means this image is not fully current at the time of its publication.

Concluding statement

Based upon these findings, we suggest that more research should be dedicated to shedding light onto what types of treatments are considered effective and/or popular in East and Southeast Asia. A survey of practitioners in these countries would be particularly interesting, given that it would allow comparisons between what is being practiced versus researched. While there are logistical challenges that would make this tricky, such knowledge would be invaluable in understanding the state of psychotherapy and counselling "on the ground" (rather than "in the journals") in these countries.

While we would like to see more research on every country in this region, we particularly recommend that researchers from places like China, Japan, Australia, North America, and Europe should partner to do research with those in the areas with the fewest published articles. This would allow more understanding about counselling practices in South Korea, Singapore, the Philippines, Thailand, Malaysia, and Vietnam. We also encourage more research focused on counselling for the elderly in these countries.

Educational questions & activities

1. Why is the majority of psychotherapy research centred on European and American populations?
2. Has psychotherapy research focusing on East and Southeast Asian countries increased in the twenty-first century?
3. What population does most East and Southeast Asian psychotherapy research focus upon?

4. How much of the East and Southeast Asian psychotherapy research focuses upon treating depressive disorders?
5. What was the most popular treatment researched in East and Southeast Asian psychotherapy Research?

References

Chung, M., Tsu, J., Kuo, C., Lin, P., & Chang, T. (2014). Therapeutic effect of dynamic interpersonal group psychotherapy for Taiwanese patients with depressive disorder. *International Journal of Group Psychotherapy, 64*(4), 537–545. doi: 2050/10.1521/ijgp.2014.64.4.537

Deng, L., Lin, X., Lan, J., & Fang, X. (2013). Family therapy in China. *Contemporary Family Therapy: An International Journal, 35*(2), 420–436. doi: 2050/10.1007/s10591-013-9273-3

Ho, R.T.H. (2015). A place and space to survive: A dance/movement therapy program for childhood sexual abuse survivors. *The Arts in Psychotherapy, 46,* 9–16. doi: 2050/10.1016/j.aip.2015.09.004

Kim, J. (2015). Music therapy with children who have been exposed to ongoing child abuse and poverty: A pilot study. *Nordic Journal of Music Therapy, 24*(1), 27–43. doi: 2050/10.1080/08098131.2013.872696

Ono, Y., Furukawa, T.A., Shimizu, E., Okamoto, Y., Nakagawa, A., Fujisawa, D., . . . Nakajima, S. (2011). Current status of research on cognitive therapy/cognitive behavior therapy in Japan. *Psychiatry and Clinical Neurosciences, 65*(2), 121–129. doi: 2050/10.1111/j.1440-1819.2010.02182.x

Pelling, N. (2013). Advertised psychologists and counsellors in Hong Kong and Singapore. *Asia Pacific Journal of Counselling and Psychotherapy, 4*(2), 185–199. doi: 10.1080/21507686.2013.824907

Pelling, N. (2021). Singaporean supervisory identity development and its relationship to supervisory experience, counselling experience, and training in supervision. *Asia Pacific Journal of Counselling and Psychotherapy, 12*(2), 186–204. doi: 10.1080/21507686.2021.1960400

Shirotsuki, K., Kodama, Y., & Nomura, S. (2014). The preliminary study of individual cognitive behavior therapy for Japanese patients with social anxiety disorder. *Psychological Services, 11*(2), 162–170. doi: 2050/10.1037/a0034781

Tuason, M.T.G., Fernandez, K.T.G., Catipon, M.A.D.P., Trivino-Dey, L., & Arellano-Carandang, M.L. (2012). Counseling in the Philippines: Past, present, and future. *Journal of Counseling & Development, 90*(3), 373–377. doi: 2050/10.1002/j.1556-6676.2012.00047.x

Zhao, J., Ji, J., Yang, X., Yang, Z., Hou, Y., & Zhang, X. (2011). National survey of ethical practices among Chinese psychotherapists. *Professional Psychology: Research and Practice, 42*(5), 375–381. doi: 2050/10.1037/a0025138

24 Research on Evidence-Based Therapies in Asian Countries

J. Kyle Haws, Yasmin Shirali, and Caleb W. Lack

Evidence-based practice (EBP) in psychology marries empirically supported research and clinical skills to provide the best possible treatment for clients (Anderson, 2006). Mental health practitioners of all kinds who use EBP typically use treatments that have been experimentally tested and for which there is strong evidence to support their efficacy. Such EBTs in counselling and psychotherapy have acquired abundant amounts of evidence demonstrating that they have the intended effect on the client (Draguns, 2013). For example, exposure therapy is intended to reduce fear and anxiety provoked by a particular stimulus by exposing the client in small steps to the feared stimulus (Foa, Gillihan, & Bryant, 2013). Abundant amounts of research have validated that exposure therapy does what it is intended to do – reduce both self-reported fear and anxiety as well as behavioural avoidance. However, despite the evidence and support, some therapists use treatments that have not been sufficiently tested or have been found not to work. This can be very damaging for a client seeking help, as they may not engage in the most effective treatment for their particular problem or may even forgo known effective treatments for untested or ineffective ones. For this reason, it is essential that therapists stay away from questionable methods and use EBTs whenever possible (Chambless & Hollon, 1998).

Currently, the majority of EBTs in psychology fall under the umbrella of cognitive-behavioural therapy (CBT), which attempts to help clients by changing maladaptive thought processes or behaviours, and often both of these, to help change emotions (Tolin, 2010; Norcross, 2001; Lyons & Woods, 1991). Depending on the client's goals, a therapist applying CBT might use various techniques that have been found to be effective for a particular problem, from cognitive restructuring to exposure with response prevention to social skills training to mindfulness. A therapist may also use a specific treatment 'package' that's been designed for a specific diagnosis or cluster of disorders. For example, exposure therapy is predominantly used to treat anxiety disorders (Parsons & Rizzo, 2008). The client makes a hierarchy of fears, and – with the therapists' support and expertise – conquers each one in order from the least severe to the most severe. Dialectical behavioural therapy combines group therapy, individual therapy, and phone therapy (Robins & Rosenthal, 2011). This EBT is mostly used for clients with borderline personality disorder, but is also effective in treating other conditions. Interpersonal therapy – the only treatment we included that is not a form of CBT – is mostly used to treat unipolar mood disorders (de Mello, de Jesus Mari, Bacaltchuk, Verdeli, & Neugebauer, 2005). The therapist focuses on the client's interpersonal problems (e.g., attachment style, social relationships, etc.) and, while building an alliance with the client, uses rationale and later encourages him to take social risks in order to turn past negative experiences into positive ones.

DOI: 10.4324/9781003490067-30

Each EBT has specific guidelines and often has manuals written to help guide treatment, but it is important to remember that each client is unique, and some adaptations must be made in order to most effectively help that client. This is often referred to as 'flexibility within fidelity,' meaning that one should implement EBTs within the context of an individualized approach that takes into account a person's unique cultural and social background (Kendall, Gosch, Jami, & Sood, 2008). For example, adaptations may be made due to cultural variations in attitudes towards diagnosis and treatment, or the inclusion of family.

Although trials examining various EBTs have been conducted in multicultural countries like the United States and with ethnically diverse client populations for many years, the effectiveness of these treatments on people with diverse cultural or ethnic backgrounds was rarely tested during the early years of the EBT movement (Nagayama Hall, 2001). Culture can act as a major mediating variable of mental health and a therapeutic experience, and can lead to two culturally different people receiving the exact same treatment to experience very different results (Bernal & Scharron-del Rio, 2001). For this reason, it is crucial that the effectiveness of EBTs be tested and verified among people of different cultures and ethnicities. Major meta-analysis studies have found that the most effective treatments typically labelled as EBTs featured the greatest amount of cultural adaptations and flexibility. For example, Rossello and Bernal (1999) found that interpersonal therapy was more effective than CBT in treating Puerto Rican adolescents with depression due to the fact that IPT addresses values that are highly important in Puerto Rican culture.

While many therapists believe in the importance of making cultural adaptations – such as adjusting for language and cultural norms – there are some who believe in the efficacy of unmodified versions of EBTs to treat culturally different clients. While there is some evidence that supports the effectiveness of unmodified versions of EBT with ethnoculturally distinct populations (e.g., Huey & Polo, 2008), it is essential that more research on unmodified versions of EBTs is conducted in order to determine whether or not cultural adaptations should be routinely integrated into EBTs.

With this overall conflict in the literature in mind, a review of research with Asian Americans specifically found that they were more responsive to culturally adapted treatments than other ethnocultural groups (Bernal & Domenech Rodríguez, 2012). Thus, culturally appropriate adaptations to EBTs could be a requirement for effective treatment of disorders in people across many different cultural groups, especially given the lack of homogeneity observed in various Asian populations. While Eastern-Asian countries have different values, beliefs, and traditions than those of the Western world, they also vary greatly amongst themselves. It is evident from research in Western countries that differences in culture can result in slightly different therapeutic needs (Griner & Smith, 2006).

So, although the therapeutic foundation can and should remain the same (fidelity), adaptations must be made to account for these differences (flexibility). Several researchers have examined exactly how to accomplish this. Seponski et al. (2020) emphasize the challenges of working from a more Western model, emphasizing that respect for and understanding of a country's mental health needs and cultural norms is paramount. Other examples include practicing cultural humility models when working with Chinese migrants (Bercean et al., 2020), understanding differences in expectations of psychotherapy between Asians and Westerners (Young & Yu, 2020), and how types of therapy can be adapted to working with Vietnamese people from a culturally sensitive model (Sumneangsanor et al., 2017). Thankfully, using conceptual models unique to an individual's culture appears to be both common in real-world practice and highly useful in engaging Asians and Asian

Americans in treatment (Hall et al., 2019). This has spurred cultural adaptations of CBT both broadly and for specific problems (such as schizophrenia; Li et al., 2017). Still, further research on EBTs using various Asian populations is required in order to best understand and make these necessary adaptations.

Recently, there have been attempts to provide an overviews of the status of psychotherapy and counselling interventions using EBTs in a number of Asian countries. Selvapandiyan (2019) described the lack of published studies using CBT in an Indian population, with a specific note a lack of efforts to ensure fidelity to best-practice standards in such research. The author even makes a call for regulation of CBT, as many published papers use non-CBT or outdated treatment interventions (although Sudhir et al., 2019 take issue with some of the methods used and critiques). Similar updates on the status of CBT have been undertaken in Japan (Ishikawa et al., 2020), as well as counselling practices (Tu & Jin, 2016) and clinical psychology (Wu et al., 2019) generally in Taiwan.

In this review, we take an overview of published research articles investigating evidence-based therapies for children, adolescents, adults, and elders living in various Asian countries. First, we identify the primary evidence-based therapies used, where the research originated, and the population. Second, we review the research to determine if it was quantitative, qualitative, a review, a meta-analysis, or a case-study. Third, we evaluate the age of the research population. Finally, we examine the specific psychopathology or diagnosis that is targeted by the EBT.

Method

A literature search was performed using the PsycINFO and PsycArticles databases for relevant publications over a 25-year period (1995–2020). Key words used for the search were *therapy, counseling, psychotherapy, cognitive behavioral, exposure therapy, rational emotive, interpersonal therapy, systematic desensitization, dialectical, biofeedback,* and names of various East Asian countries (such as *China, Hong Kong, Taiwan, Singapore, Japan, Korea, Thailand, Malaysia, Philippines, Vietnam, Cambodia, Indonesia,* and so on). After this initial search, the results were narrowed down based on a review of the abstracts (or the full article, if the abstract was unclear) to find those studies which met our criteria. Eventually, the search yielded 484 publications across these 25 years that were either research on EBTs conducted in Asian countries and/or research on EBTs applied to Asian populations.

Results

The majority of the research on EBTs with Asian populations has been published in the last ten years, with 45 per cent of the total 461 publications found being published since 2015. The year 2019 produced the most amount of published research on EBTs on Asian populations and/or published by researchers in Asian countries, followed closely by years 2020, 2018, and 2016 (see Figure 24.1). After a decline in 2008–2010, published research increased again and has maintained increasing publication rates during the last five years. This indicates a growing amount of published English-language research is being done on various types of EBTs, especially variations of cognitive-behavior therapy, with Asian populations.

The 25-year trends for research on EBTs and participants from Asian countries show that a significant amount of research is conducted with participants from China. Japan, Hong Kong, and Korea are the countries who follow China in the amount of research

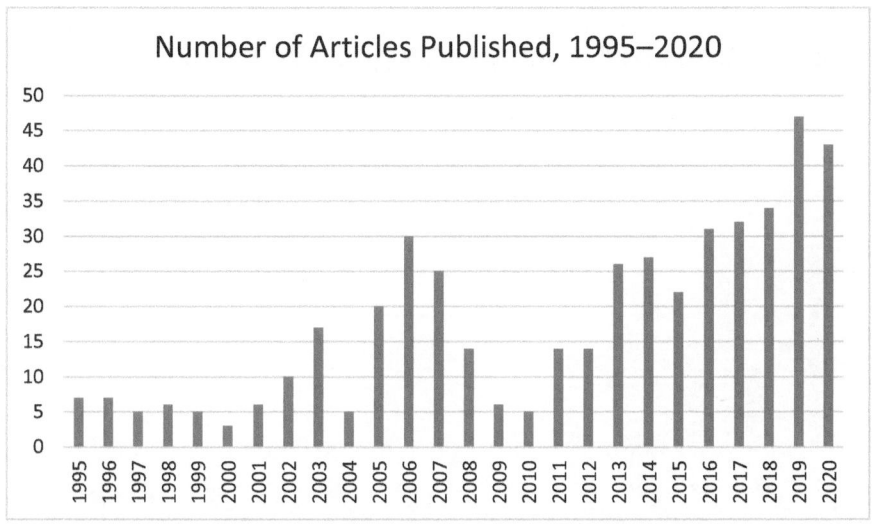

Figure 24.1 This chart illustrates the number of published, English language studies conducted with
EBTs and Asian populations or countries from 1995 to 2020

conducted on participants from those areas. There was little to no research examining populations from Indonesia, Cambodia, and Thailand, and no studies were found on populations in the Philippines, Vietnam, and Burma (see Figure 24.2). Please note that numbers in this chart and all following ones may not add up evenly to the 461 total publications due to researchers from multiple countries, multiple diagnoses, or multiple age groups being included in a single study.

The 25-year trends reveal that researchers operating out of China, Japan, Korea, Hong Kong, and the USA are producing the most research examining EBTs on Asian populations. China by itself produced almost 30 per cent of the research on the topic, with it and Japan together producing over half of the published research on the effectiveness of EBTs (see Figure 24.3).

A significant portion of the published research was quantitative in nature, using experimental methods such as random assignment, blinded or double-blinded evaluation of outcomes, and proper controls (see Figure 24.4). This is very welcome, as this indicates new, experimental data is either coming from Asian countries or tested using Asian populations rather than just relying on clinical opinion. Backing up this fact is that the number of quantitative research studies increased across the studies time period, while the number of case studies and reviews/discussions declined significantly across the 2015–2020 period. While there is some focus on other types of studies, the majority of the research studies are providing new experimental data on the effectiveness of EBTs.

The most commonly targeted population in terms of age for this research are adults. Over 71 per cent of the research conducted was with adult populations. These descriptive statistics reveal a huge gap in the literature examining the effectiveness of EBT with child, adolescent, and elder populations in Asian countries (see Figure 24.5). In many ways, this is not surprising, given that similar gaps are seen in literature in the United States.

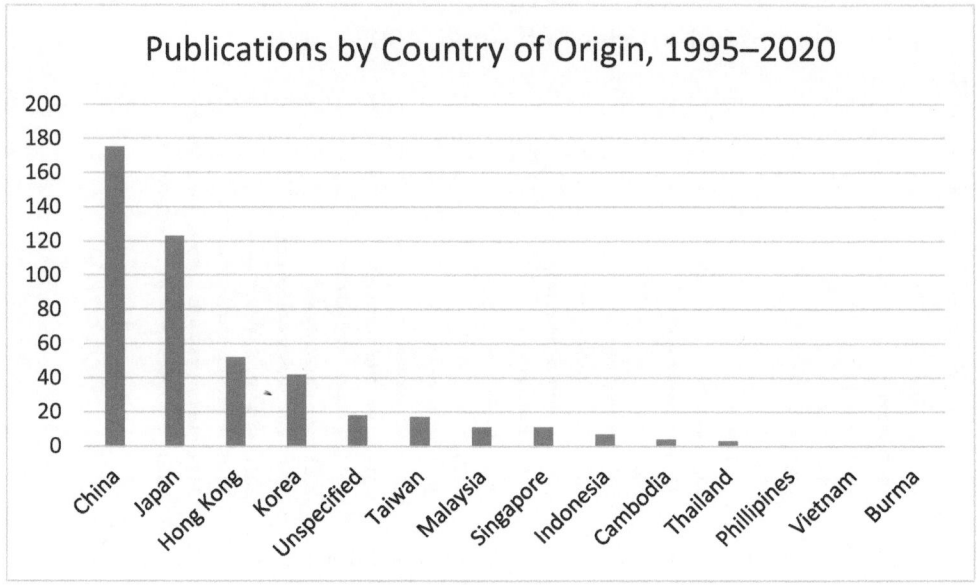

Figure 24.2 Country of origin for participants involved in the research

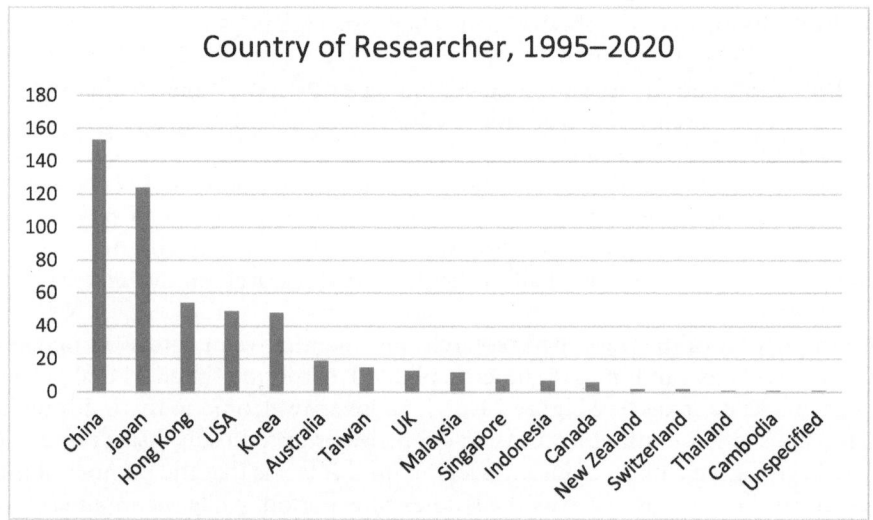

Figure 24.3 Country of origin for the researchers involved in the research

The research on EBTs was diverse and varied in regard to diagnoses (see Figure 24.6). A full half of the research found examined either anxiety (26%) and mood (24%) disorders. Inversely, there is minimal research on some relatively common diagnoses, such as schizophrenia, OCD, and eating disorders, with Asian populations. The 'other' category comprised a wide variety of issues, ranging from general quality of life in sub-clinical populations to various behavioural health issues such as weight loss.

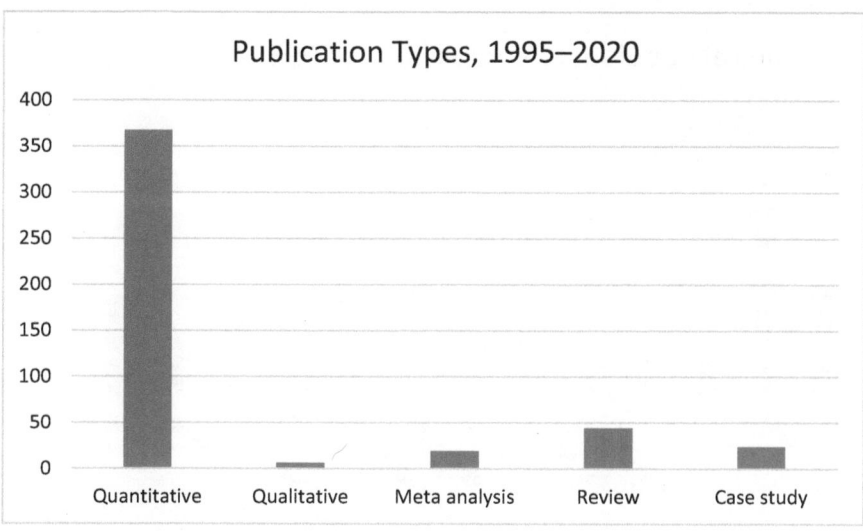

Figure 24.4 Type of research conducted on the EBTs and Asian populations

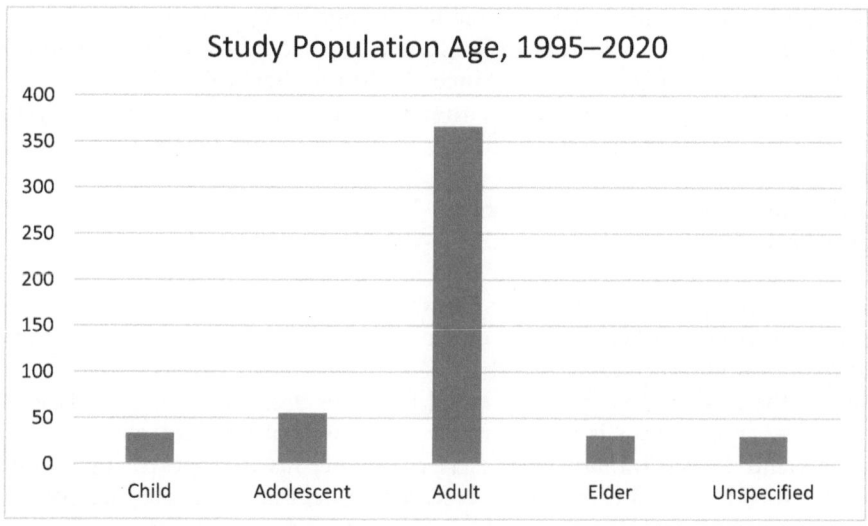

Figure 24.5 Age of the target population involved in the EBT research

Discussion

The amount of research on EBTs has oscillated some during the 25-year span, but for the most part has steadily inclined. The first sharp spike in the number of publications regarding EBTs occurred in 2005. This could be influenced in part by the fact that the APA issued a policy statement that same year showing full approval and support

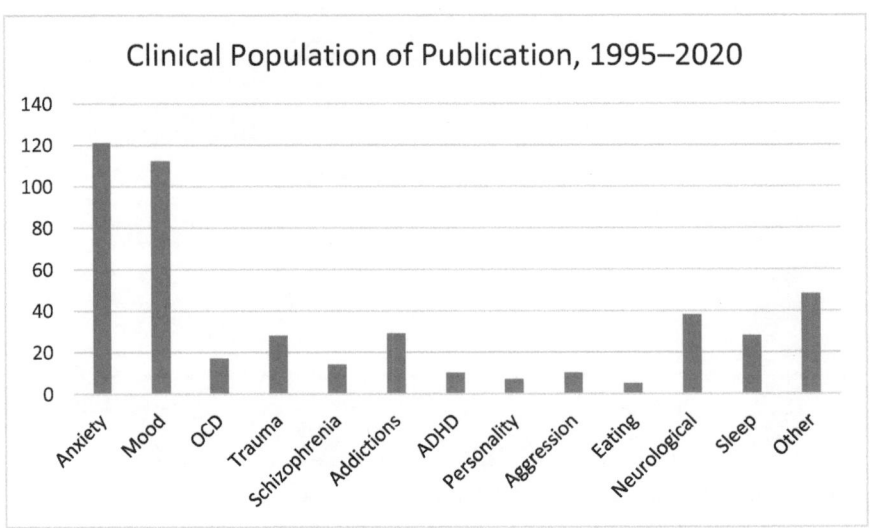

Figure 24.6 Diagnostic focus of the published research on EBTs. 'Other' represents behavioural, psychological, or emotional issues not better described by the previous categories

of psychologists using evidence-based practice in psychology, with an emphasis on research-supported treatments such as EBTs. Research wavered some in 2009 and 2010, and from there began to increase again. Since 2015, numbers of publications covering cognitive-behavior therapy, interpersonal therapy, biofeedback, and other EBTs has exploded, with 45% of the total articles for the entire study period coming out during this period.

This review covers only 461 publications on EBT from Asian countries or focused on Asian populations with a variety of diagnoses. While it is tempting to use Western EBTs directly with Asian populations, there are gaps in the research literature. We need more solid research examining evidence-based psychotherapies across cultures and with different age groups. As described earlier, when evidence is available it is promising, but there are many areas that are still in need of research.

Promisingly, the research on evidence-based practices used on Asian populations and coming out of Asian countries is rapidly increasing. Most of the research is focused on treating anxiety and depression, however, there are numerous attempts to apply evidence-based practices to other conditions. Many researchers in Asian countries are conducting exploratory studies with attempts to apply evidence-based practices to conditions such as aggression, eating disorders, and Attention-deficit/hyperactivity disorder (ADHD). Cognitive-behavior therapy is the most commonly researched evidence-based practice in Asian countries, especially in recent years. Most research is focused on adults, although there is some focus on children and adolescents. The research conducted with adolescents mostly focuses on applying evidence-based practices for aggression and at-risk teens. The elderly population is not a common focus in most studies, but it would be beneficial to conduct more studies with the elderly population, seeing as how best estimates are that 15 per cent or more of elderly people suffer from depression, anxiety, and other common mental health problems (World Health Organization, 2016).

Research on CBT is most prolific in Japan and China, with many studies attempting to apply CBT to treat other conditions, such as psychosis and aggression (Draguns, 2013). There has also been a recent wave of research applying CBT to help with insomnia. CBT has emerged as a prominent candidate of culturally modified treatment in multicultural societies. CBT is flexible enough to incorporate cultural sensitivity and the patient's cultural identity into treatment. There has been increasing research on internet-based and app-delivered CBT, especially in China. This could lead to evidence-based practices reaching a wider audience and thus helping more people, as many people fear the stigma of attending therapy or are unable to personally attend therapy sessions.

Concluding statement

The application of EBTs in Asian populations and countries is a powerful aid that can reduce distress and suffering. The advantages of EBT are the increased efficiency of treatment, a better therapeutic relationship between patient and therapist, and more extensive and validating evidence. However, it must be remembered that applying EBTs without thoroughly collecting empirical evidence can be detrimental to patient needs, cultural sensitivity, and reducing distress (Marsella, 2010). Strictly adhering to a manualized psychotherapy developed for a Western audience can give the appearance of an insensitive or an inflexible therapist. The best results of psychotherapy occur when the treatments are modified to a specific ethnocultural group. Meta-analysis reveal that the social and communicational components of psychotherapy are major predictors of a successful therapeutic outcome. While research examining the effectiveness of psychotherapy across the different nations of the world is currently small, trends from this study indicate an increasing amount of research being conducted and published, which can only be beneficial to the many individuals struggling with mental health issues.

Educational questions & activities

1. What is the largest group of evidence-based treatment (EBT)?
2. If an evidence-based treatment (EBT) has a manualised version one must apply the treatment as per the manual exactly for effectiveness. Is this statement True or False?
3. Evidence-based treatments (EBTs) are effective in all cultures. Is this statement True or False?
4. Is the research on evidence-based practices used with Asian populations and coming out of Asian countries increasing, decreasing, or remaining steady?

Selected references for further reading

Selected internet resources

Research supported psychological treatments

https://div12.org/psychological-treatments/
  • A regularly updated website that focuses on what psychological therapies have support for what types of mental health problems.

Evidence-based mental health treatment for children and adolescents

https://effectivechildtherapy.org/
- A regularly updated website that focuses on treatments for youth with mental health problems.

References

Anderson, N.B. (2006). Evidence-based practice in psychology. *American Psychologist, 61*(4), 271–285.

Bercean, A., Breen, L.J., McEvoy, P.M., Yeak, S., & Rooney, R. (2020). Improving the cultural sensitivity of cognitive–behavioral therapy for Chinese migrants with depression: Community members' and clinicians' perspectives. *Professional Psychology: Research and Practice, 51*(6), 613–622. https://doi.org/10.1037/pro0000326

Bernal, G., & Domenech Rodríguez, M.M. (2012). Cultural adaptation in context: Psychotherapy as a historical account of adaptations. *Cultural Adaptations: Tools for Evidence-Based Practice with Diverse Populations*, 3–22. Washington, DC: American Psychological Association.

Bernal, G., & Scharron-del Rio, M. (2001). Are empirically supported treatments valid for ethnic minorities? Toward an alternative approach for treatment research. *Cultural Diversity & Ethnic Minority Psychology, 7*(4), 328–42.

Chambless, D.L., & Hollon, S. D. (1998). Defining empirically supported therapies. *Journal of Consulting and Clinical Psychology, 66*, 7.

de Mello, M.F., de Jesus Mari, J., Bacaltchuk, J., Verdeli, H., & Neugebauer, R. (2005). A systematic review of research findings on the efficacy of interpersonal therapy for depressive disorders. *European Archives of Psychiatry and Clinical Neuroscience, 255*(2), 75–82.

Draguns, J. (2013). Cross-cultural and international extensions of evidence-based psychotherapy: Toward more effective and sensitive psychological services everywhere. *Psychologia, 56*, 74–88.

Foa, E.B., Gillihan, S.J., & Bryant, R.A. (2013). Challenges and successes in dissemination of evidence-based treatments for posttraumatic stress lessons learned from prolonged exposure therapy for PTSD. *Psychological Science in the Public Interest, 14*(2), 65–111.

Griner, D., & Smith, T.B. (2006). Culturally adapted mental health intervention: A meta-analytic review. *Psychotherapy: Theory, Research, Practice, Training, 43*(4), 531.

Hall, G.C.N., Kim-Mozeleski, J., Zane, N.W., Sato, H., Huang, E.R., Tuan, M., & Ibaraki, A.Y. (2019). Cultural adaptations of psychotherapy: Therapists' applications of conceptual models with Asians and Asian Americans. *Asian American Journal of Psychology, 10*(1), 68–78. https://doi.org/10.1037/aap0000122

Huey Jr, S.J., & Polo, A.J. (2008). Evidence-based psychosocial treatments for ethnic minority youth. *Journal of Clinical Child & Adolescent Psychology, 37*, 262–301.

Ishikawa, S., Chen, J., Fujisawa, D., & Tanaka, T. (2020). The development, progress, and current status of cognitive behaviour therapy in Japan. *Australian Psychologist, 55*(6), 598–605. https://doi.org/10.1111/ap.12450

Kendall, P.C., Gosch, E., Furr, J.M., & Sood, E. (2008). Flexibility within fidelity. *Journal of the American Academy of Child & Adolescent Psychiatry, 47*(9), 987–993.

Li, W., Zhang, L., Luo, X., Liu, B., Liu, Z., Lin, F., ... Naeem, F. (2017). A qualitative study to explore views of patients', carers' and mental health professionals' to inform cultural adaptation of CBT for psychosis (CBTp) in China. *BMC Psychiatry, 17*, 9. https://doi.org/10.1186/s12888-017-1290-6

Lyons, L.C., & Woods, P.J. (1991). The efficacy of rational-emotive therapy: A quantitative review of the outcome research. *Clinical Psychology Review, 11*(4), 357–369.

Marsella, A.J. (2010). Ethnocultural aspects of PTSD: An overview of concepts, issues, and treatments. *Toxicology, 16*, 17–26.

Nagayama Hall, G. (2001). Psychotherapy research with ethnic minorities: Empirical, ethical, and conceptual issues. *Journal of consulting and clinical psychology, 69*, 502–10.

Nagayama Hall, G.C., & Maramba, G.G. (2001). In search of cultural diversity: Recent literature in cross-cultural and ethnic minority psychology. *Cultural Diversity and Ethnic Minority Psychology, 7*(1), 12–26.

Norcross, J.C. (2001). Purposes, processes and products of the task force on empirically supported therapy relationships. *Psychotherapy: Theory, Research, Practice, Training, 38*(4), 345.

Parsons, T.D., & Rizzo, A.A. (2008). Affective outcomes of virtual reality exposure therapy for anxiety and specific phobias: A meta-analysis. *Journal of Behavior Therapy and Experimental Psychiatry, 39*(3), 250–261.

Robins, C.J., & Rosenthal, M.Z. (2011). Dialectical behavior therapy. In J.D. Herbert, & E.M. Forman (Eds.), *Acceptance and mindfulness in cognitive behavior therapy: Understanding and applying the new therapies*, 164–192. Hoboken: Wiley.

Rossello, J., & Bernal, G. (1999). The efficacy of cognitive-behavioral and interpersonal treatments for depression in Puerto Rican adolescents. *Journal of Consulting and Clinical Psychology, 67*(5), 734.

Selvapandiyan, J. (2019). Status of cognitive behaviour therapy in India: Pitfalls, limitations and future directions—A systematic review and critical analysis. *Asian Journal of Psychiatry, 41*, 1–4. https://doi.org/10.1016/j.ajp.2019.02.012

Seponski, D.M., Lewis, D.C., Bermudez, J.M., & Sotelo, J.M. (2020). Cambodian therapists' perspectives of western-based psychotherapy models: Addressing the challenges for service providers. *Journal of Family Psychotherapy, 31*(1–2), 36–55. https://doi.org/10.1080/08975 353.2020.1759018

Sudhir, P.M., Manjula, M., Kumar, A., & Sharma, M.P. (2019). Current status of cognitive behaviour therapy in India: The need to adopt a balanced view. *Asian Journal of Psychiatry, 44*, 158–159. https://doi.org/10.1016/j.ajp.2019.07.046

Sumneangsanor, T., Vuthiarpa, S., & Somprasert, C. (2017). Mental health disorder therapeutic modalities modified for the GMS. *Current Psychiatry Reviews, 13*(4), 259–263. https://doi.org/10.2174/1573400513666170721102543

Tolin, D.F. (2010). Is cognitive–behavioral therapy more effective than other therapies?: A meta-analytic review. *Clinical Psychology Review, 30*, 710–720.

Tu, S., & Jin, S. (2016). Development and current status of counselling psychology in Taiwan. *Counselling Psychology Quarterly, 29*(2), 195–205. https://doi.org/10.1080/09515 070.2015.1128399

World Health Organization. (2016). Mental health and older adults: Fact sheet. Retrieved from www.who.int/mediacentre/factsheets/fs381/en/ on September 12, 2016.

Wu, E., Lin, Y., Hua, M., Hsu, W., Guo, N., Yang, C., . . . Liao, Y. (2019). Scientists and practitioners: Thematic reviews and reflective perspectives in the development of clinical psychology in Taiwan. *Chinese Journal of Psychology, 61*(4), 361–392.

Young, C.B., & Yu, C.K. (2020). Hong Kong and western people have different expectations of counselling: A Hong Kong study of the expectations about Counselling—Brief form. *Asia Pacific Journal of Counselling and Psychotherapy, 11*(2), 198–219. https://doi.org/10.1080/21507 686.2020.1809480

Part 7

International Variations

Part 7, **International Variations**, contains eight chapters. This section begins with Chapter 25, outlining resources that can be used by supervisees and their supervisors to explore professional and regulatory aspects of counselling and psychology in various countries worldwide. Chapter 25 can thus serve as a starting point for supervisee and supervisor further explorations of our helping professions across the globe. The rest of this section contains Chapters 26, 27, 28, 29, 30, 31, and 32 exploring counselling and supervision in Canada, Hong Kong, Indonesia, Malaysia, the Philippines, Singapore, and the United States of America, respectively.

Chapter overview

Chapter 25, **International Counselling and Psychology Professional Organisations and Resources**, by Nadine Pelling, is a practical chapter providing a listing of professional organisations and regulatory bodies along with their contact details. This chapter also provides references for some of the existing scholarship related to descriptions of counselling and psychology as professions in various countries worldwide. Both supervisors and therapists in training will find these resources helpful in beginning to explore counselling and psychology as professions across the globe. Such a global perspective can only aid in one's broad view of counselling and psychology and is necessary for supervising trainees in a global and mobile marketplace.

Chapter themes

In this chapter you will explore the following themes:

- Professional organisations
- A limited listing of counselling & psychology organisations worldwide
- Professional resources
- A limited selection of counselling & psychology resources worldwide
- Internationalisation in counselling and psychology

Chapter 26, **Counselling regulation, education, supervision, and representation in Canada**, by Nicola Gazzola and Kate Gignac, looks at how counselling and supervision work and are regulated in Canada.

DOI: 10.4324/9781003490067-31

Chapter themes

In this chapter you will explore the following themes:

- Clinical supervision: Applied activity and research
- Counselling regulation in Canada
- Pathways to becoming a counsellor in Canada
- Counselling supervision in Canada

Chapter 27, **Strategic Approaches to Managing the Development of the Counselling Profession in Hong Kong**, by Pui Chi Tse, looks at how supervision and counselling works in Hong Kong.

Chapter themes

In this chapter you will explore the following themes:

- Contextual understanding of counselling professional development in Hong Kong
- History, culture, and changes
- Struggles, difficulties, and challenges
- Threats, dilemmas, and opportunities

Chapter 28, **An Overview of Counselling Practices in Indonesia**, by Marina Salmond, Karel K. Himawan, Jessica Ariela, and Eunike M. Himawan, looks at counselling and supervision in Indonesia.

Chapter themes

In this chapter you will explore the following themes:

- Counselling representation in Indonesia and the overlapping scope of mental health practitioners
- The diversity of counselling education in Indonesia
- The lack of counselling regulation in Indonesia
- Counselling supervision in Indonesia

Chapter 29, **Counselling Regulation, Education, and Representation in Malaysia**, by Melati Sumari, Dini Farhana Baharudin, Hartini Abdul Rahman, and Norfaezah Md Khalid, explores supervision and counselling regulation in Malaysia.

Chapter themes

In this chapter you will explore the following themes:

- Counselling regulation in Malaysia
- Registration of counsellors
- Ethical codes

- Counselling education in Malaysia
- Counselling representation in Malaysia

Chapter 30, *The Counseling Profession in the Philippines* by Ma. Teresa G. Tuason, Margaret Helen Alvarez, and Bridget Stanton, looks at how supervision and counseling work in the Philippines.

Chapter Themes

In this chapter you will explore the following themes:

- Counseling regulation in the Philippines
- Counseling education in the Philippines
- Opportunities for counseling jobs in the Philippines
- Counseling representation in the Philippines
- Supervision of counseling in the Philippines

Chapter 31, **The Professionalisation of Counselling Supervision in Singapore**, by Jeffrey Po, looks at how supervision works in Singapore. He suggests that the country's counselling workforce embrace all that supervision has to offer.

Chapter themes

In this chapter you will explore the following themes:

- Accredited counselling supervisors in Singapore
- Supervision training available in Singapore
- APACS College of Professional Supervisors

Chapter 32, **Counseling Regulation, Education, and Representation in the United States of America**, by Janeé Steele and Tiffany Lee, explores counseling regulation, education, and representation in the United States.

Chapter themes

In this chapter you will explore the following themes:

- Counseling regulation in the United States
- Counseling regulation in the United States
- Counseling representation in the United States
- Pathways to becoming a counselor in the United States
- Supervision of counseling in the United States

25 International Counselling and Psychology Professional Organisations and Resources

Nadine Pelling

Professional organisations

In counselling supervision we enhance and develop knowledge, self/other awareness, and skill. We hope that this development continues outside of supervision and that continuous lifelong learning results. One way to encourage continuous learning, as well as the development of collegial support amongst counsellors, is to promote membership in various professional organisations as beneficial. It is my firm belief that all counsellors, therapists, psychologists, and social workers should belong to at least one professional organisation for easy access to a developed code of ethics, collegial support, and continuing professional development via the availability of workshops, conferences, and the production of professional journals. I believe that active membership promotes reflective practice and continuing professional development. Professional organisations are also a valuable resource for investigating what type of training and experience are needed in various professional areas and regions. Indeed, many professional organisations have links to regulatory authorities that provide information on legislative, or voluntary, requirements when they are present.

An incomplete listing of international psychological and counselling-related professional organisations (and some regulatory bodies) is presented in Table 25.1 for your convenience. This information was as accurate as possible at the time of printing and information has come from a variety of sources, including the internet. This is an updated list based upon Pelling (2006, 2009, and 2017).

Professional resources

Students often ask me, 'What do I need to do in order to be a professional counsellor?' to which my first answer is generally a compound question, 'Where and in what capacity do you intend on working (i.e., Canada or Australia and psychology or counselling)?' because regulation differs across the globe and professions. I then refer those seeking international counselling or psychology information to the relevant country's professional organisations and regulatory bodies as previously presented. I also often offer a collection of references relating to the area and location of interest and encourage concerted self-initiated investigation by the professional involved.

It is beyond the scope of the present chapter to outline the nature of psychology and counselling across the globe. Moreover, professions (often like professionals) develop over time and any specific information presented could become dated quickly. Thus, I have chosen to simply present some of the references I have collated in the following sections

DOI: 10.4324/9781003490067-32

Table 25.1 A limited listing of international counselling and psychology organisations

Region	Discipline	Service Area	Name	WWW site	Address	Contact
North America	Counseling	United States of America	American Counseling Association (ACA)	www.counseling.org	PO Box 31110, Alexandria, VA 22310-9998	ACAMemberServices@ counseling.org
North America	Counseling	United States of America	American Association of State Counseling Boards (AASCB)	wwwaascborg. wildapricot.org	108 Wind Haven Drive, Suite A Nicholasville, KY 40356	Phone: 1 (859) 269 1802 Info@AASCB.org
North America	Counseling	United States of America	Association for Counselor Education and Supervision (ACES)	www.acesonline.net	PO Box 682, Lake Worth, FL 33460	Phone: 1 (800) 347-6647 execaces@gmail.com
North America	Counseling	United States of America	National Board for Certified Counselors (NBCC)	www.nbcc.org	3 Terrace Way Greensboro, NC 27403	Phone: 1 (336) 547-0607 Fax: 1 (336) 547-0017 nbcc@nbcc.org
North America	Psychology	United States of America	American Psychological Association (APA)	www.apa.org	750 First St. NE, Washington, DC 20002-4242	Phone: 1 (800) 374-2721 1 (202) 336-5500
North America	Counselling	Canada	Canadian Counselling and Psychotherapy Association (CCPA)	www.ccpa-accp.ca	202-245 Menten Place Ottawa, ON, K2H 9E8	Phone: 1 (877) 765-5565 Fax: 1 (613) 237-9786
North America	Counselling	Canada	Canadian Professional Counsellors Association (CPCA)	www.cpca-rpc.ca	PO Box 907 Vernon, BC V1T 6M8	Phone: 1 (250) 558-3323 Fax: 1 (250) 558-3369 info@cpca-rpc.ca
North America	Counselling	Canada	Canadian College of Professional Counsellors and Psychotherapists (CCPCP)	www.ccpcp.ca	PO Box 23045 Vernon, BC V1T 9L8	Phone: 1 (250) 558-7700 inquiry@ccpcp.ca

Region	Country	Type	Organisation	Website	Address	Contact
North America	United States of America and Canada	Psychology	Association of State and Provincial Psychology Boards (ASPPB)	www.asppb.org	PO Box 849, Tyrone GA 30290	Phone: 1 (678) 216-1175 Fax: 1 (678) 216-1176 asppb@asppb.org
North America	Canada	Psychology	Canadian Psychological Association; Societe Canadienne de Psychologie (CPA)	www.cpa.ca	141 Laurier Avenue West, Suite 702 Ottawa, Ontario K1P 5J3	Phone: 1 (613) 237-2144 Fax: 1 (613) 237-1674 cpa@cpa.ca
Europe	United Kingdom	Counselling	British Association for Counselling and Psychotherapy (BACP)	www.bacp.co.uk	BACP House 15 St John's Business Park Lutterworth, Leicestershire LE17 4HB England UK	Phone: +44 01455 883300 bacp@bacp.co.uk
Europe	United Kingdom	Counselling	United Kingdom Council for Psychotherapy (UKCP)	www.psychotherapy.org.uk	UKCP 2 America Square, London EC3N 2LU, England UK	Phone: +44 020 7014 9955 membership@ukcp.org.uk
Europe	United Kingdom	Psychology	British Psychological Society (BPS)	www.bps.org.uk	The British Psychological Society St Andrews House 48 Princess Road East Leicester LE1 7DR England UK	Phone: +44 (0) 207 330 0890 membership@bps.org.uk
Australasia	Australia	Counselling	Australian Counselling Association (ACA)	www.theaca.net.au	P.O. Box 88 Grange Qld 4051 Australia	Phone: +61 (07) 3356 4255 Fax: +61 (07) 3356 4709 memberships@theaca.net.au.

(Continued)

Table 25.1 (Continued)

Region	Discipline	Service Area	Name	WWW site	Address	Contact
Australasia	Counselling	Australia	Psychotherapy and Counselling Federation of Australia (PACFA)	www.pacfa.org.au	290 Park Street Fitzroy North VIC 3068 Australia	Phone: +61 (03) 9486 3077 Fax: +61 (03) 9486 3933 admin@pacfa.org.au
Australasia	Counselling & Psychology	Australia	The Australian Psychologists and Counsellors in Schools Association (APACS)	www.apacs.org.au		info@apacs.org.au
Australasia	Psychology	Australia	Australian Psychological Society (APS)	www.psychology.org.au	PO Box 38 Flinders Lane VIC 8009 Australia	Phone: +61(03) 8662 3300 Fax: +61 (03) 9663 6177 contactus@psychology.org.au
Australasia	Psychology	Australia	Psychology Board of Australia (PsyBA)	www.psychologyboard.gov.au	PsyBA AHPRA GPO Box 9958 Melbourne VIC 3001	Phone: +61 3 9275 9009
Australasia	Psychology	Australia	Australian Indigenous Psychologists Association	www.indigenouspsychology.com.au		contact@indigenouspsychology.com.au
Australasia	Counselling	New Zealand	New Zealand Association of Counsellors (NZAC)	www.nzac.org.nz	PO Box 25154, Wellington 6140	Phone: +64 (04) 471 0307 Fax: +64 (04) 471 1535 admin@nzac.org.nz membership@nzac.org.nz
Australasia	Psychology	New Zealand	New Zealand Psychological Society (NZPsS)	www.psychology.org.nz	PO Box 10536, The Terrace, Wellington 6143	Phone: +64 4 473 4884 Fax: +64 4 473 4889 office@psychology.org.nz
Australasia	Psychology	New Zealand	New Zealand Psychologists Board (NZPB)	www.psychologistsboard.org.nz	PO Box 9644, Marion Square, Wellington 6141, New Zealand	Phone: +64 4 471 4580 info@nzpb.org.nz

Australasia	Counselling	Hong Kong Professional Counsellors Association (HKPCA)	www.hkpca.org.hk	Room 18, Flat S-V, 6/F, Valiant Industrial Centre, No. 2-12 Au Pui Wan Street, Fotan, N.T., Hong Kong.	+852 2334 7172 enquiry@hkpca.org.hk
Australasia	Psychology	Hong Kong Psychological Society (HKPS)	www.hkps.org.hk	Room 506, Lemmi Centre, 50 Hoi Yuen Road, Kwun Tong, Kowloon, Hong Kong	Fax: +852 2852 1776 admin@hkps.org.hk
Australasia	Counselling	Asian Professional Counselling & Psychology Association (APCPA)	www.apcpa.com.hk	Department of Counselling and Psychology, Hong Kong Shue Yan University, 10 Wai Tsui Crescent, Braemar Hill Road, North Point, Hong Kong	Phone: +852 2806-7326 Fax: +825 2806-8044 admin@apcpa.com.hk
Australasia	Counselling	Hong Kong Society of Counseling and Psychology (HKSCP)	http://hkscporg.weebly.com	Room 305-306, Summit Insurance Building, 789 Nathan Road, Prince Edward, Hong Kong	Phone:+852 2790 7123 info@hkscp.org

(Continued)

Table 25.1 (Continued)

Region	Discipline	Service Area	Name	WWW site	Address	Contact
Australasia	Counselling	Malaysia	Malaysian Psychotherapy Association Persatuan Psikoterapi Malaysia (PPM)	www.malaysianpsychotherapy.net/	11-1 Wisma Laxton, Jalan Desa, Taman Desa, 58100, Kuala Lumpur	Phone: +60 3-2727 7434 Fax: +60 03 - 7982 6130 info@psychology.com.my
Australasia	Psychology	Malaysia	Malaysian Psychological Association (PSIMA)	www.psima.org.my	D/A Malaysian Psychology Department, University of Malaysia, 43600 Bangi, Selangor	membership@psima.org.my
Australasia	Counselling	Singapore	Singapore Association for Counselling (SAC)	www.sacsingapore.org	c/o Work Central Offices, 190 Clemenceau Avenue, #06-01 Singapore Shopping Centre, Singapore 239924	Phone: +65 6708 8292 Fax: +65 6252-4533 admin@sacsingapore.org
Australasia	Psychology	Singapore	Singapore Psychological Society (SPS)	www.singaporepsychologicalsociety.org	Secretariat Office 8 Eu Tong Sen Street #18-81 The Central Singapore 059818	secretariat@singaporepsychologicalsociety.org
International	Psychology		International Association of Applied Psychology (IAAP)	www.iaapsy.org		Phone: +1 317 205 9480 operationscenter@iaapsy.org
International	Counselling		International Association for Counselling	www.iac-irtac.org		ceo@iac-irtac.org

for your review. This is not an exhaustive bibliography but simply a starting point for those interested in gaining more information.

Educational questions & activities

1. As an individual or a group list all of the possible benefits and drawbacks of being a member of a professional organisation.
2. Ask a trusted colleague or supervisor what they think the benefits and drawbacks of being a member of a professional organisation entail.
3. Look up one professional organisation in your practice area and in your home country and one in a country in which you are interested. What do the respective organisations say about your professional area in those countries?
4. How much does it cost for a student or a beginning professional to join the professional organisation most relevant to your work?

Selected references for further reading

United States of America

Lichtenberg, J.W., Goodyear, R.K., Hutman, H., & Overland, E.A. (2016). Counselling psychology in the United States. *Counselling Psychology Quarterly*, 29(2), 216–224.

Munley, P.H., Duncan, L.E., McDonnell, K.A., & Sauer, E.M. (2004). Counseling psychology in the United States of America. *Counselling Psychology Quarterly*, 17(3), 247–271.

Weinrach, S.G., & Thomas, K.R. (1993). The National Board for Certified Counselors: The good, the bad, and the ugly. *Journal of Counseling and Development*, 72(1), 105–109.

Canada

Alden, L., Mothersill, K., Steffy, R., & McIlwraith, R. (1996). Priorities for professional training in the 90s: Perspectives of directors of psychology training programs. *Canadian Psychology/ Psychologie Canadienne*, 37(4), 223–228. doi:10.1037/0708-5591.37.4.223

Bedi, Robinder. (2016). A descriptive examination of Canadian counselling psychology doctoral programs. *Canadian Psychology*, Advance on-line publication. Retrieved from http://ovidsp.ovid. com/ovidweb.cgi?T=JS&PAGE=reference&D=paovftq&NEWS=N&AN=00011346-900000 000-99959. doi:10.1037/cap0000047

Bedi, R.P., Christiani, K.D., & Cohen, J.A. (2018). The future of Canadian counselling psychology: Doctoral students. *Counselling Psychology Quarterly*, 31(2), 205–222. doi:10.1080/ 09515070.2016.1277977

Bedi, Robinder, Haverkamp, Beth, Beatch, Romeo, Cave, Douglas, Domene, Jose, Harris, Gregory, et al. (2011). Counselling psychology in a Canadian context: Definition and description. *Canadian Psychology*, 52, 128–138. doi:10.1037/a0023186

Bedi, Robinder, Klubben, Laura, & Barker, Gordon. (2012). Counselling vs. clinical: A comparison of psychology doctoral programs in Canada. *Canadian Psychology*, 53, 238–253. doi:10.1037/ a0028558

Bedi, R.P., Sinacore, A., & Christiani, K.D. (2016). Counselling psychology in Canada. *Counselling Psychology Quarterly*, 29(2), 150–162. doi:10.1080/09515070.2015.1128398

Borgen, W., Robertson, S., Caverley, N., & Patterson, P. (2021). Making the case for counsellor education accreditation in Canada: A cross-jurisdictional review of emerging trends in the pre-service training of counsellors and related mental health professionals. *Canadian Journal of Counselling & Psychotherapy*, 55(1), 74–95. doi:10.47634/cjcp.v55i1.70427

Dobson, K.S., & Dobson, D.J. (2019). Professional psychology training in Canada: How did we get here and where could we go? *Canadian Psychology*, 60(4), 247–254. doi:10.1037/cap0000179

Haverkamp, Beth, Robertson, Sharon, Cairns, Sharon, & Bedi, Robinder. (2011). Professional issues in Canadian counselling psychology: identity, education, and professional practice. *Canadian Psychology*, 52, 256–264. doi:10.1037/a0025214

Hiebert, Bryan, Domene, Jose, & Buchanan, Marla. (2011). The power of multiple methods and evidence sources: Raising the profile of Canadian counselling psychology research. *Canadian Psychology*, 52, 265–275. doi:10.1037/a0025364

Janel, G. (2002). Facilitating mobility for psychologists through a competency-based approach for regulation and accreditation: The Canadian experiment. *European Psychologist*, 17(3), 203–212.

Lalande, V. M. (2004). Counselling psychology: A Canadian perspective. *Counselling Psychology Quarterly*, 17(3), 273–286.

Sinacore, Ada. (2011). Canadian counselling psychology coming of age: An overview of the special section. *Canadian Psychology*, 52, 245–247. doi:10.1037/a0025331

Sinacore, Ada, Borgen, William, Daniluk, Judith, Kassan, Anusha, Long, Bonita, & Nicol, Jennifer. (2011). Canadian counselling psychologists' contributions to applied psychology. *Canadian Psychology*, 52, 276–288. doi:10.1037/a0025549

Wada, K., Kassan, A., Domene, J.F., Bedi, R., Kintzel, F., & West, A. (2020). The future of counselling psychology education and training in Canada: A post-conference reflection. *Canadian Journal of Counselling and Psychotherapy*, 54(4), 572–594. doi:10.47634/cjcp.v54i4.70773

Young, Richard, & Lalande, Vivian. (2011). Canadian counselling psychology: From defining moments to ways forward. *Canadian Psychology*, 52, 248–255. doi:10.1037/a0025165

United Kingdom

Aldridge, S. (2006). Update on regulation. *Therapy Today*, 34–35.

Balfour, F.G.H. (2000). The statutory registration of psychotherapists. *British Journal of Guidance & Counselling*, 16(3), 311–320.

British Association for Counselling and Psychotherapy. (2005). Regulation: The mapping project. *Therapy Today*, 37–39.

British Psychological Society. (2005). Statutory regulation – Some questions answered. *The Psychologist*, 18(4), 238–239.

Denburg, M.L. (1969). Registration of applied psychologists. *Bulletin of the British Psychological Society*, 22(74), 19–20.

Dryden, W., Mearns, D., & Thorne, B. (2000). Counselling in the United Kingdom: Past, present and future. *British Journal of Guidance & Counselling*, 28(4), 467–483.

Inskipp, F., & Johns, H. (2003). A visionary in British counselling. *International Journal for the Advancement of Counselling*, 25(2–3), 115–118.

Jacobs, M. (2000). Counselling in the United Kingdom: Past, present and future. *British Journal of Guidance & Counselling*, 28(4), 451–466.

Jones Nielsen, J.D., & Nicholas, H. (2016). Counselling psychology in the United Kingdom. *Counselling Psychology Quarterly*, 29(2), 206–215. doi:10.1080/09515070.2015.1127210

Joseph, S., Murphy, D., & Holford, J. (2018). Counselling training in higher education in the United Kingdom: Challenges and opportunities for research. *Counselling and Psychotherapy Research*, 18(4), 387–394. doi:10.1002/capr.12189

Latak, K. (2006). Studying psychology in Europe. *The Psychologist*, 297. www.bps.org.uk/psychologist/students-may-2006

Walsh, Y., Frankland, A., & Cross, M. (2004). Qualifying and working as a counselling psychologist in the United Kingdom. *Counselling Psychology Quarterly*, 17(3), 317–328.

Woolfe, R. (1999). Training routes for counsellors, counselling psychologists and psychotherapists. In R. Bor, & M. Watts (Eds.), *Trainee handbook: A guide for counselling and psychotherapy trainees* (pp. 6–18). London: Sage Publications.

Australia

Brown, J., & Corne, L. (2004). Counselling psychology in Australia. *Counselling Psychology Quarterly*, 17(3), 287–299.

Davis-McCabe, C., Di Mattia, M., & Logan, E. (2019). Challenges facing Australian counselling psychologists: A qualitative analysis. *Australian Psychologist*, 54(6), 513–525. doi:10.1111/ap.12393

Di Mattia, M.A., & Grant, J. (2016). Counselling psychology in Australia: History, status and challenges. *Counselling Psychology Quarterly*, 29(2), 139–149. doi:10.1080/09515070.2015.1127208

Gonsalvez, C.J., Shafranske, E.P., McLeod, H.J., & Falender, C.A. (2021). Competency-based standards and guidelines for psychology practice in Australia: opportunities and risks. *Clinical Psychologist*, 25(3), 244–259. doi:10.1080/13284207.2020.1829943

Helmes, E., & Wilmoth, D. (2002). Training in clinical psychology in Australia: A North American perspective. *Australian Psychologist*, 37(1), 52–55.

Kavanagh, P.S. (2015). Psychology regulation, education, and representation in Australia. *International Journal of Mental Health. Special Issue: Mental Health in Australia (N. Pelling Ed)*, 44, 4–10. doi:10.1080/00207411.2015.1009742

Littlefield, L., Giese, J., & Katsikitis, M. (2007). Professional psychology training under review. *InPsych*, 29(2), 6.

Nicholson Perry, K., & Katsikitis, M. (2021). Riding on a wave: reflections on a new era in psychology training. *Clinical Psychologist*, 25(3), 241–243. doi:10.1080/13284207.2021.2010669

Norton, P.J., Norberg, M.M., Naragon-Gainey, K., & Deacon, B.J. (2022). An examination of accreditation standards between Australian and US/Canadian doctoral programs in clinical psychology. *Clinical Psychologist*, 26(2), 181–187. doi:10.1080/13284207.2021.1949944

Pelling, N. (2005). Counsellors in Australia: Profiling the membership of the Australian Counselling Association. *Counselling, Psychotherapy, and Health*, [On-line serial], 1(1), 1–18. www.cphjournal.com

Pelling, N. (2006). Getting a global perspective: Counselling Australia. *Counseling Today*, 48(7), 35.

Pelling, N. (2015). Mental health in Australia. *International Journal of Mental Health*, 44(1–2), 1–3, doi:10.1080/00207411.2015.1009741

Pelling, N.J. (Ed.) (2006). Journal special issue: Counselling in Australia (2006). *International Journal of Psychology*, 41(3), 153–215.

Pelling, N.J. (2007) Advertised Australian counselling psychologists: A descriptive survey of practice details and self-perceived competence in six counselling psychology practice areas. *Counselling Psychology Quarterly*, 20(3), 213–227.

Pelling, N.J. (2015). Counselling and psychotherapy in Australia: Cynthia's story. In Roy Moodley, Marguerite Lengyell, Rosa Wu, & Uwe P. Gielen (Eds.), *International counseling case studies handbook*. Alexandria, VA: Wiley.

Pelling, N.J., Bowers, R., & Armstrong, P. (Eds.) (2006). *The Practice of counselling (2006)*. Melbourne, Victoria: Thomson.

Pelling, N.J., & Burton, L.J. (2017a). *Abnormal psychology: The Australian and New Zealand handbook*. London, UK: Taylor and Francis.

Pelling, N.J., & Burton, L. . (2017b). *The elements of applied psychological practice in Australia: Preparing for the National Psychology Exam*. London, UK: Taylor and Francis.

Pelling, N., & Sullivan, B. (2006). The credentialing of counselling in Australia. *International Journal of Psychology*, 41(3), 194–203.

Pelling, N., & Whetham, P. (2006). The professional preparation of Australian counsellors. *International Journal of Psychology*, 41(3), 189–193.

Salter, M., & Rhodes, P. (2018). On becoming a therapist: A narrative inquiry of personal–professional development and the training of clinical psychologists. *Australian Psychologist*, 53(6), 486–492. doi:10.1111/ap.12344

Schofield, M.J. (2013), Counseling in Australia: Past, present, and future. *Journal of Counseling & Development*, 91, 234–239. doi:10.1002/j.1556-6676.2013.00090.x

Schweinsberg, A., Mundy, M.E., Dyer, K.R., & Garivaldis, F. (2021). Psychology education and work readiness integration: A call for research in Australia. *Frontiers in Psychology*, 12. doi:10.3389/fpsyg.2021.623353

New Zealand

Du Preez, E., Feather, J., & Farrell, B. (2016). Counselling psychology in New Zealand. *Counselling Psychology Quarterly*, 29(2), 163–170. doi:10.1080/09515070.2015.1128397

Furbish, D.S. (2007), Career counseling in New Zealand. *Journal of Counseling & Development*, 85, 115–119. doi:10.1002/j.1556-6678.2007.tb00453.x

Kennedy, B.J., Tassell-Matamua, N.A., & Stiles-Smith, B. (2022). Psychology in Aotearoa New Zealand. In G.J. Rich, & N.A. Ramkumar (Eds.), *Psychology in Oceania and the Caribbean* (pp. 115–132). Cham: Springer International Publishing AG. doi:10.1007/978-3-030-87763-7 (chapter 8).

Shouksmith, G. (2005). Psychology in New Zealand. *The Psychologist*, 18(1), 14–16.

Stanley, P., & Manthei, R. (2004). Counselling psychology in New Zealand: The quest for identity and recognition. *Counselling Psychology Quarterly*, 17(3), 301–315.

Hong Kong, Singapore, and Malaysia

Chan Lai Cheng, J., Bates, G., & Goh, W.Y.F. (2022). An exploratory study of student counsellors' motivations, considerations, and plans in Singapore. *Asia Pacific Journal of Counselling and Psychotherapy*, 13(1), 5–21. doi:10.1080/21507686.2022.2036785

Glamcevski, M. (2008). The Malaysian counselling profession, history and brief discussion of the future. *Counselling, Psychotherapy, and Health*, 4(1), *Counselling in the Asia Pacific Rim: A Coming Together of Neighbours Special Issue*, 1–18.

Jin Kuan Kok (2013) The role of the school counsellor in the Singapore secondary school system. *British Journal of Guidance & Counselling*, 41(5), 530–543. doi:10.1080/03069885.2013.773286

Nee, K.G., Beevi, Z., Khairudin, R., & Salem, E. (2022). Employability of the psychology community in Malaysia. *Malaysian Journal of Psychology/Jurnal Psikologi Malaysia*, 36(1), 79–96.

Pelling, N. (2013). Advertised psychologists and counsellors in Hong Kong and Singapore. *Asia Pacific Journal of Counselling and Psychotherapy*, 4(2), 185–199. doi:10.1080/21507686.2013.824907

Pelling, N. (2021). Singaporean supervisory identity development and its relationship to supervisory experience, counselling experience, and training in supervision. *Asia Pacific Journal of Counselling and Psychotherapy*, 12(2), 186–204. doi:10.1080/21507686.2021.1960400

See, C.M., and Ng, K.M. (2010). Counseling in Malaysia: History, current status, and future trends. *Journal of Counseling & Development*, 88(1), 18–22. doi:10.1002/j.1556-6678.2010.tb00144.x

Sumari, M., Baharudin, D.F., Rahman, H.A., & Khalid, N.M. (2021). Counselling regulation, education, and representation in Malaysia. *Australian Counselling Research*, 15, 8–15.

Yeo, L.S., Tan, S.Y., & Neihart, M.F. (2012). Counseling in Singapore. *Journal of Counseling & Development*, 90(2), 243–248. doi:10.1111/j.1556-6676.2012.00031.x

Yuen, M., Leung, S.A., & Chan, R.T.H. (2014). Professional counseling in Hong Kong. *Journal of Counseling & Development*, 92(1), 99–103. doi:10.1002/j.1556-6676.2014.00135.x

International Counselling and Psychology Resources

Goodyear, R., Lichtenberg, J., Hutman, H., Overland, E., Bedi, R., Christiani, K., ... & Young, C. (2016). A global portrait of counselling psychologists' characteristics, perspectives, and professional behaviors. *Counselling Psychology Quarterly*, 29(2), 115–138. doi:10.1080/09515070.2015.1128396

Hohenshil, T.H. (2010). International Counseling Introduction. *Journal of Counseling & Development*, 88(1), 3. doi:10.1022/j.1556-6678.2010.tb00140.x

Lee, Kin. (2013). Training and educating international students in professional psychology: What graduate programs should know. *Training & Education in Professional Psychology*, 7, 61–69. doi:10.1037/a0031186

Marsella, A.J., & Pedersen, P. (2004). Internationalizing the counseling psychology curriculum: toward new values, competencies, and directions. *Counselling Psychology Quarterly*, 17(4), 413–423.

Nixon, Mary. (1990). Professional training in psychology: Quest for international standards. *American Psychologist*, 45(11), 1257–1262. Retrieved from http://ovidsp.ovid.com/ovidweb.cgi?T=JS&PAGE=reference&D=paovfta&NEWS=N&AN=00000487-199011000-00012

Okorodudu, R.I. (2006). Global citizenship: Implications for *Guidance and Counselling Innovations in Developing Nations*. *International Journal for the Advancement of Counselling*, 28(2), 107–120.

Pelling, N. (2004). Counselling psychology: Diversity and commonalities across the Western World. *Counselling Psychology Quarterly*, 17(3), 239–245.

Pelling, N.J. (Ed.) (2021). Journal special issue: International counselling regulation. *Australian Counselling Research Journal*, 15(Winter), 1–44. Retrieved from www.acrjournal.com.au/resources/assets/journals/Volume-15-SW-Issue-2021/Volume15-SW-Issue-2021-FULL.pdf

Takooshian, Harold, Gielen, Uwe, Plous, Scott, Rich, Grant & Velayo, Richard. (2016). Internationalizing undergraduate psychology education: Trends, techniques, and technologies. *American Psychologist*, 71, 136–147. doi:10.1037/a0039977

References

Pelling, N. (2006). Professional counselling organisations. In N. Pelling, R. Bowers, & P. Armstrong (Eds.), *The practice of counselling* (Chapter 19, pp. 442–454). Sydney: Thomson.

Pelling, N. (2009). Professional organisations and resources in counselling and psychology. In N. Pelling, J. Barletta, & P. Armstrong (Eds.), *The practice of clinical supervision* (Chapter 3, pp. 45–55). Samford Valley, QLD: Australian Academic Press.

Pelling, N. (2017). International Counselling and Psychology Professional Organisations and Resources. In N. Pelling, & P. Armstrong (Eds.), *The practice of counselling and clinical supervision* (Chapter 4, pp. 71–84). Samford Valley, QLD: Australian Academic Press.

26 Counselling Regulation, Education, Supervision, and Representation in Canada

Nicola Gazzola and Kate Gignac

Clinical supervision: An applied activity and research focus

Canada is a geographically large country that includes ten provinces and three territories. In Canada mental health is regulated at the provincial level. There are currently five Canadian provinces that have regulation for the practice of counselling while the other five provinces and three territories are at varying levels of regulation. There are regulatory bodies at the provincial level with numerous professional associations at both the provincial and national levels. This article outlines the nature of counselling and psychotherapy in Canada, its development and regulation across various provinces, as well as related training opportunities leading to recognition of various professional counsellor titles. In addition to the practice of counselling and psychotherapy, we will also discuss clinical supervision and counsellor education within the Canadian context.

It would not be surprising that at some point during their life a person may have been referred to, or met with, a counsellor. This may have been within an educational institution, a business or employment setting, through community mental health services, or having some removed awareness of this member of the helping profession. The cautious scoping of the counsellor's office in the high-school hallway, a life altering call to a helpline, sharing the career reigns while traversing a job loss, seeking an anchor during tumultuous teen angst, or thirsting for a compassionate ear amid personal troubles were perhaps moments when we stepped onto the counsellor's pathway, so they could walk alongside us and offer support and, perhaps, some solutions.

Counselling involves the use of a skilful, ethical, and meaningful therapeutic relationship to bring about emotional growth, self-acceptance, and life enhancing awareness of personal resources that foster resilience. The counsellor is set upon the task of helping people work through developmental challenges, come to terms with life's problems, find ways to enrich important relationships, build strong coping abilities to withstand crisis, open the path to insight and self-knowledge, it would not be surprising that at some point during their life a person may have been referred to, or me with, a counsellor. disentangle emotions that fuel inner conflict. Among the many descriptions encapsulating what counsellors do, the current rendering by the Canadian Counselling and Psychotherapy Association succinctly captures its breadth and scope:

> Counselling is a relational process based upon the ethical use of specific professional competencies to facilitate human change. Counselling addresses wellness, relationships, personal growth, career development, mental health, and psychological illness or

DOI: 10.4324/9781003490067-33

distress. The counselling process is characterised by the application of recognised cognitive, affective, expressive, somatic, spiritual, developmental, behavioural, learning, and systemic principles.

www.ccpa-accp.ca/profession-and-regulation/

In Canada, and elsewhere the terms counselling and psychotherapy have traditionally been transposable as both share certain core activities (BACP, 2016; Martin, Turcotte, Matte, & Shepard, 2013). Some uphold a distinction between the two terms and the lines of difference are usually demarcated by training, professional focus, or practice setting. It is not uncommon for counselling professionals in Canada to use a number of titles such as: counselling therapist, psychotherapist, mental health therapist, clinical counsellor, career counsellor, vocational guidance counsellor, marriage and family therapist, conseiller/conseillere d'orientation, orienteur, orienteur professionnel, and psychoeducateur (www.ccpa-accp.ca/profession-and-regulation/). This plethora of title use has caused the collective counsellor identity to be viewed as elusive and unsettled while individual expressions of 'counsellorness' are a strong, daily portrayal for many (Gazzola et al., 2010; Gignac & Gazzola, 2016, p. 312). Having a clear professional identity provides those accessing mental health services with a clear understanding of the valuable role, skill set, and approach to psychological wellbeing counsellors offer.

For counsellors in Canada and other countries, knowledge and practice edges often adjoin those of other allied professions such as social work, psychiatry, and clinical psychology, making it challenging to highlight the uniqueness of these helpers. A similar overlapping of edges that warrants mention within the Canadian context occurs between counselling psychology and counselling but apparent distinction rests upon academic origins (Sinacore & Ginsberg, 2015). Counsellor education is considered the home of counsellors, while counselling psychology claims roots in psychology with practitioners licensing typically as psychologists. The lines around the counsellor identity are not definitive and as a fairly new profession this will be an evolving process going forward both provincially and nationally as the social, economic, political, and global contexts unfold (Gazzola et al., 2010).

The professional identity of counsellors in Canada has been depicted as a unique amalgam of geopolitical representation, cultural heritage, and pluralistic aspirations that continue to shape the collective persona (Gazzola, 2016). Characteristics identified through a survey of Canadian counsellors by Gazzola and Smith (2007) revealed strong altruistic values, a commitment to personal excellence, the pursuit of success, and perpetual growth as key features of their professional identity portrait. Examining how counselling professionals negotiate the identity work process within the Canadian context as regulatory frameworks unfold, Gignac and Gazzola (2016, 2018) found this milieu brought forth a strong sense of agency, craftsmanship in undertaking the identity lifelong project, protean efforts during periods of uncertainty, and a desire to uphold the integrity of their distinctiveness. Counsellor identity in Canada and within each province will certainly continue to evolve against the backdrop of unfolding regulatory initiatives.

The ability of counselling professionals to articulate who they are, their important contribution, the values they uphold, and how they are distinct is not unique to the Canadian context. Elusive and uneven recognition, subordination of the profession at times (McLaughlin & Boettcher, 2009) causing worrisome diminished relevance amid allied professions (Manthei, 1995), and exacting tireless efforts to uphold core humanistic values (Hansen, 2003), are professional identity challenges confronting counsellors around the globe. Our goal in this chapter is to articulate how counsellors are represented and become qualified professionals ready to serve the needs of clients across Canada.

Counselling regulation in Canada

In Canada, the licensing, credentialing, and registration of counsellors are undertaken by provincial regulatory bodies (www.ccpa-accp.ca/certification/). Although several key mental health professions like social work, psychology, and psychiatry are subject to statutory regulation within each of the Canadian provinces, the counselling profession has not yet achieved the same breadth of implementation. At this time, statutory regulation systems are in place in only five of these provinces or territories (see Table 26.1). Counsellors outside of these provinces undertake voluntary registration with the Canadian Counselling and Psychotherapy Association (CCPA), which offers qualifying members the Canadian Certified Counsellor (CCC) designation.

The province of Nova Scotia has established title protection through the Counselling Therapist Act (2011) which restricts the use of Registered Counselling Therapist (RCT) and all derivatives or abbreviations of this (www.ccpa-accp.ca/certification/). The Nova Scotia College of Counselling Therapists (NSCCT) regulates the practice of counselling therapy and has established definitions, professional conduct codes, and oversees matters of professional misconduct or incapacity (Nova Scotia College of Counselling Therapists, 2011).

In New Brunswick, a similar approach to regulation occurred with the implementation of title protection which permits the use of Licensed Counselling Therapist by registered members. The regulatory authority overseeing this is the College of Counselling Therapists of New Brunswick (CCTNB), which received proclamation in 2017 and is working through the initial phase of this process (Bill 30, The Mental Health Services Protection Act). The most recent province to regulate counselling is Alberta. The Mental Health Services Protection Act received Royal Assent in December 2018 via Bill 30. The Alberta College of Counselling Therapy (ACCT), part of Alberta's Health Professions Act, was formed to provide oversight, accountability, and public protection (FACT-Alberta, 2019).

With full statutory regulation (i.e., title and scope of practice) of counselling in the province of Quebec (i.e., Guidance Counsellor and Vocational Counsellor) counselling professionals are clearly identified and protected. Holding the longest and most comprehensive regulation for the profession, L'Ordre des Conseillers et Conseillieres d'Orientation du Québec (OCCOQ) is the college responsible for safeguarding professional conduct and protection of the public. Only members of the OCCOQ are permitted to use the titles: guidance counsellor, vocational guidance counsellor, conseiller d'orientation, and

Table 26.1 Regulatory status of counselling in Canada

Counselling Regulation across Canada		
Regulated	Regulation Activities Underway	Regulation Discussion Pending
Nova Scotia	Newfoundland & Labrador	Yukon
New Brunswick	Prince Edward Island	Nunavut
Quebec	Manitoba	Northwest Territories
Ontario	Saskatchewan	
Alberta	British Columbia	

conseillere d'orientation (Government of Quebec, 2013). All professions in Quebec are governed by the Office of Professions du Québec and within their code, each is distinguished by their scope of practice while benefits are recognised in having shared reserved activities across the mental health field (Martin, Turcotte, Matte, & Shepard, 2013).

In Quebec and Ontario there is statutory regulation for psychotherapy with title protection and practice restrictions. Considered a distinct practice from counselling and spiritual counselling, those wishing to practice psychotherapy in either of these provinces are required to join a college or obtain permits through a provincial order. In Ontario this is the purview of the College of Registered Psychotherapists of Ontario (CRPO), while in Quebec the issue of permits falls under the remit of the Ordre des psychologies du Québec (OPQ). Counsellors in Ontario, as of December 2017 are encouraged to verify with the CRPO whether activities they perform fall within the Controlled Act of Psychotherapy and therefore require registration with the regulatory college now that full proclamation has transpired (CRPO, 2017a).

In the five other provinces there are ongoing discussions and initiatives to put regulatory mechanisms in place with some further along on this route. The Prince Edward Island Counselling Association (PEICA) applied in 2017 to the government for title protection of Registered Counselling Therapist (RCT) under the RHPA (Regulated Health Professions Act) and will be seeking regulation in the near future. The Federation of Associations for Counselling Therapists in British Columbia (FACT-BC) continues to work towards establishing regulation of the profession (www.ccpa-accp.ca/profession-and-regulation/). In the three territories, these discussions have not seen a similar level of commitment or progress.

Counselling representation in Canada

Canada is the largest North American country, spanning roughly ten million square kilometres (Citizenship and Immigration Canada, 2012). Although Canada is a large territory, second only to Russia in geographical size, its population is relatively modest. Canada is a country that is just shy of 38 million people (Statistics Canada, 2020). Canada is part of the Commonwealth and a parliamentary democracy. The responsibility for lawmaking in Canada is shared among one federal, ten provincial and three territorial governments (House of Commons, 2000). In Canada, mental health is regulated at the provincial level.

The Canadian Counselling and Psychotherapy Association (CCPA), which was formed in 1965, is the oldest national association for professionally trained counsellors and now has close to 7,000 members. Its mandate is to provide leadership and promote the counselling profession in Canada. Individuals are eligible to become a Canadian Certified Counsellor (CCC) if they hold a university degree at the graduate or doctoral level in counselling or a related field that meets the professional standards and ethics of the CCPA. A qualified professional must also become a member of the CCPA before applying for certification.

Within the national association there are sixteen chapters that focus on different areas of specialisation or timely issues related to the profession (e.g., counsellor educators and supervisors chapter, creative arts, social justice, spirituality, school counsellors, Indigenous circle, and private practice). The CCPA also facilitates certification of counsellors and supervisors, offers live and online professional development courses or webinars, offers accreditation of counselling programmes, and hosts an annual national conference.

Another nationally recognised, self-regulated association for counsellors is the Canadian Professional Counsellors Association (CPCA), which was founded in 1990. Individuals must meet competency-based criteria for membership as a Registered Professional Counsellor (RPC) or as Master Practitioners in Clinical Counselling (MPCC). The CPCA approves several education providers and is dedicated to promoting the professionalism of counsellors.

Pathways to becoming a counsellor in Canada

A great place to begin on the counsellor pathway is with a bachelor's degree as it prepares individuals for entry to a variety of counselling career choices. Whether coming to the counselling profession after a previous career or directly from an undergraduate programme like psychology, education, or social work the pursuit of graduate level studies is typically required for professional practice. Options for specialised areas of counselling work such as school counselling, private practice, or family and couples work may be part of graduate study programmes or obtained through ongoing professional development.

Counselling education in Canada

Those interested in becoming counsellors in Canada must hold an undergraduate degree in education, psychology, or an equivalent to pursue graduate level studies. A master level degree in counselling, psychology, or social work is the minimum educational requirement for certification, registration, and licensing in most provinces in Canada (www.ccpa-accp.ca/profession-and-regulation/). School counsellors are also required to be qualified teachers in most jurisdictions. There is great variability in the standards and delivery of counsellor education in Canada precisely due to academic training being a provincial responsibility (Gazzola, 2015).

Graduate studies in counselling are traditionally situated within education faculties of universities in Canada rather than in psychology departments despite their shared historical roots (Young & Nichol, 2007). They are either referred to as counselling psychology or educational counselling programmes and vary from 14 months to two years in duration. There are several universities across Canada that offer graduate level studies for those pursuing a general counselling degree or with a specialised focus (e.g., art therapy, marriage and family, psychotherapy, and spirituality) as outlined on the Canadian Counselling and Psychotherapy Association website (www.ccpa-accp.ca/certification/) (see Table 26.2). Four of these universities have programme accreditation from the Canadian Counselling and Psychotherapy Association (CCPA) while several other academic institutions hold accreditation with the Canadian Psychological Association (CPA) at the graduate and doctoral level for their counselling psychology programmes (Gazzola, 2016).

Masters-level programmes in counselling are generally offered as a Master of Counselling/Counselling Psychology (M.A. or M.C.) with a thesis requirement or the Master of Education (M.Ed.) which is a terminal degree for professional practice. For those entering a master's in counselling psychology programme, a four-year B.A. in psychology (honours) is necessary and the completion of pre-requisite courses in psychology (abnormal, developmental, personality), statistics, research design, and basic counselling skills. A master's in educational counselling programme often does not require an honours B.A. in psychology but may call for similar pre-requisite courses upon entry (Government of Canada, 2018). Students can also complete their graduate studies in counselling

Table 26.2 Graduate-level academic and professional counsellor training programmes across Canada

Province	University
Alberta	Athabasca University; City University; St. Stephen's College; University of Alberta; University of Calgary; University of Lethbridge
British Columbia	Adler School of Professional Psychology; City University; Gonzaga University; Simon Fraser University; University of British Columbia; Trinity Western University; University of Northern British Columbia; University of Victoria
Manitoba	Brandon University; Université de Sainte-Boniface; University of Manitoba; University of Winnipeg; Providence Theological Seminary
New Brunswick	Université de Moncton; University of New Brunswick; Yorkville University
Newfoundland	Memorial University of Newfoundland
Nova Scotia	Acadia University
Ontario	Saint Paul University; University of Western Ontario; University of Guelph; University of Ottawa; University of Toronto; Wilfred Laurier University; Canada Christian College & School of Graduate Theological Studies; Tyndale Seminary
Quebec	Concordia University; McGill University; Université de Laval; Université de Montreal; Université de Quebec a Montreal; Université de Quebec a Rimouski; Université de Québec a Trois-Rivieres; Université de Sherbrooke; Université Québec en Abitibi-Temiscamingue; Université du Québec en Outaouais
Saskatchewan	Briercrest College and Seminary; University of Regina

*Source: Canadian Counselling and Psychotherapy Association (2018b)

through two online programmes that combine online coursework with a practicum-based experience. The first is Yorkville University, which offers a Counselling Psychology (M.A.) programme and the second option is the Counselling (M.C.) at Athabasca University.

The Canadian Counselling and Psychotherapy Association (CCPA) has worked steadfastly to set standards and procedures for accreditation of counselling programmes in Canada. The Council on Accreditation of Counsellor Education Programs (CACEP) is the body responsible for overseeing the accreditation process, which was established in 1987 to ensure quality, consistent training. Counsellor education programmes are required to achieve established standards of CACEP within their institutional setting, ensure certain programme content and objectives are met, provide quality practicum experiences, adhere to student selection and advising protocols, and attend to faculty qualifications, instructional support, and self-evaluation in master's level programmes (Robertson & Borgen, 2016). There are currently four universities in Canada that hold CACEP accreditation for their counselling programmes (see Table 26.3).

Counselling supervision in Canada

Clinical supervision is an important requirement for counsellors in Canada and one which has historically been conducted by experienced clinicians with varying degrees of formal training (Johnson & Stewart, 2000). This apprenticeship approach has increasingly come under review (Peake, Nussbaum, & Tindell, 2002; Watkins, 2012) and the move toward solidifying more formal, compulsory training for supervisors has gained international momentum (Milne & James, 2002; Scott, Ingram, Vitanza, & Smith, 2000). A similar

Table 26.3 CACEP-accredited Master's-level counselling programmes in Canada

University and Year of Accreditation

University of British Columbia
- M.A. Counselling Psychology (2006)
- M.Ed. Counselling Psychology (2006)

Acadia University
- M.Ed. in Counselling (2009)

Trinity Western University
- M.A. Counselling Psychology (2012)

University of Victoria
- M.A. Counselling Psychology, Thesis Route (2017)
- M.A. Counselling Psychology, Project Based (2017)

shift toward mandatory training through accredited counselling programmes or at the behest of regulatory colleges overseeing the mental health professions has begun to take shape in Canada (Hunsley & Barker, 2011).

Clinical supervision is provided to counsellors-in-training as part of their degree completion and also to supervisors-in-training, often at the doctoral level while they establish supervision competency. These are the primary levels of competency formation being addressed across the mental health field within accredited programmes and by professional associations (e.g., Canadian Psychological Association, Canadian Counselling, and Psychotherapy Association). Both the provision of clinical oversight and training of supervisors within academic settings remains uneven, under evaluated, and emergent as core requirements across provincial jurisdictions are independently established in the Canadian context (Hadjistavropoulos, Kehler, & Hajistavropoulos, 2010).

This desire to articulate the academic training requirements during degree capture and forward into perpetuity through continuing education for clinicians has been recently evidenced in the province of Quebec. Clinicians providing counselling and psychotherapy services in Quebec following passage of Bill 21 by the National Assembly of Quebec (2009) will now be required to have completed six hours of supervision training to demonstrate competency if not obtained during postdoctoral training and ongoing mandatory continuing education. This move has set precedent for supervision to become a specialty area beyond counselling and psychotherapy practice (Gonsalvez & Milne, 2010), which in time may move Canada closer to international supervision standards. In particular, the requirement for supervision of supervision by other professional associations like the British Association for Counselling & Psychotherapy, which has shown merit in approaching protection of the public and perhaps elevating professional credibility (Wheeler & King, 2000).

This shift in the view of clinical supervision occurring well beyond the formal training periods of clinicians requires a solid grounding in research evidence to delineate competencies and build capacity to support this endeavour (DeAngelis, 2014). Preliminary steps toward this longer-term objective are evidenced by a recent move in the province of Ontario to make formal training of supervisor's mandatory. According to the College of Registered Psychotherapists of Ontario (2017b) a supervisor must possess five or more years of experience in the practice of psychotherapy and demonstrate competence as well as completing 30 hours of directed learning in clinical supervision (i.e., course work, supervised practice as a supervisor, individual/ peer/group learning, or independent study). Not only are provincial regulatory bodies like the CRPO starting to establish guidelines to mandate supervisory training in lieu of lifelong requisites, there is another broader movement underway for counselling supervision in Canada.

At the national level the Canadian Counselling and Psychotherapy Association (CCPA) has established the Canadian Certified Counsellor-Supervisor (CCC-S) designation to credential professional supervision competency. The requirements for obtaining the CCC-S designation include:

- CCC Designation – Canadian Certified Counsellor in good standing with CCPA
- Attestation – ethical and professional conduct, commitment to CCPA Code of Ethics and Standards of Practice, possession of professional liability insurance, annual documentation of continuing education and clinical supervision requirements
- Clinical Experience – minimum of 5 years post-graduate degree clinical experience within the last 10 years [800 hours/year]
- Employment History and Supervision Training – providing documentation summaries
- Supervision Experience – evidence of provision of 20 hours minimum clinical supervision over last two years or equivalent supervisory designation from another recognised professional association
- Supervision Education – confirmation of graduate-level training in supervision
- Annual Renewal – CE credits and supervision practice hours

With the aim of promoting the professional credibility of clinical supervisors, the CCPA is working to establish a recognised national credential of professional supervision and build capacity for quality professional development opportunities both online and at national conferences. Graduate-level courses in clinical supervision are offered at the introductory, intermediate, and advanced levels to support annual renewal requirements, which include twelve hours of documented supervision work and four continuing education credits in the area of clinical supervision. The current movement toward establishing supervisory competencies and training requirements will undoubtedly influence not only professional development but also the unfolding identity of counsellors in Canada (Gazzola & De Stefano, 2016).

Concluding statement

In Canada, as in other countries around the globe, there is considerable overlap between the work of counsellors and that of other allied mental health professionals. Within counselling, there are numerous occupational titles that are used (e.g., guidance counsellor, counselling therapist, mental health counsellor, etc.). Counselling and psychotherapy are becoming increasingly regulated in Canada, a process that falls under the jurisdiction of provincial governments. The province of Quebec has the most comprehensive statutory regulation of counselling (i.e., guidance counsellor/vocational guidance counsellor) with several other provinces in various stages of statutory regulation underway. Both Quebec and Ontario currently regulate 'psychotherapy', which is considered distinct to counselling in those provinces.

One of the cornerstones to counselling practice is clinical supervision. In the past supervision mainly occurred within the educational process, specifically during the master's level counselling practica that most counselling programmes require. Further, the typical supervisor has traditionally been a seasoned practitioner whose qualifications as a supervisor have been exclusively years of practice as a counsellor. This has been gradually shifting and the requirements for becoming a supervisor now include some formal training in clinical supervision in addition to a minimum number of years in the field practicing as a counsellor. In general, counselling, and to some degree supervision, is increasingly becoming regulated in Canada. Because mental health falls under the jurisdiction of the provinces, counselling regulation currently exists at varying levels across Canada and the regulatory process is a dynamic one.

Final Note: Please address correspondence regarding this chapter to Nick Gazzola, Professor, Counselling Psychology, Faculty of Education, University of Ottawa, Ottawa, Ontario, K1N 6N5, Canada. Email: gazzola@uottawa.ca

References

British Association for Counselling & Psychotherapy (BACP). (2016). Retrieved 10 March 2016, from www.bacp.co.uk/crs/ Training/whatiscounselling.php

Citizenship and Immigration Canada. (2012). Discover Canada: The rights and responsibilities of citizenship. Retrieved from www.cic.gc.ca/english/pdf/pub/discover.pdf

College of Counselling Therapists of New Brunswick (CCTNB). (2018). Constitution. Retrieved from www.ccpa-accp.ca/ constitution-bylaws/

College of Registered Psychotherapists of Ontario (CRPO). (2017a). Legislation. Retrieved from www.crpo.ca/ legislation-by-laws/

College of Registered Psychotherapists of Ontario (CRPO). (2017b). Supervision. Retrieved from www.crpo.ca/ supervision/

DeAngelis, T. (2014). Fostering successful clinical supervision. *APA Monitor*, 45(8), 42–45.

FACT-Alberta. (2019). Update on the regulation of counselling therapists, addictions counsellors, and child and youth care counsellors in Alberta. Retrieved from www.fact-alberta.org/files/ Regulation%20Update%20Document_Final.pdf

Gazzola, N. (2015). Professional identity of counselling and the regulation of the profession in Canada. In L. Martin, B. Shepard, & R. Lehr (Eds.), *Canadian counselling and psychotherapy experience: Ethics-based issues and cases* (pp. 117–144). Ottawa: Canadian Counselling and Psychotherapy Association.

Gazzola, N. (2016). Is there a unique professional identity of counselling in Canada? In N. Gazzola, M. Buchanan, S. Nuttgens, & O. Sutherland (Eds.), *Canadian handbook of counselling and psychotherapy* (pp. 1–12). Ottawa, ON: Canadian Counselling and Psychotherapy Association.

Gazzola, N., & De Stefano, J. (2016). Training and supervision of clinical supervisors. In B. Shepard, L. Martin, & B. Robinson (Eds.), *Handbook of counselling supervision* (pp. 99–118). Ottawa, ON: Canadian Counselling and Psychotherapy Association.

Gazzola, N., & Smith, J. (2007). Who do we think we are? A survey of counsellors in Canada. *International Journal for the Advancement of Counselling*, 29, 97–110. doi:10.1007/ s10447- 007-9032-y

Gazzola, N., Smith, J.D., King-Andrews, H.L., & Kearney, M.K. (2010). Professional characteristics of Canadian counsellors: Results of a national survey. *Canadian Journal of Counselling*, 44(2), 83–99.

Gignac, K., & Gazzola, N. (2016). Negotiating professional identity construction during regulatory change: Utilizing a virtual focus group to understand the outlook of Canadian counsellors. *International Journal for the Advancement of Counselling*, 38(4), 298–318. doi:10.1007/ s10447-016-9273-8

Gignac, K., & Gazzola, N. (2018). Embracing counsellor professional identity work: Experiential accounts of transformation and transition. *Canadian Journal of Counselling and Psychotherapy*, 52(3), 205–228.

Gonsalvez, C.J., & Milne, D. (2010). Clinical supervisor training in Australia: A review of current problems and possible solutions. *Australian Psychologist*, 45, 233–242. doi:10.1080/00050067.2010.512612

Government of Canada. (2018). Educational counsellors. Retrieved from http://noc.esdc.gc.ca/English/noc/ProfileQuickSearch. aspx?val=4&val1=4033&ver=16&val65=counsellor

Hadjistavropoulos, H., Kehler, M., & Hadjistavropoulos, T. (2010). Training graduate students to be clinical supervisors: A survey of Canadian professional psychology programmes. *Canadian Psychology*, 51(3), 206–212. doi:10.1037/a0020197

Hansen, J. (2003). Including diagnostic training in counseling curricula: Implications for professional identity development. *Counselor Education and Supervision*, 43, 96–107.

House of Commons. (2000). Parliamentary institutions. In R. Marleau and C. Montpetit (Eds.), *House of Commons procedure and practice*. Retrieved from www.parl.gc.ca/marleaumontpetit/DocumentViewer.aspx?Sec=Ch01&Seq=2&Language=E

Hunsley, J., & Barker, K.K. (2011). Training for competency in professional psychology: A Canadian perspective. *Australian Psychologist*, 46, 142–145. doi:10.1111/j.1742-9544.2011.00027.x

Johnson, E.A., & Stewart, D.W. (2000). Clinical supervision in Canadian academic and service settings: The importance of education, training, and workplace support for supervisor development. *Canadian Psychology/Psychologie Canadienne*, 41(2), 124–130. doi:10.1037/h0086862

Manthei, R. (1995). Should we be concerned about this? Or, have you ever wondered about...? *New Zealand Association of Counsellors Newsletter*, 16, 33–36.

Martin, L., Turcotte, M., Matte, L., & Shepard, B. (2013). The counselling and psychotherapy profession in Canada: Regulatory processes and current status. *British Journal of Guidance & Counselling*, 41, 46–57. doi:10.1080/03069885.2012.750271

McLaughlin, J.E., & Boettcher, K. (2009). Counselor identity: Conformity or distinction? *Journal of Humanistic Counseling Education and Development*, 48, 132–143. doi:10.1002/j.2161-1939.2009.tb00074.x

Milne, D.L., & James, I.A. (2002). The observed impact of training on competence in clinical supervision. *British Journal of Clinical Psychology*, 41(1), 55–72. doi:10.1348/014466502163796

Peake, T., Nussbaum, B., & Tindell, S. (2002). Clinical and counseling supervision references: Trends and needs. *Psychotherapy: Theory, Research, Practice, Training*, 39(1), 114–125. doi:10.1037/0033-3204.39.1.114

Robertson, S.E., & Borgen, W.A. (2016). CCPA accreditation of counsellor education programs in Canada: An historical perspective. *Canadian Journal of Counselling and Psychotherapy*, 50(3), 259–277.

Scott, K.J., Ingram, K.M., Vitanza, S.A., & Smith, N.G. (2000). Training in supervision: A survey of current practices. *The Counseling Psychologist*, 28, 403–422. doi:10.1177/0011000000283007

Sinacore, A.L., & Ginsberg, F. (Eds.) (2015). *Canadian counselling and counselling psychology in the 21st century*. Montreal, QC: McGill-Queen's University Press.

Statistics Canada. (2020). Table 17-10-0009-01 Population estimates, quarterly. doi:10.25318/1710000901-eng

Watkins, C.E. Jr. (2012). Psychotherapy supervision in the new millennium: Competency-based, evidence-based, particularized. *Australian Counselling Journal of Contemporary Psychotherapy*, 42(3), 193–203. doi:10.1007/s10879-011-9202-4

Wheeler, S., & King, D. (2000). Do counselling supervisors want or need to have their supervision supervised? An exploratory study. *British Journal of Guidance and Counselling*, 28, 279–290.

Young, R.A., & Nichol, J.J. (2007). Counselling psychology in Canada: Advancing psychology for all. *Applied Psychology: An International Review*, 56, 20–32. doi:10.1111/j.1464- 0597.2007.00273

27 Strategic Approaches to Managing The Development of the Counselling Profession in Hong Kong

Pui Chi Tse

Clinical supervision: An applied activity and research focus

The counselling profession in Hong Kong has developed for nearly half a century, but it is still like a young child. The lack of government and public recognition has created a lot of difficulties. The demand for counselling is continuously increasing while its recognition as a unique profession remains low due to its generic nature and the cultural context. This chapter discusses the strategic approaches appropriate for the Hong Kong Chinese culture in the development of the counselling profession. I begin with a historical review of Hong Kong's counselling development as the ground for further examination. The related concepts in management, such as strategic thinking and planning, values, power, and training, are put forth as stimulation for thoughts and action plans for counselling leaders. Managing the strategic plans and options for successful development demands clearer attention and strategic commitments from the leaders and professionals.

Managing counselling professionalization

Professional status and identity are critical developmental issues for many professionals. Deliberately long discussions on professional identity within the counselling profession have taken place in the United States since the 1980s (Fitzgerald & Osipow, 1986; Watkins, 1983; Watkins, Lopez, Campbell, & Himmell, 1986). Promotion of a core identity as a counsellor has been the prominent challenge for decades. Professionalization is an evolutionary process for occupational groups to improve their social professional status (Pavalko, 1971) for the protection and security of professional members (Goode, 1960). The word 'profession' carries esteemed and privileged connotations associated with social and occupational status (Pavalko, 1971). Professional issues, including training and education, accreditation and licensing, professional membership, and identity are all crucial for the advancement (Romano, 1992; Simpson, 1993).

The training of counselling professionals is a marvellously complex process. It possesses a pedagogical nature which provides counsellors platforms and/or shelters to strengthen their competitiveness and competencies by continuous refreshment of their skills and knowledge through formal training. Counselling professional development in Hong Kong is even more sophisticated because of the constraints from Eastern culture on a Western health discipline and other specific stumbling blocks in the past years.

Before moving on to the discussion of the applicability of strategic management of development in this field, begin the discussion with the historical development of counselling education in Hong Kong for a contextual understanding. The pace of historical

DOI: 10.4324/9781003490067-34

change constitutes the unique rhythm of professional development. I then use some of the essential components of the strategic approach in counselling education to assist in the discussion of counselling education management here in Hong Kong.

Contextual understanding of counselling professional development in Hong Kong

History, culture, and changes

Hong Kong was a British colony for almost 150 years. 'As many historians acknowledge, Hong Kong was not a typical colony' (Sweeting, 2007, p. 91). Hong Kong, in terms of its roots, has a deep, long-standing, and well-established Chinese culture. In the early days, Hong Kong was mainly a Chinese migrant society, with most of its population coming from the South China region. The Chinese have their own means of sustaining and enhancing mental health. There is no concept of counselling in Chinese culture. At first, counselling was a totally imported product. Foreigners played a dominant role in the procurement of early counselling services. The development of counselling in Hong Kong currently reaches back only 40–50 years.

Although the history of counselling in Hong Kong is short, the emerging profession of counselling and psychotherapy was unique in this community. In order to understand the development of counselling education in Hong Kong, a look at the historical and socio-political context is needed.

The Chinese still embrace collectivism, while the West clings to individualism, although the effects of globalisation have brought forth the erosion of boundaries. The basic value orientation of the two cultures is different. Western individualistic worldviews and the collectivistic Eastern worldviews clash with each other and this is the foundation for the difficulty in counselling education in Hong Kong. Individualism stresses individual initiatives, a greater focus on the self, and emotional independence (Hofstede, 1980). It also emphasises self-reliance and freedom of choice, rights and duties, and personal growth. In contrast, collectivism emphasizes group goals over personal goals, stresses conformity and in-group harmony, and defines the self in relation to the group (Triandis, 1995). There is no emphasis on personal growth, but only group fame. It is difficult for the individual to survive in isolation. Social pressure, such as family and peer groups, will attack a person when he or she strives for his or her own growth.

Besides, seeking help may reveal one's inadequacy and dependency (Nadler, 1990). There is a Chinese adage: 'Problems within the family should not be discussed outside the family.' It hurts the 'Mianzi' if one's psychological problems are revealed to others. Social stigma attached to mental health service needs to be taken into consideration in Chinese culture. 'Mianzi' literally means face in the Chinese language. Symbolically, having mianzi is the representation of one's access to power and privileges. Losing mianzi undermines one's power and social network. 'Mianzi' serves the function of perceived social position and prestige within one's social network (Hwang, 1987). To talk to a stranger, a so-called counsellor, about one's own personal issues can be very threatening to a Chinese person. To gain mianzi is a common important goal among Chinese people. This is one of the major causes of the difficulties in counselling development in Chinese assimilated Hong Kong culture. If a culture does not openly accept counselling, there will be less demand in the market and counselling education thus has a poor ground to grow from.

Furthermore, Chinese people often downplay the severity of mental illness and choose to focus on the situations that generate the condition rather than the problem itself (Kleinman & Lin, 1981). It takes a very long time to cultivate the concepts of counselling among Chinese people. Culturally speaking, the efficacy of counselling and psychotherapy needed a long process of integration with Chinese traditions for local people to accept it. These cultural barriers have had an adverse effect on counselling development in the Chinese community. However, the trend of globalisation could also facilitate the process of connection of this profession in the Hong Kong Chinese culture.

Huy and Mintzberg (2003) stated that there are three types of change: dramatic, systematic, and organic. Dramatic change descends from the top management, systematic change is generated laterally, and organic change emerges from the grass roots. These three forces interact dynamically. 'Change has no meaning unless it is juxtaposed against continuity' (Huy & Mintzberg, 2003, p. 79). Changes sometimes facilitate but sometimes hinder its development. The rise of globalisation, aside from the expansion of trade and investment across borders, has opened the door to cultural interchange.

Globalisation is not the product of a single action, like switching on a light or starting a car engine. It is a historical process that has undoubtedly sped up enormously in the last ten years, but it is a permanent, constant transformation (Sadler, 1993, p. 29). The influx of Western knowledge as well as Western social movements has sped up the opportunity to provide counselling services for local needs.

Struggles, difficulties, and challenges

The counselling movement began as an attempt to meet society's developmental needs to resolve the widespread social discontent originating from two social uprisings and disturbances, which were spawned by the Cultural Revolution in China in 1966 and 1967 (Leung, 1999; Yu et al., 2010). These changes precipitated a series of social and political reforms instigated by the British government. The Hong Kong Government started to rely on voluntary organisations to provide related services for the community and crisis intervention. 'Links between politics and education provide the bases for many of the mysteries of this period' (Sweeting, 2007, p. 13). The disturbances in the 1960s paved the way for expansion of social services to meet the social needs. According to Leung (1988), the first informal counselling service in Hong Kong was offered in 1967 at the Yang Memorial Social Service Center. In 1969 the Hong Kong Federation of Youth Groups started an experimental counselling programme staffed by an American-trained counsellor in Hong Kong. We can say that organic change emerged from the grass roots in the community, which provided fertile ground for the birth of counselling in Hong Kong. Organic change, which often proceeds as a challenge to authority, involves messy processes and tends to arise from the ranks without being formally managed (Huy & Mintzberg, 2003). However, Leung (1988) stated that at that time counselling was like an adopted child who came from a very different background trying to fit into a new family in Hong Kong. Counselling faced a lot of challenges at this earliest stage. This child had not been nurtured properly. Publicizing counselling services was major work of the early counsellors in the 1970s (Leung, 1988).

In addition, with regard to the issue of professional identity, the role of counsellor in Hong Kong had no clear demarcation from social workers, clinical psychologists, and psychotherapists. The functions of a counsellor, however, are shared by various types of helping professionals, such as teachers, clinical psychologists, educational psychologists, and social workers (Goodyear, 1984). They also provide counselling services in a variety of settings. Striving for a collective identity is not an exclusive issue for Hong Kong counsellors. The counselling identity confusion acts as a great hindrance to its development as a unique profession.

Counselling education in this early stage was scattered, unsystematic and Westernized. Prior to 1971 there were no formal training programmes on counselling in Hong Kong. The first formal counselling course was offered in 1977 at master's degree level at the Chinese University. The programme was academically oriented rather than focused on professional training (Leung, 1988). The government lacked a proactive strategy to face the changes in society and had not made any effort to assist the professional growth of counselling. Of course, the government's ignorance of the professional identity was one of the major factors. The government only recognized the discipline of social work and registered social workers as part of the social service system. The professional identity of counselling graduates has not been recognized by the social service agencies. They could not find jobs and even when the government or an NGO employed them, they would be allocated to the social work system and positioned as lower than social workers. This discriminatory practice indeed affected the morale and professional esteem of counsellors.

In Hong Kong, education policy is usually subsequently developed from relevant economic developments, and the policymakers' foresights are often questioned (Sweeting, 2007). Long-term planning in the field of education is devalued, and counselling education is no exception. Counselling services are time-and money-consuming. Counsellors spend hours and hours listening and serving individuals, which is not economical use of resources in such a pragmatic society like Hong Kong. The provision of counselling services is regarded as very expensive. The government therefore neglected counselling education. All these struggles and difficulties have been significant contributors to the slow development of the counselling profession in Hong Kong.

Threats, dilemmas, and opportunities

Change is a natural process in society. Crises, blows, and distress are general features of the changing world and symbolise hardship and distress. Crises and threats can sometimes be viewed in functional terms as facilitators (Rosenthal et al., 2001).

Since its return to China, Hong Kong has undergone more changes, and the confusion over the professional identity of counselling has seen no major improvement under the government's social service hierarchy. A few critical policy changes have brought benefits as well as threats to counselling development since 1997.

Social services encountered a great change when entering into the year 2000. The reform consisted of three parts: a Service Performance Monitoring System (SPMS), the Lump Sum Grant subvention policy (LSGS), and opening up service contracts to business enterprises for competitive bidding alongside non-profit organisations (NPOs) (Lee, 2005). The essential features of the LSGS for subsidising social welfare, which became effective on 1 April 2000, are a flexible funding model based on a one-line vote, in which NPOs have the flexibility to decide their staffing structures, salary levels, and other items of expenditure. NPOs can carry over unused funds to the next financial year (Social Welfare Department, 2000). Ninety percent of the social services in Hong Kong are offered by NPOs that are largely subsidized by the government. About 346 NPOs receive 70 per cent of their major funding from the government, with the total public funding amounting to 2.4 per cent of the total public expenditure, or 0.5 per cent of GDP (Lee, 2005). These government-subsidised NPOs employ many staff, including trained professionals, welfare workers, and childcare workers. The launching of this governmental subvention policy has brought a dramatic change to social service agencies, and among social service agents there are voices both for and against their resource management. This alternative structural implementation of resources certainly brought chances and opportunities for counsellors. It created a lot of worries for social work training staff but rekindled hope for counselling graduates. The flexible funding model allows more freedom of choice in staffing. Counsellors thus have more chances to be employed and receive fair pay according to their competence and effort.

Prior to 2004, all counselling training programmes held by universities were master's degree level. Hong Kong Shue Yan University is the only university to offer the Honours Diploma in Counselling and Guidance, since 1977. In 2004, Hong Kong Shue Yan University was successfully accredited the proficiency to provide undergraduate training in counselling psychology in Hong Kong. It was a great stride forward in the history of counselling education in Hong Kong.

Although this big leap is an indicator of the better acceptance and recognition of the need for counselling training in the community as well as the community urge for counsellors, Yu and his colleagues conducted a survey on the public's understanding of counselling in Hong Kong in 2010 which revealed that the majority of respondents had no knowledge of counselling and no interest in this service. The counselling profession has undergone slow evolvement in Hong Kong. Their research result

> confirms the tough reality that the counselling profession in Hong Kong is still in an early stage of development and faces a number of challenges. The next step is to use our findings to identify opportunities and devise strategies to remedy some of these issues.
> (Yu et al., 2010, p. 48)

The increasing employment rate as counsellors in schools and agencies as reported by the graduates from the Counselling and Psychology programme is evidence that contributes to the success of accreditation. However, primary school counsellors, who are hired by tender and posts, are often awarded to the lowest bidders (Ngo & Zhao, 2016). The counsellors are critically underpaid with overloaded work. This is a total contradictory phenomenon.

Entering 2018, another sudden blow occurred in the counselling profession. This was of major concern regarding the development of the counselling profession. The Education Bureau of the Hong Kong Special Administrative Region has recently issued a memorandum to primary schools about the implementation of the 'one school social worker for each school' policy (Secretary for Education of the Education Bureau, 2018), leading to the termination of the financial allowance to hire school counsellors. Only social workers are instead employed to handle the counselling cases in school. This policy has not only aroused the attention of many existing school counsellors but also social workers who anticipate a far greater workload than they are currently facing (Ngo & Zhao, 2016). The relevant policies ignore the role and opinions of the counselling industry and are not moving towards optimising the 'comprehensive student guidance service.'

Positively speaking, challenges can either be viewed as burdensome and oppositional but also as opportunities. On the one hand, this policy has caused a great blow to the counselling profession especially for those who are working in schools; on the other hand, this is a chance to attract public attention to the counselling profession. In response to this change, the Asian Professional Counselling and Psychology Association (APCPA) has initiated the gathering of scholars, counsellors, teachers, principals and school counsellors, and the leaders of social services together to hold discussions in an open forum on 'Guardian Counselling, Professionalism, and comprehensive school Counselling System.' This also united counsellors together to hold press conferences and make noise in society, expressing the importance of the role of counselling services. As a result, this movement attracts more social attention. The journey of professional recognition is tough and there is still a long way to go.

Instead of feeling upset and frustrated about the development of the counselling profession, good strategic plans with proactive actions to tackle these challenges have been developed.

Strategic approaches to counselling education management in Hong Kong

Management is a business concept which refers to the process of administration or the people who perform the act of management. It has its primary function of getting things done in a properly effective way. 'Management' was a very bad word for voluntary non-profit organisations (Drucker, 1990). Similar reactions are found in the education field. Management means 'business' to them, but educators and social service providers did not want to treat such a meaningful mission as 'education' or 'social service,' as 'a business'; thus, most of them believed that they did not need 'management.' Actually, the functions of management consist of indispensable aspects such as creating policy, organizing, planning, and regulating resources and human behaviour in the organisation. The economic, social change, and political developments do affect counselling education, creating opportunities or constituting threats. Educational management is a field of study and practice concerned with the operation of educational organisations (Bush, 2003). Bolam (1999, p. 194) defines educational management as 'an executive function for carrying out agreed policy.'

Strategic management is a concept about how to improve profitability and competitiveness in the business field. The original meaning of the word derives from the Greek 'strategia,' which is the ability to employ available resources to win a military conflict (Mitreanu, 2006). Planning, formulation, and implementation of strategies are primary tasks of leaders and administrators. The concept of 'strategic approach' is not new in counselling and psychotherapy fields – we have strategic approaches in treatment and intervention for difficult cases or paradoxical situations.

As is revealed in the history of the counselling development in Hong Kong, the trajectory has encountered a lot of difficulties. Lack of resources has been a cause of the slow development, matching the notion of strategy in management which implies a strong focus on competition or struggles for resources.

'Strategy is a highly complex concept and attempts to define it adequately within the compass of a sentence or two are almost certainly going to miss out some key elements' (Sadler, 1993, p. 3). Hofer and Schendel (1978, p. 4) delineate strategy as 'the basic characteristics of the match and organisation achievers with its environment.' Successful management requires a clear link between aims, strategies and operations (Bush, 2003). To maximise the available community resources and cultivate new resources, strategic management may open up new horizons for counselling educators.

The notion of strategy is a means to a specific end and goal; it implies temporary success and becomes arguably inappropriate when success has to be indefinitely sustained (Mitreanu, 2006). Counselling education is the breeding ground for novices in the profession to continuously grow and serve the community. Besides, they function to create the counselling culture of sustainability. In order to achieve true sustainability, continuing education plays a significant role in the participatory processes, and forms a crucial part of the general strategy (Wong, 2003). But how to enhance the professionalism and sustainability and how to put these into practice and transformation are important topics to be considered. Ultimately, development of professionalism is a long-term strategy which runs contrary to business. However, strategic management is to be operated differently across stages and situations. Short-term strategy may be operated simultaneously for the purpose of long-term strategy.

How can we strategically change the trend of counselling development? This is a good question. No matter how difficult it is, instead of being the 'prisoner of the past' (Williamson, 1999), bound by the limitations and realities, strategic management has been recognised as the critical approach of survival in a tumultuous environment.

The rapid social and political reform in Hong Kong is a critical moment in spreading its development. The leaders in counselling education could create a portfolio of options strategically, starting with a broader vision of the counselling profession, set goals by creating meanings, and direct actions through eliminating uncertainty or ambiguity. Williamson (1999) suggested that with strategic options on the future, one will be able to reposition oneself faster than the competitors that have focused all their investments on 'doing more of the same.' This requires alteration of the traditional processes and inputs of new thinking about how planning and opportunism interact with each other in determining strategies. Below are five dimensions for consideration in strategic management to be discussed:

Strategy as leadership strengthening

Leadership is one of the frequently discussed and significant topics in the social sciences (Bass, 1990; Bennis, 2007). Leadership is generally agreed as a process of influencing group activities towards the achievement of goals (Khanka, 2006).

Rosenbach, Taylor, and Youndt (2012, p. 2) state, 'Leadership is all about getting people to work together to make things happen that might not otherwise occur or to prevent things from happening that would ordinarily take place.'

Actually, a consequence of globalisation is the emergence of generic or ubiquitous expectations of leaders (Brundrett, 2003). 'A central element in many definitions of leadership is that there is a process of influence' (Bush, 2003, p. 5).

Basically, counselling professionals are more competent in their counselling room with therapeutic practice. The scope of counselling training focus falls mainly on how to facilitate individuals to resolve their personal or interpersonal issues. The knowledge, formal qualification and skill-set are not formative on the dimensions of professional and organisational management. Counsellors' influences largely target the individual level or small group level. The inclusion of the essential element of 'concept of Leadership' in the mindset of counsellor educators was prominent in the twentieth century. The competency of drawing people together to develop social strength should be another dimension of the attention of the leaders in the counselling field. This serves significant constructions of relationships in the community and society, which are not recognized by the public and government.

A huge amount of theories, models, and approaches were propounded to help leaders to understand how to achieve different goals with different leadership styles (Sajjadi, 2014). 'Over the last 30 years, transformational leadership has become one of the most prominent theories of organisational behavior' (Sajjadi 2014, p. 11). Hodgetts and Luttans (2000) point out that transformational leaders are capable of motivating their people to work together to achieve goals.

At this stage of counselling professional development in Hong Kong, the major imperatives of the leaders are to (1) share their counselling vision among counsellors, such as promoting the mental health of the community; (2) develop professional identification, including ethical, culturally-inclusive and quality-assurance practices among counsellors; (3) attract public attention and understanding of the counselling profession and its idiosyncratic nature and powerful contributions to the community's psychological health; and (4) master political practice in government and political settings as well as administrate conducive social policy for psychological welfare. These are strategically significant tasks for counselling leaders; thus, the inseparable relationship between leadership and management needs to be implemented. Planning guides action and management towards their mission. Effective strategic planning articulates goals with action to make progress successful.

Strategy as thinking and planning

Leaders are expected to be more proactive in both leading and managing resources. Cuban (1988) provides one of the clearest distinctions between leadership and management. He linked leadership to change and management to maintenance activity. How to plan? What to plan? How long should the plan be? Who are the planners? The government, or the counsellor educators? Who are the leaders among these? The counsellor educators? The processing of laying out a planning model focuses on setting objectives, external and internal analysis, strategy evaluation and operationalisation and planning. Haines (1995, p. 1) states, 'We must become architects of the future, not defenders of the decline.'

According to Tracy (2014), leaders have roles as strategists and planners, which enables their engagement in long-term vision and big picture planning. Mintzburg (1994, p. 107) distinguished the difference between strategic planning and strategic thinking. He suggested that strategic planning often spoils strategic thinking, causing managers to confuse real vision with the manipulation of numbers and this confusion lies at the heart of the issue: the most successful strategies are vision, not plans. He claimed that, 'Strategic planning isn't strategic thinking. One is analysis, and the other is synthesis' (Mintzburg, 1994, p. 107). The breaking down of a goal or set of intentions into steps, and formalising those steps for implementation is 'analysis.' On the contrary, strategic thinking involves intuition and creativity, which is an integrated perspective on strategies. He also stated that sometimes strategies must be left as broad visions, not precisely articulated, so as to adapt to a changing environment.

Facing a scarcity of resources, the most central strategic question, whether using a competition or corporate strategy, has to be considered among universities, associations and other counselling education providers. For instance, an identity problem is the 'twice-told' issue of the counselling field. Counsellors have always been frustrated by not having a clear and distinct professional identity. This kind of primitive/outdated disturbing thought also discourages leaders from planning ahead. Thoughts guide direction of reaction. Strategic thinking strengthens intellectual capacity. It enhances the exploration of opportunities and future planning.

How to open new capabilities and opportunities is one major task of strategic management. To think strategically, there are two notable dimensions: first of all, whether anybody can become counsellors, such as the clergy, teachers, social workers, and peers. What does this mean for the counselling profession? From a strategic point of view, the counselling culture has already been built up all through the strata in society. Acceptance by the general public demonstrates that there is a market. This market naturally evolved from customers' needs which created the demand for counsellors. This widespread adoption to popularise the profession is a medium which counselling educators can utilise in the process of bettering the profession. In addition, instead of making alignment with medical or pathological models, we could also maximize the worthiness of the 'growth model' which has always been our focus in counselling. The market for enhancing healthy 'normal growth' is much greater (Gale & Austin, 2003). To enhance personal growth and a healthy relationship are parts of the eco-awareness. Using a growth model to empower deficits/pathologies are significantly beneficial to the community. Environmental consciousness is a current trend in this global age. This is a connection with the world trend. Why do we have to stick to the bitterness of having confused boundaries with other mental health professions? Counselling has many more resources and capabilities to create contributions beyond our expectations if we can think out of the box. This is strategic thinking in counselling education and what Gale and Austin (2003) called 'work to create market demand.'

People may argue about the gatekeeping functions of counselling educators or supervisors. To open the door to the public means the popularisation, or 'secularisation' of the profession. It would affect its professional image in a negative way. Chandler (1962) identified four stages in the life cycles of companies and institutions. The first stage is the initial acquisition of resources, i.e., vertical integration. The second is the drive for the efficient use of these resources through a functional organisational structure. The third is another period of growth involving new product lines and/or diversification. Finally, there is a second shift in structure to a divisionalised form. This developmental approach to understanding the growth of a company clarifies the stages/circumstances of development for the counselling profession. Acquisition of resources as well as setting up of markets and channels is the very fundamental stage in an organisation's development. The control of quality and enrichment through more and more education comes after people's understanding and recognition.

Client education, such as promotion of health, is a set of planned educational activities separate from clinical patient care. The primary focus of these activities includes acquisition of information, skills, beliefs, and attitudes, which impact on health status, quality of life, and possibly healthcare utilisation (Burckhardt, 1994, p. 2, cited in Coates, V., 1999).

Strategic thinking in management of the counselling profession enables the realisation of a growth model and releases us from becoming prisoners of existing constraints. We need to build new capabilities. 'Real strategic change requires inventing new categories, not rearranging old ones' (Mintzburg, 1994). The radical changes have permeated every aspect of our life in the dynamic era; we have to seek new ways to unleash new perspectives.

Strategy as a value implementation process

Bush (1998, p. 328) links up leadership to values or purposes while management relates to implementation or technical issues. When we talk about strategic management in counselling development in Hong Kong, we must ask: 'Why do people choose to enter into the field of counselling and not other professions?' People's decisions and choices are largely determined by values. 'Planning represents a calculating style of management, not a committing style' (Mintzburg, 1994, p. 109). Nowadays, commitment is not enough for counselling leaders. They need to spend time on focused strategic thinking and planning on a regular basis. It leads counselling educators to think about the meaning and value of counselling to the community.

Kluckhohn (1951, p. 395) states that 'a value is a conception, explicit or implicit, distinctive of an individual or characteristic of a group, of the desirable which influences the selection from available modes, means and ends of action.' The spirit of the counselling profession lies in its honour of human values, and its recognition as a 'deep need within human development' (Stripling, 1983, p. 206). Carl Rogers' necessary and sufficient conditions – respect, unconditional positive regard, and empathy – carried the most profound influence in the counselling movement. Rogers (1957) identified that a congruent and integrated relationship is one of the core conditions for constructive personality change to occur. This highlights the value of relationship.

The commitment to professional development originates from the sharing of its values. The sociologist Philip Selznick (1957, cited in Mintzburg, H., 1994) claimed that strategies take on value only as committed people infuse them with energy. It is a matter of how to communicate the mission lively. With an attempt to arouse the attention of the counselling value and its significance to modern society, Tse (2010) delineates the value of counselling in terms of the concepts of human capital. She mentions four dimensions of the counselling nature: developmental, curative, relationship enhancement, and psychoeducation, which are crucial to the formation of human capital. She alerts governments and economists to pay special attention to the role of counselling in terms of human capital development. A huge amount of money is put into it each year by the government in an attempt to decrease the mental health problems in the community. These are extremely valuable to the community and organisation in the twentieth century for enhancing self-understanding, facilitating problem-solving life issues, enabling human relationships, and the provision of knowledge relating to psychological health. Prevention is always more strategic and cost-effective than intervention.

How do the leaders in counselling education exert influence on the community? To talk about strategic management and the facilitation of the growth of the counselling profession, we must not neglect its substance of value. The collective value of the Chinese emphasizes that an effective way to get things done is through interpersonal relationships. And it is more effective to resolve disputes through negotiation and compromise rather than confrontation. 'Counselling relationship is the heart of counselling process. It supplies the vitality and the support necessary for counselling to work' (Nystul, 2003, p. 54). Counselling can also be named the 'Relationship profession,' to help people build intrapersonal and interpersonal relationships through professional helping relationships. Relationship building is perceived as the capacity to relate to others, which is a necessary domain in counselling. Crucially, the individual must develop the capacity to relate to the external world. How do the counselling educators and leaders cultivate a counselling culture and communicate these values of the counselling profession in Hong Kong? The art and heritage of relationships in the Chinese culture will facilitate the integration and promotion of counselling education. Multicultural compatibility is certainly an important topic in strategic management.

Understanding the cultural and sociopolitical context of the value system is essential. The strategy for implementation of counselling values somehow is the implication of the integration of the Western and Eastern cultural connotation of mental health.

Strategy as a commitment to lifelong learning

Strategy is an emergent process. People other than members of top management can trace strategies back to a range of actions and decisions. After a process of learning over time, formulation and implementation start to emerge. Strategies are found as patterns from the past, and later as plans for the future or as perspectives to guide overall behaviour. Strategies therefore are found throughout the organisation. The role of leadership is to manage the process of strategic learning (Sadler, 1993).

Learning is truly a self-reinforcing, self-regenerating dynamo (Samoff, 1996). The process of learning is exhilarating and energizing. As referred to as concepts by Ellyard (1998), counsellor educators can promote a learning culture to monitor the development of the profession. Ellyard's model of learning comprises eight elements which are (1) lifelong learning; (2) learner-driven learning; (3) just-in-time learning; (4) customized learning; (5) transformative learning; (6) collaborative learning; (7) contextual learning; and (8) learning to learn. This model sheds light for counsellors in the widening of their learning horizons.

To manage the counselling profession, we need to activate learning modes in both trainers and trainees by setting up systematic planning for the acquisition of knowledge or promoting the mindset of lifelong learning. Counselling educators or supervisors act as the facilitators of the learning culture, and the provision of different learning strategies is a form of management of the qualities of the profession. Learning can be customized to the individual needs of different learners. Learning can be collaborative as a way to learn from fellow counsellors, other professionals from other disciplines, or other organisations. Learning can also be found from exposure to different contexts and situations. Transformative learning is practised through a consistent revision of the working experience or the experiences of supervisors.

With reference to the medical profession in Hong Kong, the implementation of the Hong Kong Doctors Union (HKDU) Continuing Medical Education (CME) programme, which was launched in July 2000, aimed at maintaining a credible and equitable record of GPs/FPs participation in approved quality assurance education activities. CME points can be earned from attending talks, reading articles and also doing distance-learning courses. Under this programme, each doctor has to earn a minimum of 90 CME points in a three-year cycle before he/she can obtain the CME certificate.

In the counselling profession, supervision is one of the critical lifelong learning components across the professional trajectory (Falender & Shafranske, 2004). After institutional formal training has been completed, in-service training in the form of seminars and the tradition of ongoing clinical supervision is the major emphases and heritage in lifelong counselling education. Norcross, Prochaska, and Farber (1993) found that clinical supervision was the second most frequently reported activity among members of the APA's Division of Psychotherapy. Meyer (1978) found that counselling skills decline after training without supervision. Usually, the reasons given for low levels of supervision relate primarily to budget constraints, high workloads of staff and supervisors, higher priorities, and lack of available supervisors (Ladany, Ellis, & Friedlander, 1999). Employers, registration boards, and professional bodies are increasingly acknowledging the importance of good supervision in contributing to the maintenance and enhancement of high-quality clinical practice. Both hours of attending counselling-related talks and seminars, and hours of supervised counselling are elements for credible adjudication for quality assurance.

Learning is a permanent process which results in opportunities, challenges, unexpected situations at work, and any previous experience being turned into a learning experience (Torokoff & Mets, 2005). Ellyard (1998, p. 62) claims that a learning culture is necessary for success in the twenty-first century and learning is the 'most powerful instrument for shaping the future.' Grey (2004, p. 21) said, 'Yesterday's knowledge and skills are vulnerable to obsolescence, and future success requires flexibility, responsiveness and new capabilities.' Fong (1997) stated that it is not ethical to practise counsellor education and supervision without updated knowledge (Shen, 2008). The first step in commitment to professional development is the recognition of areas needing growth. She stated that, ethics aside, being current and contemporary is a necessary requirement of our careers. Counsellors have to continuously focus on professional development. Facing clients from various strata, diversified problems and issues in different life stages and lifelong as well as life broad learning will equip counsellors with the tools to deal with all kinds of clients. Counsellors are challenged by a constantly changing world. Their learning needs are increasing.

Through commitment to lifelong learning practice, counsellors progressively increase their self-awareness, acquire more advanced counselling skills and techniques, and master theoretical knowledge. Learning schools can be said to be the groundwork of management. All learning is integrated into a personal and professional identity as a counsellor – a growth process that is continuous and ongoing across the counsellor's professional lifespan (Borders, 1989, p. 9). A good foundation for the profession lies in ongoing learning attitudes.

Strategy as power administration

Power can be said to be the ability to influence. 'The concept of power is as ancient and ubiquitous as any that social theory can boast' (Dahl 2007, p. 201). 'Everyone recognises the need to be organised in order to plan activities, assign responsibilities, and identify a common goal to be reached. Once everything is in place, power must be used to give direction and control the process' (Seperich and McCalley, 2006, p. 14). This is a central concept in social and political fields which can explain many different social phenomena (Menge, 2018).

Dahl (2007, p. 201) defines power as 'a relation between people, and is expressed in simple symbolic notation.' Power can be said to be 'the driving energy' (Seperich and McCalley 2006, p. 15) of an organisation or community. The process of power execution in management is always complex. Different powers have different sources and different consequences. Social psychologists French and Raven (1959) proposed a classic study in regard to five categories of power, reflecting the different resources and influence that power holds: coercive, reward, legitimate, expert, and referent power.

'Expert power' to the community is the typical 'power' addressed in a profession. This means the person's power, which derives from one's skills or expertise. This type of power is specific and limited to a particular trained area. Achieving professional status has always been a significant issue in the counselling profession. Professional status and social recognition is a form of expert power. Max Weber (1968, as cited in Rosenbach, Taylor, & Youndt, 2012) delineated an influential distinction between different sources of authority. According to Weber, tradition is one of the identified sources that represents power and authority based on what has been inherited, established, and practised in the past. Leaders in the counselling field mostly follow this practice. The leadership power comes mainly from the experience and expertise in the profession. However, it does not mean that people who are an authority in the counselling profession are good administrators or competent leaders.

With regard to strategic management, Sadler (1993, pp. 20–21) distinguishes two types of power, 'micro power' and 'macro power.' He states,

> The former relates to the exercise of power within the organisation in connection with the processes of strategic management. The latter is to do with the exercise of power by the organisation in its external relationships.

Within an organisation, there are battles among managers and staff for resources, power, status, and promotion. Externally, it may involve rational or illegitimate means to create pressure on the government over policy making or resources. Strategy formulation is shaped by organisational and political powers. Other than professional knowledge, counselling educators have to deal with many other management-related issues which require the skilful use of the earned or unearned power in the social position.

The expertise and experience of counsellors help counsellors to establish their own professionality and identity, as well as related authority within the counsellor circle. But it is also important to consider one social dimension: who has the power to recognise professional status? Professional bodies or the government? Certainly, recognition from both sides is of the same importance. Professional identity confusion will likely be found if professional bodies are not recognised or their work is ignored by the government. The leaders could utilize strategies to face these problems.

Lukes (1974), the political theorist, developed a three-dimensional model of political power as something overt, covert, or latent. The government has the overt power to offer recognition to a profession but actually may not have the knowledge for credentialing the profession. They may employ a professional body and set standardised criteria for assessment and codes of ethics for professional guidelines, to offer accreditation. The most commonly noted criteria used to evaluate whether an occupation has evolved to the status of a profession include there being (1) a specialized body of knowledge and theory-driven research, (2) the establishment of a professional society or association, (3) control of training programmes, (4) a code of ethics to guide professional behaviour and (5) standards for admitting and policing practitioners (Caplow, 1966). The covert power to determine the status lies in the hands of the professional body. Thus, it is very important for professional leaders to develop clear guidelines and ethics for practitioners before it can become a trustworthy profession. Professional education shares the common aim of providing membership of a professional body and indicating capability in a professional role.

However, simply by obtaining the certificates or membership of a professional body does not guarantee expertise. Gale and Austin (2003, p. 3) argued,

> Differences in training, specialisation, professional affiliations, and credentialing have challenged professional counsellors' sense of collective identity ... Paradoxically, achieving professional status has done little to promote professional counsellors' sense of collective identity or to distinguish counsellors from other mental health professionals.

They pointed out that the achievement of professional status has led to the creation of greater diversity and less unity among persons who identify themselves as professional counsellors. One of the reasons for such diversity is counsellors' lack of confidence to secure their professionalism owing to the generic nature of this helping profession. Besides, different orientations of training, licenses, and membership from different professional bodies may contribute to conflicting codes of ethics. There are two sides of the coin. More effort should be devoted to solving the potential problem in this area. The rationale for strategic management is vitally important. Firstly, thinking out of the box is a form of cognitive power, which will help us to find our way whenever we are blocked. Power devoted to strategic thinking is crucial to leaders. Counsellor leaders, as strategic leaders, need to engage in strategic thinking and planning with the big picture in mind and anticipate crises and potentials in the professional field. Secondly, counsellors' ongoing effort in the self-development of counselling competence and high-quality counselling practice will enhance the professional self-esteem as well as accumulation of expertise power. Thirdly, counsellors who join together as a union will form a strong, united voice to effect real changes in their workplaces, their profession, and even the broader community. The famous Gestalt saying, 'The whole is greater than the sum of the parts,' reminds us that what one can do, many can do better. Collection of power that comes from within will help us to utilise the external resources.

Conclusion

Counselling educators, in order to meet the speedy changes, progressive challenges of the world's demands, new standards, and prevalent good quality service delivery, must be well prepared. In Hong Kong, the emerging counselling profession has gone through a series of difficulties. It is pragmatically expected that market demand influences the development of a profession in a situation like Hong Kong. Financial stringency in the public, education, and non-profit sectors poses constant constraints on development plans. The input of the strategic approach in education management has triggered a huge controversy owing to its loaded concepts from the business world. However, the business of being counselling educators is both complex and exposing. The counselling profession requires strategic leadership, thinking, planning, marketing and cultural awareness of the implicit and explicit values and development skills. Success in counselling management depends on various endogenous and exogenous factors. Counsellor educators and leaders have a responsibility to promote professional growth in terms of lifelong learning and engagement in high-quality supervised professional practice. The atmosphere of changes can be transformed into more options with opportunism through strategic management. A positive attitude to strategic approaches and good use of potential power in counselling development and management is like having an important tool. Whether we can use it or not depends on how much we know about it. All the difficulties and challenges are parts of the journey along the professional evolution.

References

Bass, B.M. (1990). *Bass and Stogdill's handbook of leadership* (3rd ed.). New York, NY: Free Press.

Bennis, W.G. (2007). The challenges of leadership in the modem world—Introduction to the special issue. *American Psychologist, 62*, 2–5.

Bolam, R. (1999). Educational administration, leadership and management: Towards a research agenda, in T. Bush, L. Bell, R. Bolam, R. Glatter, & P. Ribbins (Eds.). *Educational management: Redefining theory, policy and practice.* London: Paul Chapman Publishing.

Borders, L.D. (1989). Facilitating supervisee growth: Implications of the developmental models of counselling supervision. *Michigan Journal of Counselling and Development, 17*, 9–14.

Brundrett, M., Burton, N., & Smith, R. (2003). *Leadership in education*. London: Sage.

Burckhardt, C.S., Moncur, C., & Minor, M.A. (1994). Exercise tests as outcome measures. *Arthritis & Rheumatism*, 7, 169–175.

Bush, T. (1998). The National professional qualification for headship: The key to effective school leadership? *School Leadership and Management*, 18(3), 321–334.

Bush, T. (2003). *Theories of educational leadership and management*. London: GBR Sage Publications.

Caplow, T. (1966). The sequence of professionalization, in H.M. Vollmer, & D.L. Mills (Eds.). *Professionalization*. Englewood Cliffs, NJ: Prentice Hall.

Chandler, A.D. (1962). *Strategy and structure: Chapters in the history of the industrial enterprise*. Cambridge, MA: MIT Press.

Coates, V. (1999). *Education for patients and clients*. Florence, KY, USA: Routledge.

Cuban, L. (1988). *The managerial imperative and the practice of leadership in schools*. Albany, NY: State University of New York Press.

Dahl, R.A. (2007). The concept of power. *Behavioral Science*, 2(3), 201–215. https://doi.org/10.1002/bs.3830020303.

Drucker, P.F. (1990), cited in Courtney, Roger (2001). *Strategic management for voluntary non-profit organizations*. Florence, KY, USA: Routledge.

Ellyard, P. (1998). *Ideas for the new millennium*. Melbourne, Australia: Melbourne University Press.

Falender, C.A., & Shafranske, E.P. (2004). *Clinical supervision—A competency-based approach*. Washington, DC: American Psychological Association.

Fitzgerald, L., & Osipow, S. (1986). An occupational analysis of counseling psychology. *American Psychologist*, 41, 535–544.

Fong, M.L. (1997). Presidential address: Making professional development a priority. *Counsellor Education and Supervision*, 37(2), 82–88.

French, Jr., J.R.P., & Raven, B.H. (1959). The bases of social power, in D. Cartwright (Ed.), *Studies in social power* (pp. 150–167). Ann Arbor, MI: Institute for Social Research.

Gale, A.U., & Austin, B.D. (2003). Professionalism's challenges to professional counsellor's collective identity. *Journal of Counselling and Development, Winter*, 81(1), 3–10.

Goode, W.J. (1960). A theory of role strain. *American Sociological Review*, 25, 483–496.

Goodyear, R.K. (1984). On our journal's evolution: Historical developments, transitions, and future directions. *Journal of Counselling and Development*, 63, 3–8.

Grey, C. (2004). *Essential readings in management learning*. London, GBR: Sage Publications Ltd. http://site.ebrary.com/lib/ marmara/Doc?id=10076759.

Haines, S.G. (1995). *Successful strategic planning*. Menlo Park, CA, USA: Course Technology Crisp.

Hodgetts, R.M., & Luthans, F. (2000). *International management: Culture, strategy, and behavior*. USA: McGraw Hill Companies, Inc.

Hofer, C.W. Schendel, D. (1978). *Strategy formulation: Analytical concepts*. St. Paul: West Publishing Company.

Hofstede, G. (1980). *Culture's consequences: International differences in work-related values*. Beverly Hills, CA: Sage Publications.

Huy, Q.N. & Mintzberg, H. (2003). The rhythm of change. *MIT Sloan Management Review*, 44(4), 77–84.

Hwang, K.K. (1987). Face and favor: The Chinese power game. *The American Journal of Sociology*, 92(4), 944–974.

Khanka, S.S. (2006). *Organisational behaviour*. New Delhi: S. Chand & Company Ltd.

Kleinman, A., & Lin, T.Y. (1981). *Normal and abnormal behavior in Chinese culture*. Dordrecht, Holland/Boston: Reidel publishing company.

Kluckhohn, C. (1951) Values and value-orientations in the theory of action: An exploration in definition and classification, in T. Parsons and E. Shils (Eds.). *Toward a general theory of action*. Cambridge, MA: Harvard University Press, 388–433. https://doi.org/10.4159/harvard.9780674863507.c8.

Ladany, N., Ellis, M.V., & Friedlander, M.L. (1999). The supervisory working alliance, trainee self-efficacy, and satisfaction. *Journal of Counseling and Development*, 77, 447–455.

Lee, W.Y. (2005). Nonprofit development in Hong Kong: The case of a Statist–Corporatist Regime. *Voluntas: International Journal of Voluntary and Nonprofit Organizations*, 16, 1.

Leung, S.A. (1999). The development of counselling in Hong Kong: Searching for professional identity. *Asian Journal of Counselling*, 6, 77–95.

Leung, T.M. (1988). *History of counselling service in Hong Kong*, Doctoral dissertation, University of North Texas.

Lukes, S. (1974). *Power: A radical view*. London: Macmillan.

Menge, T. (2018). The role of power in social explanation. *European Journal of Social Theory*, 21(1), 22–38. https://doi.org/10.1177/1368431017714426.

Meyer, Jr., R.J. (1978). Using self-supervision to maintain counselling skills: A review. *Personnel and Guidance Journal*, 57, 95–98.

Mintzburg, H. (1994). The fall and rise of strategic planning. *Harvard Business Review (January–February)*, 107.

Mitreanu, C. (2006). Is strategy a bad word? *MIT Sloan Management Review*, 47(2), 95–96.

Nadler, A., 1990, cited in Kung, W.W. (2003). Chinese Americans' help seeking for emotional distress. *The Social Service Review*, 77(1), 110–134.

Ngo, J., & Zhao, S. (2016, 15 March). 'Extremely problematic': Hong Kong education and counselling professionals slam authorities over insufficient staff support. *South China Morning Post*. Retrieved from www.scmp.com/news/hong-kong/ education-community/article/1925694/ extremely-problematichong-kong-education-and.

Norcross, J.C., Prochaska, J.O., & Farber, J.A. (1993). Psychologists conducting psychotherapy: New findings and historical comparisons on the psychotherapy division membership. *Psychotherapy*, 30, 692–697.

Nystul, M.S. (2003). *Introduction to counselling: An art and science perspective* (2nd ed.). Boston: Allyn & bacon.

Pavalko, R. (1971). *Sociology of occupations and professions*. Itasca, IL: F. E. Peacock Publishers, Inc.

Rogers, C.R. (1957). The necessary and sufficient conditions of therapeutic personality change. *Journal of Consulting Psychology*, 21, 95–103.

Romano, G. (1992). The power and pain of professionalization. *American Counselor*, 1, 17–23.

Rosenbach, W.E., Taylor, R.L., & Youndt, M.A. (2012). Part I-HEART, in *Contemporary issues in leadership* (7th ed.). New York: Routledge.

Rosenthal, U., Boin, A., & Comfort, L.K. (2001). *Managing crises: Threats, dilemmas, opportunities*. USA: Charles C. Thomas Publisher, Ltd.

Sadler, P. (1993). *Strategic management*. Milford, CT, USA: Kogan Page Limited.

Sajjadi, A. (2014). New emerging leadership theories and styles. *Technical Journal of Engineering and Applied Sciences*, 4(3), 180–188.

Samoff, J. (1996). Which priorities and strategies for education? *International Education Development*, 16(3), 249–271.

Secretary for Education of Education Bureau, H. K. S. A. R. G. (2018, 27 April). The policy of 'one school social worker for each school' in primary schools. Education Bureau Circular Memorandum No. 36/2018. Retrieved from https://applications. edb.gov.hk/circular/upload/EDBCM/ EDBCM18036E.pdf.

Seperich, G.J., & McCalley, R.W. (2006). Overview of the power sources, in *Managing power and people*. New York: M. E. Sharpe.

Shen, Y. (2008). The effect of changes and innovation on educational improvement. *International Educational Studies*, 1(3), 73–77.

Simpson, E. H. (1993). Professional identity of counselling and counselling psychology in Canada (M.Sc., The University of Calgary (Canada). Retrieved from http://0.search.proquest.com/ docview/304039607/abstract/6CBDC446038B4C81PQ/3.

Social Welfare Department (2000). *Social welfare services lump sum grant manual* (2nd ed.). Hong Kong: Government Printer.

Stripling, R.O. (1983). Building on the past—A challenge for the future, in G.R. Walls, & L. Benjamin (Eds). *Shaping counsellor education programs in the next five years: An experimental prototype for the counsellor of tomorrow.* Ann Arbor: Eric/Caps, 205–209.

Sweeting, A. (2007). Education in Hong Kong: Histories, mysteries and myths. *History of Education*, 36(1), 89–108.

Torokoff, M. and T. Mets (2005). The learning organisation and learning in the organisation: The concept for improving the labour quality in a school. *Management of Organizations: Systematic Research*, 35, 203–216.

Tracy, B. (2014). The leader as strategist, in *Leadership*. USA: American Management Association.

Triandis, H.C. (1995). *Individualism and collectivism*. Boulder, CO, Westview Press.

Tse, P.C. (2010). The counselling profession: An important resource for enhancing human capital development. *Asia Pacific Journal of Counselling and Psychotherapy*, 1(1), 15–27. https://doi.org/10.1080/21507680903570425.

Watkins, Jr., C.E. (1983). Counseling psychology versus clinical psychology: Further explorations on a theme or Once more around the 'identity' maypole with gusto. *The Counseling Psychologist*, 12, 76–92.

Watkins, Jr., C.E., Lopez, E, Campbell, v., & Himmcll, C. (1986). Contemporary counseling psychology: Results of a national survey. *Journal of Counseling Psychology*, 33, 301–309.

Williamson, P.J. (1999). Strategy as options on the future. *Sloan Management Review*, 40(3), 117–127.

Wong, E.O.W. (2003). Analyzing the contribution of continuing education and leadership empowerment to sustainable development-experience from a Hong Kong tertiary institution. *International Journal of Sustainability in Higher Education*, 4(4), 364–374.

Yu, C., K. C., Fu, W., Zhao, X., & Davey, G. (2010). Public understanding of counsellors and counselling in Hong Kong. *Asia Pacific Journal of Counselling and Psychotherapy*, 1(1), 47–54. https://doi.org/10.1080/21507680903574310. Australian Counselling Research Journal | www.acrjournal.com.au.

28 An Overview of Counselling Practices in Indonesia

Marina Salmond, Karel K. Himawan, Jessica Ariela, and Eunike M. Himawan

Introduction

Compared to other similar mental health practices, such as: psychiatry and psychology, counselling practices in Indonesia is arguably a newly practised area. Currently, there are no government regulations in place to control and protect counselling practices in Indonesia, while psychologists and psychiatrists have been formally recognised by the government as mental health professionals since 2014, as written in the Law Number (No.) 18 of 2014 on Mental Health (Republik Indonesia, 2014). More recently, the introduction of the Law Number (No.) 23 of 2022 on Psychological Services and Education even gives more structures towards psychological services, including the scope of practices of psychology graduates, that involves providing counselling in non-clinical setting. Many sources indicate that Indonesia has recognised psychologists as health workers since 2008 (i.e., Sebayang, Mawarpury, & Rosemary, 2018). Indonesia also seems to follow an international path (i.e., Frances, 2014; Himawan & Lestari, 2021), wherein the understanding, and thus the treatment of mental health, tends to be reduced to the physiological aspect. As a result, there is a tendency to misdiagnose and mistreat psychological issues as physical illness (Maramis, Pantouw, & Lesmana, 2021). At the same time, individuals reporting mental health issues are at risk of being stigmatised (Hartini et al., 2018). Displaying negative emotion is also considered a sign of weakness, especially among men – a typical cultural issue in a patrilineal society.

As a newly practised area, the lack of systematic education, regulation, and supervision of counselling practices in Indonesia certainly impacts the profession. On one hand, such situation provides flexibility for counsellors to have a professional practice. On the other hand, that flexibility comes with a likely consequence of unstandardised counselling quality, even malpractice, as individuals who receive only short training of basic counselling declare themselves to be counsellors and manage their own practices with little to no accountability to anyone else. The absence of licensure regulations of counsellors in Indonesia adds to the complexities, in which individuals graduated in counselling education (primarily from international institutions) are not able to have their practice acknowledged in the society.

This chapter will systematically describe the current landscape of counselling practices in Indonesia, including how counselling is represented, educated, regulated, and supervised. Our discussion is based on the review of literature, regulations, and current practices to provide an overall look of the field.

DOI: 10.4324/9781003490067-35

Counselling representation in Indonesia

In a society with rich and diverse cultural beliefs and traditions, mental health issues in Indonesia are often associated with superstitious belief, such as demonic possession, or a curse of past wrongdoing (Thee, 2019). As a result, individuals experiencing mental health issues are often maltreated, blamed, and in the case of psychotic issues, experience physical constraints and neglect (Himawan & Lestari, 2021). Furthermore, with mental issues being linked to spiritual matters, counselling services often become non-existent as they are considered irrelevant.

In the last two decades, however, public attention to the mental health issues has been constantly growing, especially among younger generations, and in the urban population. A major government initiative was the introduction of a law that formally governs mental health practices in 2014 in the Law Number (No.) 18 of 2014 on Mental Health (Republic of Indonesia, 2014), which acknowledges mental health as a distinct concept from physical health. The younger generation acts as the agent of change in introducing mental health issues to the society (United Nations Children's Funds [UNICEF], 2020). A government hotline counselling centre (*layanan SEJIWA*; stands for '*sehat jiwa*' or 'psychological health services') was introduced in May 2020 to respond to mental health issues as the secondary impact of the Covid-19 pandemic (Ministry of Women Empowerment and Child Protection, 2021).

Meanwhile, in the field of counselling, the Association of Christian Counsellors Indonesia (AKKI) recently had an audience with the Christian Division of the Indonesian Ministry of Religious Affairs to raise awareness of the presence of Christian counsellors, opening the path for formal recognition of their service in the society (AKKI, personal communication, 2021).

Amidst the increasing public awareness about mental health, there are at least three factors that contribute to the blurry representation of counselling in the society: the overlapping scope of practices, the lack of specialised counselling education, and the lack of regulation of the profession.

The overlapping scope of mental health practitioners

The scope of practices across mental health practitioners appears to be overlapping. The blurred scope of practice is actually not only found in Indonesia, but also tends to be a global phenomenon (Holmes & Lindley, 2019; Tudor, 2013) due to the fact that the practitioners share similar focus in their practices. Psychologists, psychiatrists, and counsellors declare themselves to be the most appropriate professionals for handling mental health issues. Rather than collaborating, nuances of competition are often observed across professions, but primarily between psychologists and psychiatrists, the recognised profession in the society. Counsellors seem to operate within social- and religious-based settings as there is currently no licensing system that regulates counselling practices for counsellors in Indonesia. Compared to psychologists and psychiatrists, counsellors tend to have a more distinct field in dealing with non-clinical issues. However, without clear boundaries or scope of practice across professions, counselling practices appear to be less grown as there are no explicit government regulation recognising the profession as it does psychologists and psychiatrists.

Currently, formal counselling practices in Indonesian society are done by psychologists, professional counsellors, religiously-affiliated counsellors, or guidance counsellors.

Informally, especially in rural areas, traditional healers, religious leaders, village or district leaders, or sometimes, medical doctors are still the go-to people for consultation about mental health concerns. In urban population, professional counselling is conducted in settings such as: hospitals, psychology clinics, or counselling centres. Aside from guidance counsellors, some psychologists and religiously-affiliated counsellors also provide their services in academic settings. Many religiously affiliated counsellors, however, also set up private counselling practice and receive clients from all kinds of religious backgrounds. This practice, certainly, poses ethical and multicultural competency issues. Lastly, lay counsellors, whose number grows the fastest amongst counselling service providers in Indonesia, provide lay counselling in churches or religiously-affiliated schools or counselling centres.

The second factor that contributes to the underrepresentation of counselling activities in the society is the unavailability of standardised and regulated counselling education programmes in Indonesia, which is the focus of our next section.

The diversity of counselling education in Indonesia

Counselling training and programmes offered in Indonesia vary, ranging from short-term counselling training to master's degree programmes in counselling offered by certain religious education institutions. There is also an undergraduate degree programme for guidance counselling, usually offered by the Department of Education of secular universities.

Currently, the master's degree programmes in counselling are offered by few renowned Christian theology seminaries. The focus of these programmes is the integration of psychology and Christian teachings, with the main goal of providing religious-based counselling services to the Christian mass. On top of the counselling skills and psychology classes, students of these programmes also study theology and various aspects of Christian ministry. Some of the programmes require their students to undergo personal counselling, and require a certain number of supervised counselling practicum hours. A certain seminary offers an additional certification programme which includes counselling supervision practice, after the completion of the master's programme, which apparently did not include supervision as graduation requirement. Alumni of such programmes are known to provide counselling services in churches, Christian schools, universities, or private counselling centres.

Short-term counselling training is usually offered by counselling centres or the aforementioned seminaries. Trainees, who may be considered as lay counsellors, normally receive certificates of completion after a minimum of six-months training. There is no reliable data on the number of lay counsellors completing these types of short-term training, who then continue on to provide formal counselling services. The majority may do counselling in the context of religious-based, pro-bono ministry. They are usually very passionate about helping and serving those in need.

The more structured counselling education in Indonesia is 'Bimbingan Konseling' (Guidance Counselling), which is a specialised track of undergraduate degree programme under the Department of Education, which mainly covers counselling in the academic or career settings. The graduates of this programme – guidance counsellors – can continue their training to earn the license to practise as professional counsellors. This training comprises two semesters of Counselling Professional Education, including 600 hours of supervised practice. The association for these counsellors, called IKI (Ikatan Konselor Indonesia [Indonesian Counsellor Association]), mentions that they serve in private practice and in settings such as: schools; government or private institutions of higher education; industries and businesses; or other agencies; with clientele comprising of individuals, families, or groups (https://konselor.or.id/). There are also graduate and post-graduate degree programmes for guidance counsellors, focusing mainly on counselling in academic settings. Counsellors with such professional trajectory have an established association they can join, namely the ABKIN (Asosiasi Bimbingan dan Konseling Indonesia [The Indonesian Guidance and Counselling Association]). Despite their training and availability of services, however, counsellors from the guidance counselling path are not generally known in other settings.

With little recognition from the government, it is not surprising that a formal counselling degree programme which offers specialised counselling training from psychology and counselling perspective (e.g., clinical mental health counselling) is lacking in Indonesia, despite the high interest. In comparison, many international universities offer such programme under the Department of Psychology or Behavioural Sciences. This presents one of the challenges in the counselling field in Indonesia, as the available counselling programmes only train counsellors for narrow segments – educational or religious settings.

Having discussed the two factors contributing to the underrepresentation of counselling activities in Indonesia, we now turn to the third, which is the lack of regulation of the profession.

The lack of counselling regulation in Indonesia

As previously mentioned, there is currently no nation-wide law or standard of counsellor competence and professionalism regulating counselling practice in Indonesia. There are standards at the association level, albeit with minimal coordination amongst associations. These associations are set up by the different 'groups' of counsellors, mainly to support and share resources with their own 'kind.' For example, Indonesian Counselling Association (ICA) was formally established in 2016 by a group of mental health practitioners, including professional psychologists, to respond the need for a professional avenue to network, share materials, and gather with similar professions to provide counselling services that are relevant to the Indonesian cultures. ICA also has a set of code of conduct, which acts as a standard that is applied for all practising counsellors who are members of ICA. There are other associations for Christian counsellors, pastoral counsellors, guidance counsellors, and professional counsellors.

Amongst the different associations, ABKIN (Asosiasi Bimbingan dan Konseling Indonesia [The Indonesian Guidance and Counselling Association]) is by far the most established. It was founded in 1975 under the name of IPBI (Ikatan Petugas Bimbingan Indonesia [The Indonesian Guidance Officer Association]), and it is primarily focused on counsellors in the educational setting (ABKIN, 2018). It is not surprising that the majority of their members are educational counsellors (career guidance teachers), and most – if not all – of their committee members have educational background in education rather than professional counselling. They have the standard academic qualification of counsellors and counsellor competence as a regulation issued by the Ministry of Education and Culture, as written in the Ministerial Decree No. 27 of 2018 on Counsellor's Academic Qualification Standard and Competence (Ministry of Education and Culture, 2008).

Even for an established association like ABKIN, implementing the ethical code they draft is challenging. It is expected that a counsellor does not only master the theoretical and practical aspects of counselling, but must have good personality as well (ABKIN,

2018). Any violation to the ethical code can cause harm to the counsellors themselves and the party involved. The ABKIN emphasised that any violation of the code of ethics is subject to sanctions based on the provisions set by them. But in practice, this ethical code of conduct has not been implemented fully well (Sujadi, 2018). For example, a school counsellor assigned to a particular school did not understand the ethical code s/he must adhere to as a counsellor. There is also a survey which shows that many school counsellors are recognised as mean persons by the students and the students have negative impression of school counsellors (Wardani & Hariastuti, 2009).

A recent effort of recognising a standard of counsellor competence through module-based training and certification was proposed by Lembaga Konseling Keluarga Kreatif (LK3), a nation-wide Christian counselling institution and one of the providers of counselling training and education, to Indonesia's national professional certification institution (Badan Nasional Sertifikasi Profesi/BNSP). LK3 was granted licensure to conduct training and issue certification for counsellors in March 2023 (BNSP, 2023). BNSP is a relatively new independent institution in Indonesia, appointed to authorise various certifications to prepare 'ready-to-use' and high-quality workforce. Unfortunately, this certification has not been paired with government regulation regarding who can provide counselling services, unlike for other mental health practitioners such as psychologists or psychiatrists. Although currently this counsellor certification merely serves the purpose of recognising counsellor's competence, it is a stepping stone to a more structured regulation for professional counselling practices in the future.

This lack of overarching and unifying standard of counsellor competence and professional conduct is an area of concern, which also stems from the lack of recognition of the profession. Although efforts to get the different associations to come together are underway, full collaboration is still a long shot. Formulating a minimal standard of competence for counselling practice is, therefore, a huge undertaking.

Counselling supervision in Indonesia

As the counselling field in Indonesia is still in its infancy, supervision of counselling practices is also in its very early stage of development. In formal counselling education programmes previously discussed, supervision is usually done by lecturers who are practising counsellors with years of experience, but who are nonetheless not certified as supervisors. One provider of the religiously affiliated counselling programme – LK3 – however, has recently started to collaborate with a US psychology graduate school to have licensed supervisors provide regular group supervision sessions for its practicing alumni (T. Watson, personal communication, 29 March 2022), a step in the right direction.

In professional practice, directors of the counselling centres usually provide general supervision of cases, but very few are formally trained as supervisors. Others choose to utilise peer supervision model, in which counsellors regularly meet their colleagues, share counselling cases, and give input to each other. However, this peer supervision model varies from structured to non-structured, formal to informal supervision sessions.

Different counselling associations also have their own system of supervision. Some, for example ABKIN, provide more formal and structured supervision than others (Ulfa, Sugiyo, & Purwanto, 2014). Given the importance of good supervision for the effectiveness and professional development of counsellors, this is an area in great need of improvement.

Recommendation

Considering the diversity of the culture and the broad geographical areas of Indonesia as a country, a unique approach to counselling practices, education, regulation, and supervision is imperative. In response to this challenge, lay counselling, with proper training, regulation, and supervision might be a more appropriate and feasible option. With numerous counselling training programmes provided independently by counselling organisations or associations, many lay people (those without prior formal counselling education/background) may have the basic skills and concept of counselling. Therefore, they become potential helpers for people in their community to live mentally healthier, thus, creating a more resilient society and nation.

Strengthening lay counselling services is also a strategic approach to provide basic mental health services to people living in remote areas in Indonesia. Most mental health professionals live and work in bigger cities or provincial capitals and mental health services are almost non-existent in remote areas. Through lay counselling, selected locals can be trained in basic counselling skills to serve their respective communities, even those in remote places.

However, a system needs to be established to prevent potential issues, namely the issues of ethics and competence. As lay counsellors are often passionate about helping people, but operate independently and are not part of any associations, they might not be aware of the professional, ethical aspects of counselling. Therefore, lay counsellors should be equipped with the knowledge of counselling ethics and have to be affiliated with a counselling association which provides training and supervision for them. With regards to competence, although lay counsellors often serve at the frontlines of counselling services in the field, the expectation of services they provide is different compared to those of professional counsellors. For example, they are not equipped for treating clinical cases and are not as updated about the recent development in counselling techniques or interventions as the professionals. Affiliation to a counselling association will provide them with the resources to update their knowledge and skills, as well as network of referrals and guidance about when to make referrals. Hence, counselling associations can play a critical role in lay counselling services. These associations will serve as trainers, mentors, certifiers, accountability partners, referrals, as well as community builders for the nation's mental health.

Counselling associations in Indonesia need to meet and join forces in establishing regulation for counselling practices in Indonesia. Each counselling association's representatives can serve as the task force to draft the regulation, both for professional counselling and lay counselling practices. Later, this cross-association initiative could also offer diverse counselling programmes (i.e., training, certification) for members from joining associations. Therefore, each individual association retains its uniqueness and mission, and hopefully can better equip more counsellors in Indonesia through diverse approaches.

Lastly, besides equipping the counsellors themselves, it is also a huge task for counselling associations, counsellors, and other mental health professionals in Indonesia to inculcate a positive image towards counselling practices in Indonesia. Although awareness about mental health issues is rising among the younger generation, raising public awareness about the need for counselling and benefits offered by counselling is still an ongoing task. The society needs to be informed that other than helping those who have issues, counselling can foster the positive development and growth of individuals and communities. Hopefully, with proper understanding, there will be greater recognition of the counselling practices and professionals serving the Indonesian society.

Selected references for further reading

Selected internet resources

Asosiasi Bimbingan dan Konseling Indonesia (ABKIN) – Association of Guidance and Counseling Indonesia. https://abkin.org/.

Asosiasi Konselor Kristen Indonesia (AKKI) – Association of Christian Counselors Indonesia. https://akkindo.org/.

Ikatan Konselor Indonesia (IKI) – Indonesian Counselor Association. https://konselor.or.id/.

Indonesian Counseling Association. https://indo-counseling.org/.

Lembaga Konseling Keluarga Kreatif (LK3).www.keluargakreatif.com/.

References

Asosiasi Bimbingan dan Konseling Indonesia. (2018). *Anggaran Dasar dan Anggaran Rumah Tangga*. Yogyakarta: Pengurus Besar ABKIN.

Badan Nasional Sertifikasi Profesi (BNSP). (2023, 25 March). Ketua BNSP Menyerahkan Sertifikat Lisensi LSP Konselor Keluarga Kreatif. https://bnsp.go.id/detail.php?id=400.

Frances, A. (2014). DSM, psychotherapy, counselling and the medicalisation of mental illness: A commentary from Allen Frances. *The Professional Counsellor, 4*, 282–284. DOI:10.15241/afm.4.3.282.

Hartini, N., Fardana, N.A., Ariana, A.D., & Wardana, N.D. (2018). Stigma toward people with mental health problems in Indonesia. *Psychology Research and Behavior Management, 11*, 535–541. DOI:10.2147/PRBM.S175251.

Himawan, K.K., & Lestari, M.D. (2021). Perkembangan dan tantangan kesehatan mental dalam konteks global dan lokal. In M. D. Lestari & K. K. Himawan (Eds.), *Kesehatan Mental Perspektif Indonesia* (pp. 1–14). Jakarta: Rajawali Pers.

Holmes, J., & Lindley, R. (2019). *The Values of Psychotherapy*. Milton: Routledge.

Maramis, M.M., Pantouw, J.G., & Lesmana, C.B.J. (2021). Depression screening in Surabaya Indonesia: Urgent need for better mental health care for high-risk communities and suicide prevention for men. *International Journal of Social Psychiatry, 67*(5), 421–431. DOI:10.1177/002076-64020957359

Ministry of Education and Culture. (2008). *Permendiknas No. 27 Tentang Standar Kualifikasi Akademik dan Kompetensi Konselor*. Jakarta: Depdiknas.

Ministry of Women Empowerment and Child Protection. (2021). Layanan SEJIWA lindungi kesehatan mental masyarakat di masa pandemi COVID-19. www.kemenpppa.go.id/index.php/page/read/29/3178/layanan-sejiwa-lindungi-kesehatan-mental-masyarakat-di-masa-pandemi-covid-19.

Republik Indonesia. (2014). Undang-Undang Republik Indonesia Nomor 18 Tahun 2014 tentang Kesehatan Jiwa. https://peraturan.go.id/common/dokumen/ln/2014/uu18-2014bt.pdf.

Sebayang, S.K., Mawarpury, M., & Rosemary, R. (2018, 6 November). Less than 1,000 psychiatrists for 260 million Indonesians. *The Jakarta Post*. www.thejakartapost.com/academia/2018/11/06/less-than-1000-psychiatrists-for-260-million-indonesians.html.

Sujadi, E. (2018). Kode etik profesi konseling serta permasalahan dalam penerapannya. *Jurnal Tarbawi: Jurnal Ilmu Pendidikan, 14*(2), 69–77.

Thee, M. (2019, 6 November). 'You're not religious enough': pain of Indonesia's mentally ill and the online group bringing sufferers and carers together. *South China Morning Post*. www.scmp.com/lifestyle/health-wellness/article/3036343/youre-not-religious-enough-pain-indonesias-mentally-ill.

Tudor, K. (2013). Be careful what you wish for: Professional recognition, the statutory regulation of counselling, and the state registration of counsellors. *New Zealand Journal of Counselling*, *33*(2), 44–69.

United Nations Children's Funds (UNICEF). (2020). Young people take the lead on mental health. www.unicef.org/indonesia/coronavirus/stories/young-people-take-lead-mental-health.

Ulfa, Sugiyo, & Purwanto, E. (2014). Model Pengembangan Instrumen Supervisi Bimbingan dan Konseling. *Journal of Educational Research and Evaluation*, 3(1): https://journal.unnes.ac.id/sju/index.php/jere/ article/view/4396.

Wardani, I.K., & Hariastuti, R.T. (2009). Mengurangi persepsi negatif siswa tentang konselor sekolah dengan strategi pengubahan pola pikir (*Cognitive Restructuring*). *Jurnal PPB UNNESA*, *10*(2), 1–10.

29 Counselling Regulation, Education, and Representation in Malaysia

Melati Sumari, Dini Farhana Baharudin,
Hartini Abdul Rahman, and Norfaezah Md Khalid

Clinical supervision: An applied activity and research focus

Over time, counselling in Malaysia has grown from the stage of infancy (Ng & Stevens, 2001) to pubescence (See & Ng, 2010). While its historical origin has some influences from the counselling profession in the United States (Lloyd, 1987), counselling in Malaysia has become an important mental health profession with its own uniqueness and strength. Feit and Lloyd (1990) defined 'a recognized counselling profession' as comprising 'ethical standards, licensure, accreditation, specialized training, and a strong identity.' This was supported by Johari (2001), who added that 'professional bodies' to the existing criteria. The purpose of this chapter is to provide a brief overview of counselling in Malaysia. It is divided into five sections beginning with the counselling regulation and legislation, followed by counselling education, description of counselling representations through associations, some explanations on the pathway to becoming counsellors in Malaysia, and finally, counselling supervision.

Counselling regulation in Malaysia

Registration of counsellors

Counselling in Malaysia has moved towards professionalism and prominence with the introduction of the Counsellors Act 1998 (Act 580, Act 580; Commissioner of Law Revision and Percetakan Nasional Malaysia Bhd, 2006 (kpwkm.gov.my; Othman, Che Din, & Sipon, 2000; See & Ng, 2010). As a result, Malaysia is regarded as one of the first countries in the South East Asian and Australasian region to have a specific Act to regulate the profession. This Act provides an advantage over many other Asian countries because it safeguards professional standards and provides a legal and social framework for counselling in Malaysia (Glamcevski, 2008).

As an Act that applies only to Malaysian practising counsellors regarding their practice, it aims to regulate the practice of professional counselling in Malaysia (Mohd Ishak, Amat, & Abu Bakar, 2012). The Malaysian Counsellors Advisory Council was established under the Act. It acts as an advisory body to the Minister on matters pertaining to the Act and matters referred to it by the Board.

The Board of Counsellors is seen to hold more critical functions. The Act dictates that the Board is to (1) oversee the provision of counselling services; (2) to evaluate the need for counselling services in Malaysia; (3) regulate the training of counsellors and determine the types and levels of counselling that can be made available; (4) determine

DOI: 10.4324/9781003490067-36

the qualifications entitling a person to be registered under the Act; (5) determine the standard of counselling training programmes; (6) make recommendations to the government in relation to the standard of counselling services; (7) register counsellors and make them qualified; (8) regulate chargeable fees by a registered counsellors for his services; (9) appoint members to sit on any board, committee, or body formed for any purpose affecting the counselling profession; to regulate the conduct of the counselling profession including prescribing the code of ethics for the counselling profession; and (10) to perform other activities as deemed necessary to enable it to carry out its functions effectively.

Under the Act, counselling is defined as 'a systematic process of helping relationships based on psychological principles performed by a registered counsellor in accordance with the counselling code of ethics to achieve a voluntary favourable holistic change, development, and adjustment of the client, such that the change, development, and adjustment will continue throughout the lifespan of the client' (Act 580; Commissioner of Law Revision and Percetakan Nasional Malaysia Bhd, 2006).

Based on the definition above, it can be understood that counselling can only be performed by a registered counsellor. Sub-section 22(1) of the Counsellors Act 1998 mandates that individuals must register for the practice as a counsellor in order to use the title 'registered counsellor' or to use displays on any form of devices representing that he or she is a registered counsellor. Additionally, they must also hold a valid practicing certificate issued under this Act (Sub-section 23(1). To register, a person must be a Malaysian citizen or a Malaysian permanent resident, aged 21 years and above, entitled and suitable to be registered as a counsellor, and hold qualifications as listed in the Counsellors Act 1998. Failure to do so causes one to be guilty of an offense and shall on conviction be liable to a fine not exceeding thirty thousand ringgit or imprisonment for a term not exceeding three years or both as stated in Sub-section 22(2) of Act 580.

The Malaysian Board of Counsellors also has regulations for non-Malaysian citizens and non-Malaysian permanent residents wishing to practise as counsellors in Malaysia. According to the Counsellor Act 1998, they may apply for temporary registration. The Malaysian Board of Counsellors will consider the registration of a person who is registered or licensed as a counsellor in the country where he or she ordinarily practises counselling, has counselling expertise, and physical presence in Malaysia for not less than one hundred and eighty days in a calendar year to conduct counselling services (Act 580; Commissioner of Law Revision and Percetakan Nasional Bhd, 2006).

Ethical codes

The issue of unethical conduct of counsellors is provided in Sections 6 and 7 of the Act. A committee will hold an investigation for every complaint against any counsellors. If found guilty, the counsellor's name will be removed from the registry, and the counsellor will be suspended or ordered to be fined, or they may also be reprimanded for the misconduct. Disciplinary authority is given exclusively to the Board, which exercises disciplinary control in respect of all such counsellors in accordance with the Act. Offensive practices (such as fraud and forgery) and their related penalties are also clearly provided in the Act.

To further strengthen the professionalism in the delivery of the counselling services, a specific code of ethics was developed, following an adaptation of the American Counseling Association (ACA) Code of Ethics (American Counseling Association, 2014) as a result of the joint effort between the Malaysian Board of Counsellors and the Malaysian Counselling Association. Hence, the Counsellors Act 1998 and the Code of Ethics (Malaysian Board of Counsellors, 2016) provide guidelines for Malaysian counsellors to have ethical and professional practices. In many circumstances, the content in the Code of Ethics matches or complements the Act. Nevertheless, in cases where conflict arises between the two, the content of the law prevails. An example of such conflict is when the counsellor finds that his or her colleague has wrongfully practised or claimed (in an advertisement) his expertise in the area that he is not an expert or was trained in (Mohd. Ishak et al., 2012). The code of ethics outlines the steps that the counsellor needs to take to avert and correct any unethical conduct displayed by his or her peers. It is further reinforced in the Counsellors Act 1998 that a disciplinary punishment shall be imposed if the counsellor acts fraudulently, dishonesty, or moral turpitude.

Other than this, the functions of the Code of Ethics (Malaysian Board of Counsellors, 2016) are to provide guidelines to assist counsellors to act professionally so that services can be provided effectively and values can be nurtured, to create principles that determine ethical behaviour and best practices, to enable the Board to clarify ethical responsibilities of counsellors registered with the Board, and to be the basis for processing complaints and inquiries on counsellors' ethics.

The Code of Ethics (Malaysian Board of Counsellors, 2016) comprises only eight sections as opposed to the nine of the ACA Code of Ethics. Sections A, B, C, and D of this code outline the responsibilities of counsellors towards their clients, other professionals, and the community. The elements of confidentiality, privileged communication, and privacy are highlighted to help build healthy relationships and avoid ones that may impair professional judgment or increase harm to the clients (Mohd. Ishak, 2012). Section E provides details about testing and evaluation issues. This is followed by Section F on supervision, training, and teaching, which relates to the counsellor–client as well as the supervisor/educator–student relationships. Aspects of multicultural competencies are also mentioned. The code also outlines counsellors' conduct when conducting research and publishing in Section G. Finally, Section H covers standards and laws pertaining to the resolution of ethical issues. This includes adherence to five basic moral principles: autonomy, nonmaleficence, beneficence, justice, and fidelity (Mat Rani et al., 2017; Mohd. Ishak et al., 2012).

As the mental health field is diverse, with counsellors and the client population varying in degrees in terms of the roles they play, the existing Code of Ethics (Malaysian Board of Counsellors, 2016) must be broad enough in scope to accommodate application in many different situations (Mat Rani et al., 2017). Another limitation of the code is that the guidelines provided may not always be clear. Thus there is a call for a more systematic manner of decision-making. There may be a need to fall back on the court's decisions for interpretation in some circumstances.

Both the Counsellors Act 1998 and the Code of Ethics (Malaysian Board of Counsellors, 2016) provide ample guidelines for counsellors to function effectively in the profession. However, there may be a need to update and revise the existing documents from time to time as they must adapt to changes as new issues or situations arise. For example, the ACA Code of Ethics has already included a new section on distance counselling, technology, and social media. Another example is in terms of counsellors' qualifications. Even though more institutions are providing counselling programmes, they are not yet listed in the Counsellors Act 1998; and this may later cause difficulties for graduates from those programmes to be registered under the Act. Hence, by keeping track of current development and revision of the existing guidelines, the counselling profession will maintain its relevance and further enhance the high standards of professionalism in the counselling profession within society.

Counselling education in Malaysia

The Malaysian Ministry of Education has been working on producing quality graduates in guidance and counselling. At present, counselling programmes are offered by various Malaysian public and private institutions of higher education. The early development of counselling in Malaysia began in schools and public institutions of higher learning in the late 1960s. During its inception, the field of counselling in Malaysia was heavily influenced by the counselling profession in the United States (Lloyd, 1987). The first two areas of emphasis were school guidance and drug abuse prevention. University of Malaya (UM) was the first to offer a guidance and counselling major as part of its Master's in Education programme in 1976, and Universiti Kebangsaan Malaysia (UKM) offered a Diploma in Psychology (Counselling), which was later changed to the Diploma in Counselling Psychology in 1979. By 1980, more Malaysian public universities began offering guidance and counsellor education programmes focusing on their specialisations to fulfil the Ministry of Education's goal of providing full-time school counsellors by the year 2000.

Concurrently, several Malaysian universities began by offering counselling services to their own university students to support them in navigating university life. MARA Institute of Technology was the first institution to offer counselling services to support its students, followed by the University of Malaya, Universiti Kebangsaan Malaysia, and other universities (Nasir, 2008). Currently, all public and private higher education institutions are required by the Malaysian Qualification Agency (MQA) to provide counselling services to their students, which must be performed by registered counsellors only (MQA, 2018).

Counsellor education

The Malaysian counsellor education incorporates multiple counselling and psychological components. In Malaysia, institutions offering counselling in the undergraduate and graduate levels include: Universiti Kebangsaan Malaysia (UKM), Universiti Putra Malaysia (UPM), Universiti Pendidikan Sultan Idris (UPSI), Universiti Sains Malaysian (USM), Universiti Malaya (UM), Universiti Teknologi Malaysia (UTM), Universiti Utara Malaysia (UUM), Universiti Malaysia Sabah (UMS), Universiti Malaysia Sarawak (UNIMAS), Universiti Malaysia Terengganu (UMT), Universiti Sains Islam Malaysia (USIM), Kolej Universiti Insaniah, and HELP University College.

At present, there are ten public universities offering counselling programmes at the Bachelor's level and Master's level, one public university offering a counselling programme at the Bachelor's level only, three private universities offering counselling programmes at the Master's level only, and ten public universities offering doctoral-level counselling programmes. At the Master's level, nine public universities offer coursework-based programmes, two offer a combination of coursework and research programmes, and one public university is currently offering a research-based programme (Malaysian Board of Counsellors, 2017b). All doctoral counselling degrees are currently offered in the research-based mode except the University of Malaya who began to offer a doctoral degree in a combined research and coursework mode. However, the research and coursework combination does not intend to produce counsellors who specialise in a particular area.

Curriculum and delivery

Overseen by the Malaysian Ministry of Education and the Malaysian Board of Counsellors, each counsellor education programme incorporates four components: knowledge, skills, research and assessment, and area of specialisation. Only some public higher education institutions have their own emphasised areas of specialisation (e.g., educational, management and organisation, marriage and family counselling, and drug and substance use/abuse). For example, the University Putra Malaysia is known for producing school counsellors, while the Universiti Sains Islam Malaysia offers Master's in Counselling (Family Counselling or Drug Abuse) specialisations. The other universities offer counselling programmes that train future counsellors in any setting without an area of specialisation.

Most programmes are delivered on-site through lectures and clinical training (practicum and internship). Practicum training is a required programme component and needs to be completed before the internship. Practicum is typically offered in-house at the programme's institution for one academic semester (4 months), accruing 253 contact hours. Practicum experience may include simulations, live or recorded sessions in counselling labs, case consultation, and clinical reports through supervision by a qualified supervisor. Counselling labs are specifically developed for individuals and group experience, allowing students to perform practicum and enhance their counselling competencies and experiences.

Experiential learning is a unique learning experience offered by counselling programmes in the form of counselling retreats, professional development, seminars, and professional counselling forums, social and community outreach projects, as well as client-centredcentred programmes. These programmes are designed to expose and create awareness to the counselling students on current societal and mental health issues faced by Malaysians.

Internship in this field is typically carried out by an outside organisation offering counselling services, lasting between 14 and 24 weeks, with 504 hours (192 direct contact hours of individual and group counselling). Students are supervised by a primary supervisor and an on-site supervisor based on recorded sessions and case studies. Their skills are evaluated based on specific areas, namely, administration, individual group counselling, and psychological assessment skills. They also have opportunities to involve rehabilitation and prevention.

Issues in counsellor education

The demand for counselling education continues to rise as mental health awareness increases among the Malaysian authorities and society. About four decades ago, public universities were satisfying the increasing demands for counsellors by offering quality programmes and specialisations aimed at responding to the current social and mental health needs of Malaysian society. However, despite numerous advances made by the Malaysian counselling profession, some challenges remain.

As the number of training programmes continues to grow in the country, more counsellor educators will be needed to teach these programmes. However, at present, there are no standardised educational, clinical, or research requirements to become a counsellor educator in these institutions other than the requirement to register with the Malaysian Board of Counsellors. As a result, information on the varying educators' educational and research backgrounds, teaching and pedagogical methods, and clinical skills remain unregulated. One significant implication is the difficulty in measuring the qualification of the area of specialisation being offered by the counsellor educators.

In addition, there is no existing database or mechanism to track the current human resource, educators, researchers, research projects, and area of specialisations of the Malaysian counselling professionals. With the increased number of research-based doctoral counselling programmes, the existence of a national counselling database with vital information on the progress of the profession will allow for cross-cultural, international research opportunities.

Counselling representation in Malaysia

The first national professional counselling association in Malaysia was established on 16 January 1982, called the Malaysian Counselling Association (PERKAMA). Originally known as the Malaysian Counsellor Association, it was founded by a group of school counsellors, counsellor educators, and welfare officers interested in counselling (Othman & Abdullah, 2015; See, Othman, Salim, & Che Din, 2009). The name was later changed to the Malaysian International Counselling Association (PERKAMA International) in 2011 (Mohamad Hanafi & Jusoh, 2015).

The association's primary purpose is to provide a professional base for Malaysian counsellors or those in related professions in terms of professional orientation and esprit de corps (Mohd Ishak et al., 2012). Other aims of the organisation include: enabling the development of the profession, encouraging learning, professionalism, and competency of counsellors, enhancing identity, harmony, and collaboration among members from various disciplines through the exchange of knowledge and experiences, as well as providing a resource of counselling professionals to help social and mental health issues in the society (Jusoh, 2015; Mohd Ishak et al., 2012).

Beginning as a small association with about 500 to 1,000 members (Glamcevski, 2008; See et al., 2009), this association now has over 7,000 members (Malaysian Board of Counsellors, 2016). Membership of PERKAMA International is open to those who are qualified in counselling and related fields. Those who do not have the required qualifications are accepted as associate members or student members (Mohd Ishak et al., 2012; Zambri, 2012).

PERKAMA has played a massive role in lifting the dignity of professional members of the community. Upholding the belief that professionalism among counsellors requires identification of professional norms with peers, PERKAMA had taken the initiative to formulate a code of ethics in 2008 before it was accepted and revised as the Code of Ethics by the Malaysian Board of Counsellors in 2011 (Mat Rani et al., 2017; Mohd. Ishak et al., 2012). Other roles played by PERKAMA include providing services related to social issues, implementing professional development programmes to enhance the level of counsellors' competencies, expanding the scope of community service in the society, creating community counselling to meet current social needs, mobilising all counselling practitioners to actively engage in community development professionally and becoming a prominent advocate for the Malaysian Board of Counsellors to ensure that every counselling practitioner is qualified and registered (Mohammad Hanafi & Jusoh, 2015).

The association is active in organising conferences, seminars, and workshops to help increase Malaysian counsellors' professionalism and competencies (Mohamad Hanafi & Jusoh, 2015; Mohd Ishak et al., 2012). In other words, PERKAMA supports the life-long learning initiative as implemented by the Malaysian Board of Counsellors (Mohd. Ishak et al., 2012). The Malaysian Board of Counsellors promotes life-long learning by introducing Continuing Professional Development (CPD) points to ensure that counsellors are up-to-date with the latest development in counselling.

The association also encourages its members to be involved in research and publications. In 1984, the association published the first issue of its official journal, which covered both the theoretical and practical aspects of counselling (Glamcevski, 2008). Besides that, books, articles, and magazines such as Suara PERKAMA International and other publications have also been distributed to advance the field of counselling in Malaysia (Othman & Abdullah, 2015; Zambri, 2012). PERKAMA has also sought the accreditation of counselling services as a guideline in providing monitoring procedures on practitioners on any premise that carries out counselling services (Mohamad Hanafi & Jusoh, 2015).

Members of PERKAMA are also active in the community and consultative work in order to strengthen the counselling services and professionalism in the community (Zambri, 2012). PERKAMA members were involved in providing crisis intervention and counselling services during the MH370 and MH17 airplane tragedies and various natural disasters throughout the country and abroad (Mat Rani et al., 2017).

Previously, counsellors had only one local counselling association to enhance their professionalism through participation in activities, which is PERKAMA (Mohd. Ishak et al., 2012). However, given the rapid development and social changes in the country, new counselling associations have emerged. Among these associations include the Association of Education Counsellors Malaysia (PEKA), the Association of Syar'ie Counselling Malaysia, the Malaysian Registered Professional Counsellor Association (PAKARMALAYSIA), and the National Association of Christian Counsellors (NACC Malaysia).

Even though this growth can be seen as a positive effort among counsellors, Abu Bakar (2016) was of the view that there is a need for stakeholders such as the Malaysian Ministry of Women, Family, and Community Development, the Malaysian Board of Counsellors, and the Malaysian Public Service Department (Counselling and Psychology Division) to coordinate the associations related to counselling profession as well as the counselling activities to ensure that the services provided are well-regulated and beneficial to the society. In contrast, the authors view that having divisions organised around specific interest and practice areas such as those developed by the American Counseling Association (ACA) would better enhance counsellors' professional identity.

Pathways to becoming a counsellor in Malaysia

The most straightforward way to become a practising counsellor in Malaysia is to pursue a bachelor's degree in counselling in an accredited institution, which takes four years to complete. With the qualification, a person is eligible to apply to be a registered counsellor once he or she passes the interview conducted by the Malaysian Board of Counsellors. Once registered, the person is also eligible to apply for the Certificate of Practice, which allows him or her to practise as a counsellor. A person can also be a registered counsellor by pursuing a Master's degree in any accredited institution. The primary academic qualification to pursue a Master's degree is a Bachelor's degree in any field. Some public universities have strict entrance requirements to a Master's degree level. For instance, the University of Malaya requires applicants to have at minimum a 3.0 CGPA at the Bachelor's level in any human-related field and documented experience in the helping field. The Universiti Kebangsaan Malaysia requires applicants to have a strong background in psychology. If accepted, the person may be required to take and pass several pre-requisite psychology courses. Public universities usually have stricter requirements due to the limited places offered and the lack of training staffing.

Work setting

Registered counsellors in Malaysia are employed in different and various fields. They are mostly available in public sectors such as schools, hospitals, rehabilitation centres, and higher education institutions. Counsellors are also available in limited private sectors, mainly because private sectors are unwilling to invest in mental health care. Some government-listed companies appoint consultants to be their counsellors who are called if the service is needed.

Other than the public and private sectors, some counsellors choose to work with non-government organisations that provide support services for free. Some religious institutions like mosques and churches also offer counselling services. However, the counselling services at these settings are usually not regulated because the job is performed voluntarily. In addition, some professional helpers are not trained counsellors, yet they claim that they are counsellors.

Supervision of counselling in Malaysia

Supervision of practicum

There are two stages of supervision of counselling in Malaysia. First, supervision during the practicum hours, and second, supervision of internship experience. Students taking practicum courses are advanced Bachelor's and Master's degree, students. According to the Standard and Qualification of Counsellor Training (Malaysian Board of Counsellors, 2016), only students who have completed core courses, including the Life Span, Counselling Theories of Career Development, and Group Counselling courses, are allowed to register for the practicum course. As discussed in the earlier section, the counselling profession in Malaysia is regulated by the Malaysian Board of Counsellor. The Board's responsibility is not limited to monitoring the registration of counsellors. Together with the Malaysian Qualification Agency, the Board is also responsible for monitoring the local institutions in Malaysia, which offer counselling programmes. This is to ensure that the curriculum is in line with the Board's standards. During their practicum training, student counsellors are required to complete supervised practicum hours. A qualified practicum supervisor must obtain at least a Master's degree from an accredited institution, either locally or abroad, and he or she must also be registered with the Board. The supervisor can be assisted by a Registered Counsellor with a minimum qualification of a Bachelor's degree in counselling, with a valid Certificate of Practice issued by the Malaysian Board of Counsellors.

In terms of the practicum sites, the Malaysian Board of Counsellor requires the site to have the necessary facilities for clinical training. In addition, the practicum supervision is held on campus. Therefore, institutions that offer counselling programmes must have counselling training facilities. The facilities provide conducive environments for individual and group counselling, audio-video equipment for supervision purposes, and support staff responsible for taking care and handling the equipment.

A supervised practicum consists of three-credit hours, which is held for 14 weeks or a semester. During this period, the students are expected to complete 252 hours, of which

96 hours should be spent in direct contact with clients. Students accumulate their direct contacts with clients through counselling sessions. These sessions can be in the form of individual, group, couple, marriage, or family counselling.

Practicum supervision procedure

The Malaysian Board of Counsellors provides four aspects that a counselling programme needs to follow. The four procedures are:

(1) Practicum supervision requirements – In order to fulfil the 252 hours of practicum, the Malaysian Board of Counsellor, in its Standard and Qualification of Counsellor Training, set six rules and requirements for the students. The six rules are: (1) Official registration in practicum course; (2) Practicum students need to conduct sessions from the beginning towards the termination; (3) Each student needs to be supervised at least three times by the practicum supervisor; (4) The practicum site must meet the Malaysian Board of Counsellor's requirement as discussed in the previous section; (5) Practicum students need to conduct a minimum of 3-sessions with each client; (6) The handling of the administration and supervision of the practicum must conform to the requirement set by the Standard and Qualification of Counsellor Training.

(2) Evaluation criteria – The practicum supervisors need to evaluate specific criteria set by the Malaysian Board of counsellors. The criteria to be supervised include: (a) A application of theory; (b) Application of counselling techniques' skills; (c) Case conceptualisation; (d) Intervention plan; and (e) Compliance to ethical codes.

(3) Record keeping – All hours collected during the practicum training need to be documented. The purpose of documentation is to protect both counsellors and clients. Counsellors are responsible for keeping and managing the record and documentation of daily activities in the logbooks, treatment intervention plans, counselling session reports, standardised tests, and any other documents that are deemed necessary for counselling.

(4) Counselling-related activities – Lastly, the practicum supervisors are also responsible for supervising cases requiring referral, consultation, guidance activities, testing and measurement in counselling, professional growth activities, and educational psychology.

Although the Board has set standards that institutions and students need to follow, there is no specific explanation on how the 252 hours can be met. The guidelines provided in the Standard and Qualification of Counsellor Training (Malaysian Board of Counsellor, 2016) only provide general recommendations. Institutions that offer counselling programmes often set their own rubric in addition to the general guidelines to ensure that their practicum students meet the requirement. For example, Universiti Malaya, which is the pioneer in counselling programmes in the country, has a very rigorous procedure to meet the Board's requirements. Students are to conduct 24 hours of individual counselling, 30 hours of group counselling, and 42 hours of supervision. These three activities contribute to 96 hours of direct contact. The remaining hours are fulfilled through 36 hours of peer supervision, 20 hours of programme management, 48 hours of the preparation of clients' reports, 36 hours of administrative work, and 16 hours of counselling promotional activities. Judging from the hours, it can be summarised that the total supervision hours received by the practicum students are 78 hours.

In conclusion, the supervision practice during the practicum training is a tedious and challenging job. Although the course consists of only 3 credit hours, the practicum students need to accrue 252 hours in total within one particular semester. At the same time, the students undergoing practicum usually have not finished some courses. This means that they are usually registered in other courses while in practicum. The main aim of the practicum is to prepare students for internship experiences. Therefore, this period is also known as a pre-internship experience.

Supervision of internship experience

While doing practicum training on campus, students are strongly recommended to find a suitable internship site. Students are required to find internship sites by themselves. They may choose to do their internship in educational, mental health, rehabilitation, or any other settings approved by the academic supervisor. In order to maintain the supervision standards, the students are assigned, two supervisors. Firstly, the academic supervisor, and secondly, the site supervisor. Both supervisors must be registered counsellors and are registered with the Malaysian Board of Counsellors.

Students need to complete a minimum of 504 hours of internship that consists of six credits. Of 504 hours, 192 hours must consist of direct contact with clients either in individual, group, couple, or family settings. The remaining 312 hours need to be dedicated to other counselling related-activities such as administrative work, mental health promotions, and outreach programming.

In order to ensure that interns are academically and mentally prepared for internship training, the Malaysian Board of Counsellors (2016b) requires that they finish all the courses listed in the curriculum in which they enrol. This will equip the interns with all the knowledge necessary in understanding the clients, from introductory psychology courses to counselling practice. In addition, during the internship, they conduct a minimum of three counselling sessions and receive a minimum of five supervision sessions.

Internship supervision guidelines

The Malaysian Board of Counsellors provides general guidelines in internship supervision. They can be divided into internship supervision requirements, internship evaluation criteria, record keeping, and counselling related-activities.

1. Supervision requirement. In their guidelines, it is noted that supervision can be face to face, either in an individual or group supervision. The ratio between the supervisors and students in individual supervision is one supervisor to a maximum of five interns. Besides face-to-face supervision, the Board also recommends group supervision. An academic supervisor can supervise a maximum of ten interns in a group. Each intern must receive individual supervision or in groups at least five times during their internship training period. Since the interns are supervised by two supervisors, academic and site supervisors, both must rate, evaluate and assess the interns' work. The academic supervisor contributes a maximum of 80 per cent marks, while the site supervisor contributes the remaining 20 per cent. Both supervisors supervise and evaluate their interns' competencies regarding their direct contact with clients, record keeping, and organisation of counselling-related activities.

2. Evaluation criteria. The Malaysian Board of Counsellors lists six areas to be evaluated during the internship. Those areas are (1) Application of theory, (2) Using skills and techniques in counselling, (3) Case conceptualisation, (4) Treatment intervention and planning, (5) Compliance to ethical standards, and (6) Reflection. Area 6 is the only area that is not included for practicum students.

3. Record keeping. Interns are responsible for preparing documentation for each activity, direct contact, and the programme they organise as proof of accumulated hours. Record keeping tasks include the preparation and maintenance of a logbook, intervention planning, counselling report, the use of test and measurement, and any related documents.

4. Counselling-related activities. Supervisors play an active role in helping interns to do necessary referrals, consultations, organise guidance programmes and the professional growth of the counsellors, and test and measure while increasing their exposure to psychology.

In summary, the internship experience allows the students to have life experience as professional helpers in a natural setting. The period is crucial because it allows them to polish their knowledge and skills before graduation. However, the Malaysian Board of Counsellors only provides general guidelines on the number of required supervisions each intern must receive. The rubric and specific guidelines of supervision are not mentioned in their standard. Thus, it is up to the individual supervisor to interpret the standard. There is no uniform standard that all accredited institutions can follow and refer to. This leads to a question of whether the interns receive enough supervision or otherwise. Another question is the qualification of the supervisor. The standards of counselling training only mention the minimum academic qualification of supervisors, which is a Master's degree in counselling from an accredited institution. This implies that any supervisor who graduated with a Master's degree or a PhD without prior counselling experience is qualified to supervise the students as long as they are academicians. The supervisors' experience in counselling sessions is not noted in the Standard and Qualification of Counsellors' Training.

Current trends and future needs

Since the enactment of the Act of Counsellor in 1998 (Act 580; Commissioner of Law Revision and Percetakan Nasional Malaysia, 2006), counselling in Malaysia has exceedingly developed and is gradually accepted as a professional field. Before the enactment, counselling is like any other helping field that is not regulated. The rapid development of counselling is evidenced by the increasing number of higher education institutions offering counselling programmes and the increasing number of registered counsellors. With the increasing number of institutions that offer counselling programmes and the number of registered counsellors, there is a need to look at future trends. Based on the recent report issued by the Malaysian Board of Counsellors (2018b), the urban areas, particularly in the state of Selangor and the main capital city of Kuala Lumpur, recorded the highest number of registered counsellors. At the end of 2017, there were 7,765 registered counsellors in Malaysia. The report also shows that 68 per cent of the counsellors are female, and 69 per cent are Malays.

Malaysia is a multi-racial society. Even though multicultural counselling is a compulsory course in all counselling programmes offered by accredited higher education institutions, the fact remains that counselling clients from diverse backgrounds are challenging. Most

Malay counsellors work in government sectors, in which the majority of the population they serve is Malay. Examples of these sectors are schools, public hospitals, government departments, rehabilitation and detention centres, and prisons. The service is provided free to people who are part of the sectors and members of the public. More counsellors from other ethnicities are needed to improve the counselling service, especially in the government sector. Higher education institutions may play a role in recruiting more students from minority groups. More outreach programmes are also needed to introduce the field to the public. One of the reasons behind a large number of registered counsellors in urban areas is the awareness of the importance of mental health among the urban population, who are mostly educated. The government agencies such as the health clinic need to take the initiative to introduce the service. Currently, the government sectors that offer the service are usually located in big cities.

Another issue that needs attention is the need to introduce areas of specialisation in counselling. Of all the counselling programmes offered by Malaysian higher education institutions, only one offers programme specialisation. The Malaysian Board of Counsellors (2016c) has prepared the Standard and Qualification of Counsellor Training (with specialisation). The Board suggests six specialisation areas. Unfortunately, most universities choose not to offer any specialisation areas due to the lack of human resources. The biggest challenge is the lack of uniform standards and qualifications for counsellor education.

The Board only requires counsellor educators to be registered with the Board and have a Master's degree from accredited institutions. Most of these educators graduated from Malaysian public universities that do not have any concentration areas. Counsellor educators in Malaysia also completed their doctoral degrees from different institutions. Some graduated from foreign universities and come from local public universities. A majority of them graduated from institutions in Commonwealth countries, which focus on research. Commonwealth countries such as the United Kingdom, Australia, and New Zealand. A small number of educators in this field graduated from American universities that offer more concentration in counselling.

The limited number of counsellor educators who receive training in certain specialisation areas becomes a challenge to institutions that intend to offer specialisation areas. Due to this fact, there is a need for the Malaysian Board of Counsellors to review their standards and qualifications of counsellor educators because counselling is a field that requires practical training under proper supervision. A counsellor cannot claim that he or she is a specialist in a particular area just by doing empirical research in one particular area. Counsellor educators in Malaysia focus their work on research and teaching. Thus, they need proper practical training in specialised areas if they want to teach and train counsellors who intend to be specialists.

Regarding the areas of specialisation, the Malaysian Board of Counsellors may also introduce the Continuing Education (CE) programme. Specialists in particular areas can handle the CE programme, and they may consist of Malaysians or foreign experts. In addition, qualifications obtained from CE can be added to existing credentials to indicate the counsellors' and counsellor educators' qualifications.

Supervision after graduation is another critical issue in the field of counselling. Malaysian Board of Counsellors under the Counsellor Act 1998 only requires individuals to register with the Board. Once individuals finish their degrees, they are eligible to apply. Once registered, they can offer and perform counselling services without supervision. The Counsellor Act 1998 does not mention post-graduation supervision. This may lead to situations where inexperienced counsellors conduct counselling. Without proper supervision, there may be inexperienced counsellors who harm clients. Counsellor educators without experience in counselling may also have issues in teaching practical courses. Since there is no post-graduation supervision of counselling, some counsellor educators may never practise in a natural setting, yet they train future counsellors. Due to this limitation, it is strongly recommended that the Malaysian Board of Counsellors review the standard and qualifications of counsellor educators to improve the counsellor's education training.

Conclusion

Counselling in Malaysia has gone through many developmental stages. During the infancy stage, counselling was only available in selected educational institutions such as schools and a small number of higher education institutions. The service was performed by anybody who may have personal characteristics that make them suitable for helping others. With no act and standard to regulate the profession, anybody may call themselves counsellors and claim that they were doing counselling jobs. With the enactment of the counsellor Act in 1998 and the establishment of the Board of Counsellors, counselling has gradually been accepted and became well-known. Awareness to seek counselling services from professionals who are registered also increased. Today, counselling is the only helping field in Malaysia with an Act and Board that regulates the service and the practitioners offering the service. The Act and the Board also regulate the training of counsellors. Other fields like psychology and social work are still not regulated by any act.

Despite this positive development, there are many limitations that the authors have discussed and highlighted in this chapter. Continuous improvements are needed to ensure that the counselling profession remains a respected helping profession in the country.

Final Note : Please address correspondence regarding this chapter to Dr Melati Sumari, Department of Educational Psychology and Counselling, Faculty of Education, University of Malaya, 50603 Kuala Lumpur. Email : melati@um.edu.my

References

Abu Bakar, A.Y. (2016). 'Merakyatkan' khidmat kaunseling. Retrieved 4 November 2018 from www. utusan. com.my/rencana/utama/8216-merakyatkan-8217-khidmatkaunseling-1.331513

American Counseling Association. (2014). ACA code of ethics. Retrieved November 9, 2018, from www.counseling.org/ resources/aca-code-of-ethics.pdf

Commission of Law Revision and Percetakan Nasional Malaysia Bhd. (2006). Laws of Malaysia: Act 580 Counsellors Act 1998. Retrieved 2 November 2018, from www.agc.gov.my/agc/ Akta/ Vol.%2012/Act%20580.pdf

Feit, S.S., & Lloyd, A.P. (1990). A profession in search of professionals. *Counselor Education and Supervision*, 29, 216–219.

Glamcevski, M. (2008). The Malaysian counselling profession: History and brief discussion of the future. *Counselling, Psychotherapy, and Health*, 4(1), Counselling in the Asia Pacific Rim: A Coming Together of Neighbours Special Issue, 1–18.

Johari, M.J. (2001). *Etika professional [Professional ethics]*. Skudai: Penerbit Universiti Teknologi Malaysia Press.

Lloyd, A.P. (1987). Counselor education in Malaysia. *Counselor Education and Supervision*, 26, 221–227.

Malaysian Board of Counsellors. (2016). *Standard and qualification of counsellor training*. Putrajaya: Lembaga Kaunselor Malaysia.

Malaysian Board of Counsellors. (2017). *Laporan Tahunan 2016 [Annual report 2016]*. Putrajaya: Kementerian Pembangunan Wanita, Keluarga dan Masyarakat

Malaysian Qualification Agency. (2018). Assuring quality. Retrieved November 9, 2018, from www. mqa.gov.my/ portalmqav3/red/en/qa.cfm

Mat Rani, N.H., Wan Jaafar, W.M., Mohd. Noah, S., Mohd Jais, S., & Bistamam, M.N. (2017). An overview of counselor ethical code and ethical principles in Malaysian setting. *International Journal of Academic Research in Business and Social Sciences*, 7, 862–868.

Mohammad Hanafi, N., & Jusoh, A.J. (2015). Sejarah PERKAMA dan kepimpinan Tan Sri Dr. Nordin Kardi (2005-2013). *Jurnal PERKAMA*, 19, 91–109.

Mohd Ishak, N., Amat, S., & Abu Bakar, A.Y. (2012). Counseling professional ethics from the viewpoint of counselor educators. *Journal of Educational Psychology and Counseling*, 5, 71–80.

Nasir, R. (2008). *Kaunseling Kerjaya: Anjakan daripada Konvensionalisme*. Bangi, Selangor: Penerbit UKM.

Ng, K.S., & Steven, P. (2001). Creating a caring society: Counseling in Malaysia before 2020 AD. *Asian Journal of Counseling*, 8, 87–101.

Othman, A. & Abdullah, S.S. (2015). Counselling in Malaysia: Trend and practice with the Malays. *International Journal of Business and Applied Social Science*, 1, 1–10.

Othman, A.H., Che Din, M.S., & Sipon, S. (2000). Latihan kaunseling di Malaysia: Satu ulasan dan cadangan. *Jurnal PERKAMA*, 8, 137–151.

See, C.M., & Ng, K.M. (2010). Counseling in Malaysia: History, current status, and future trends. *Journal of Counseling and Development*, 88, 18–22.

See, C.M., Othman, A.H., Salim, S., & Che Din, M.S. (2009). Multicultural approaches to healing and counseling in Malaysia. In Gerstein L.H., Heppner, P., Aegisdottir, S., Leung, S.A., and Norsworthy, S. (Eds). *International handbook of cross-cultural counseling: Cultural assumptions and practices worldwide* (pp. 221–233) Melbourne: Sage.

Zambri, M.I. (2012). Ketahui Sejarah PERKAMA. Retrieved 4 November 2018 from https:// gerbangilmukaunseling.blogspot. com/2012/12/ketahui-sejarah-perkama.html

30 The Counseling Profession in the Philippines

Ma. Teresa G. Tuason, Margaret Helen Alvarez, and Bridget Rose Stanton

In the following few pages, the counseling profession in the Philippines is reviewed. Regulation of counseling in the Philippines advanced drastically due to the Guidance and Counseling Act of 2004, RA 9258 (Republic Act No. 9258). Counseling education and employment opportunities in counseling in the Philippines are also presented. Similarly, counseling representation and the ways in which people can become counselors in the Philippines are outlined.

Counseling regulation in the Philippines

Counseling in the Philippines has drastically advanced due to the Guidance and Counseling Act of 2004, RA 9258 (Republic Act No. 9258), which in a short matter of time, professionalized the practice of guidance and counseling. Because of RA 9258, the Professional Regulatory Board of Guidance and Counseling (PRB) was created, and in collaboration with the Accredited Professional Organization (APO), which is the Philippine Guidance Counseling Association, Inc. (PGCA) had the mandate to formulate the rules and regulations (referred to as the Implementing Rules and Regulations or the IRR for the Guidance and Counseling Act of 2004) that govern the profession of counseling. The IRR were written, formulated, adopted, and took effect in September 2007 (House Resolution No. 2057). Prior to this time, there were no legal or statutory means by which the practice of counseling was regulated. What may have existed was a voluntary regulation of the profession, where only people who were trained in guidance and counseling, counseling education, and counseling psychology identified as counselors and practiced the profession. Before the Guidance and Counseling Act of 2004, no movement precluded anyone who claimed to have had any training in counseling whatsoever to identify and practice as a counselor, nor was there any regulation, laws, or rules to ensure adequate training and ethical practice. In essence before 2004, the guidance counselor had no professional identity (Santamaria & Watts, 2003).

Judging by the nationwide regulation and the Republic Act on the profession, counseling practice was regulated much earlier than the practice of psychology, such that the Guidance and Counseling Act became a law in 2004 (Republic Act No. 9258), while the Philippine Psychology Act (Republic Act No. 10029), regulating the practice of Psychology and creating a Professional Regulatory Board of Psychology, was approved in March 2010 (Professional Regulatory Board of Psychology, 2012). The Guidance and Counseling Act of 2004 defined a guidance counselor as a Filipino (natural born or naturalised) who has been registered and issued a valid Certificate of Registration and a valid Professional Identification Card, and who performs the functions of guidance and counseling. It is a

DOI: 10.4324/9781003490067-37

monumental action that, because of the Guidance and Counseling Act, no person can practice guidance and counseling and call himself or herself a counselor without a valid Certificate of Registration and a valid Professional Identification Card.

Counseling, interchangeably referred to as guidance and counseling, is defined as 'the profession that involves the use of an integrated approach to the development of a well functioning individual primarily by helping him/her to utilise his/ her potentials to the fullest and plan his/her present and future in accordance with his/her abilities, interests, and needs' (Republic Act No. 9258). The functions of a guidance counselor identified in Republic Act 9258 are counseling, psychological testing (personality, career, interest, mental ability, aptitude, achievement, learning and study orientation), research, placement and group processes, and teaching guidance and counseling courses, specifically those covered in the licensure examinations, and other services related to human development.

Article III of the Guidance and Counseling Act mandates that individuals register for the practice of guidance and counseling primarily through licensure examination. Individuals are eligible to take the licensing exam with these three criteria: a) citisen of the Philippines or a foreigner whose country enjoys reciprocity, b) has no convictions of any offense, c) a Bachelor's degree and a Master's degree in guidance and counseling from an institution recognised or accredited by the Commission on Higher Education. Passing the licensure exam means to have a weighted general average of 75 per cent and to have no grade lower than 60 per cent in any of the five subjects: Philosophical, Psychological, and Sociological Foundations of Guidance; Counseling Theories, Tools, and Techniques; Psychological Testing; Organization and Administration of Guidance Services; and Group Process and Program Development. Out of the individuals who took the exam, the licensure examination pass rates have ranged from a low of 41.12 per cent in 2013 to a high of 72.2 per cent in 2009, and an average rate of per cent in the years 2008 to 2017 (Republic of the Philippines Regulation Commission, n.d.). According to Valdez (2018), the Philippines has a shortage of registered guidance counselors: from 2008 to 2017, there were only 3,220 in the entire nation, with about half of those (1,528) passing the licensing exam, while the other half (1,692) were grandfathered in by March 2009. Individuals could also register for the practice without examination (i.e., be grandfathered) within a two-year window, by submitting credentials before the Act took effect. Those eligible included: a) those who have doctoral and Master's degrees and evidence of at least three years teaching and/or counseling practice, b) those who had passed 18 units of Master's level courses in counseling, with evidence of at least seven years of counseling practice, and c) those who had completed academic requirements for a Master's degree, with evidence of five years of guidance and counseling experience.

Counseling education in the Philippines

Counseling education in the Philippines can occur at the undergraduate, master's, and doctoral levels. Individual programmes determine their curriculum and most include applications of counseling theories and models to Philippine society and current issues through research theses and dissertations (e.g., Garabiles, 2010; Nisperos, 1994). The requirement for registering to practice guidance and counseling is a Bachelor's degree in Guidance and Counseling or other related discipline, and a Master's degree in Guidance and Counseling. It is most usually the norm that students who pursue the study of counseling at the graduate level hold a Bachelor's degree in Psychology. Some Guidance and Counseling undergraduate programmes do exist, but they are not many (e.g., AB in

Guidance and Counseling, BSEd in Guidance and Counseling). The Bachelor's degree takes four years to complete and the AB/BS Psychology degree includes internship and practicum requirements as mandated by the Commission on Higher Education (CHED). The practicum is in the form of on-the-job training and has permission to train at government or non-government organisations for a mandatory 200 hours.

The Master's degree in Guidance and Counseling that is ultimately required in registering to practice as a counselor, abound in the Philippines. Across all regions of the Philippines, there are a total of 162 Master's degree programmes varying between Guidance and Counseling, Counseling Education, and Counseling (https://ched.gov. ph/). (The Master's degree that does not lead to registration as a counselor, but instead as a psychologist, is the Master's degree in Counseling Psychology. A Master's degree in Psychology, which also last two years, is the minimum requirement to take the licensing exam and register as a psychologist, along with having 200 hours of supervised clinical experience or practicum/internship work [Republic Act No. 10029]). As a consensus, Master's in Guidance and Counseling programmes in the Philippines take roughly two years to complete average 42 credits. Most of the programmes require an undergraduate degree in Psychology BS/BA or related field to enter and require a thesis and 200 hours of practicum/internship to complete. Similar to programmes in western countries, many job placements after licensure prefer hands-on experience, although a specific number of supervised counseling hours is not a requirement for registration and licensure. Programmes, therefore, design the Practicum course as a way to gain some experience in the field prior to entry, to allow some training in counseling, with close supervision of professors (Santamaria & Watts, 2003).

Although the terminal degree to register as a counselor is a Master's degree, the Philippines also has some (fewer than ten) doctoral programmes (e.g., EdD in Guidance and Counseling; PhD in Guidance and Counseling; PhD in Psychology and Guidance, PhD in Counseling). These programmes that focus on counseling, provide advanced studies in technique and innovative intervention practices that respond to trends and relevant issues in counseling, opportunities for research and empirical work in counseling, and advocacy projects to improve Philippine society as a whole. Most doctoral programmes consist of 60+ credits and require a dissertation.

Universities in the Philippines are accredited by boards that are authorised by the Commission on Higher Education (CHED). To strengthen and increase the quality of higher education, numerous accrediting agencies for both private (Association of Christian Schools and Colleges Accrediting Agency, Inc. [ACSC-AAI], the Philippine Accrediting Association of Schools, Colleges and Universities [PAASCU], and the Philippine Association of Colleges and Universities Commission on Accreditation [PACUCOA]) and public (the Accrediting Agency of Chartered Colleges and Universities of the Philippines [AACCUP] and the Association of Local Colleges and Universities Commission on Accreditation [ALCUCOA]) institutions exist to certify the levels of accredited programmes (Ching, 2012). Although a requirement of registration for the practice of counseling is a Master's degree in Guidance and Counseling from an institution recognised or accredited by CHED, there is no accreditation for the specific counseling programme, unlike in the US (e.g., CACREP, n.d.). To date, there are no accrediting boards specifically upholding the standards of guidance and counseling programmes because there are no standardised policies identified by CHED. As of January 2018, regulatory guidelines and standards for graduate programmes are said to be in progress by a technical committee led by CHED with identifying curriculum standards for guidance and counseling programmes (Valdez,

2018). This development is due to the observation that license examination pass rates have been low. Although according to the National Economic and Development Authority (NEDA) there are 162 institutions nationwide that offer guidance and counseling courses, there are no CHED-mandated policies, standards, and guidelines for guidance and counseling programmes and this may have contributed to the low pass rates (Valdez, 2018).

Opportunities for counseling jobs in the Philippines

Article II of the Implementing Rules and Regulations for Guidance Counselors (Professional Regulatory Board of Guidance and Counseling, 2007) describes their scope of practice as a) designated or appointed guidance counselors or counseling psychologists in educational institutions, rehabilitation centres, non-governmental organisations, community-based agencies, hospital and other workplace, b) faculty members who teach in the counselor education programme or who conduct training for guidance counselors, and c) administrators involved in the supervision and management of guidance services or programmes at the basic education, tertiary level and non-formal sectors as community, hospital, church, industry and private practice. While the PGCA lobbied for the recognition of licensed guidance counselors in the academe (Professional Regulatory Board of Guidance and Counseling, 2007), it appears that many of them may be working in other contexts, yet still adding to the shortage of guidance counselors. In addition, the PGCA also lobbied with both CHED and the Department of Education (Department of Education 2007) to have a guidance counselor in all schools. In particular, in 2006, CHED issued a memorandum CMO No. 21 (Commission of Higher Education, 2006) entitled 'Guidelines on Student Affairs and Services Program,' indicating the provision of such guidance services as counseling, appraisal, follow-up, and referral – all of which licensed guidance counselors are trained for. This resulted in a need for 10,000 Registered Counselors (RGC's), but such need was not fulfilled. Being that there are only 3,220 RGC's in the entire nation, and a great breadth of job opportunities and contexts that is under Article II of the IRR (Professional Regulatory Board of Guidance and Counseling, 2007) and lobbied by the PGCA, there is a disequilibrium, where RGC's are in low supply, but the demand for them is quite high. On the other hand, another kind of disequilibrium, is also experienced among Registered Psychometricians (RPm's). Coming on the heels of the Guidance and Counseling Act of 2004 has been the Psychology Act of 2009 for the licensing of psychometricians and psychologists. The accredited professional organisation, the Psychological Association of the Philippines (PAP) is lobbying for the appointment of these licensed professionals in schools. More specifically, 'Psychology Practitioners in Public Service,' a special interest group in PAP, was created to help lobby for staff positions for RPm's in government (including public schools) and to elevate the status of RPsy's (i.e., higher pay) in public service (Psychological Association of the Philippines, n.d.). Currently, there are about 15,000 RPm's (with just a little over a thousand registered psychologists) since the enactment of RA 10029 (Psychological Association of the Philippines, n.d.). Unlike the Implementing Rules and Regulations for Guidance Counselors (Professional Regulatory Board of Guidance and Counseling, 2007), that of Registered Psychologists (RPsy) were identified in terms of job placements and opportunities, but those for RPm's were not. Plans are underway with the PAP in lobbying to the Civil Service Commission and to CHED about job opportunities for psychometricians, specifically to work in academe (Psychological Association of the Philippines, n.d.). In essence, RPm's could potentially fill the need for RGC's in public schools if an item were granted them to work in public or private schools or in government, however, RPm's being holders of Bachelor's degrees in Psychology, could not work without supervision from a RPsy (Republic Act No. 10029).

Another issue that is at play here is that although RGC's are licensed to work in academe (for testing and guidance and counseling), there is a real limitation that RGC's enter private practice nor work in other clinical applications like testifying in court, unless they work in collaboration with a RPsy. Because of all these issues and circumstances and unintentional consequences of regulation, many seek licensure in both fields, as Registered Counselors and Registered Psychologists, so that they have the flexibility to work where there are opportunities and where their interests lie, such as working in more clinical settings or supervising RPm's in testing and assessment. In the current state, holding a Bachelor's degree in Psychology, and with 15,000 other RPm's, there are no job opportunities without obtaining a Master's degree in either the Counseling or Psychology route, sitting for both licensing exams, and registering in both fields.

If, however, this state of affairs continues without changes in the IRR for both fields – that is, the disproportionately low number of guidance counselors for the high demand and a disproportionately high number of RPm's for the lack of regulated job opportunities – the state of counseling as a profession and its progress may be disrupted. Moving the profession forward may necessitate that the respective rules and regulations (Republic Act No. 9258 & Republic Act No. 10029) adjust to the current state of affairs (e.g., workforce available, low passing rates of licensing examinees, regulated Master's degree in Counseling holders vs. Bachelor's in Psychology degree holders, staff positions in public schools).

Counseling representation in the Philippines

There are two sets of counseling organisations in the Philippines: one that is primarily counseling focused (e.g., PGCA, PACERS, IPCAP) and another where counseling is associated with a spiritual/religious orientation (e.g., PACC, FPCA). The main counseling organisation in the Philippines is the Philippine Guidance and Counseling Association (PGCA), which is the Accredited Professional Organization of the Professional Regulation Commission (Republic of the Philippines Regulation Commission, n.d.)—the government agency that regulates the status of professional licensure and status of various professions in the Philippines.

The PGCA, formerly known as the Philippine Guidance and Personnel Association (PGPA), is not only the Accredited Professional Organization of the PRC, but it has been the first to be PRC-accredited as a provider for Continuing Professional Education (CPE) (Philippine Guidance and Counseling Association, Inc., 2017). The PGCA is also a member branch of the American Counseling Association (American Counseling Association, n.d.). The PGCA held its first conference at the University of the Philippines in 1965, where it was conceived by 25 original members. Since this time, the PGCA holds conventions, has expanded its chapters across multiple regions, created international affiliation with the American Personnel and Guidance Association (APGA) and publishes Guidance Journal annually (Philippine Guidance and Counseling Association, Inc., 2017). The PGCA aims to be the 'premier Philippine professional organization of counselors with international recognition' (Philippine Guidance and Counseling Association, Inc., 2017). Members of the PGCA are one of three categories: Regular (licensed or non-licensed who are grandfathered in), Associate (who have not yet graduated or have no license yet) and Junior (hold a Bachelor's degree). The PGCA works to develop counselors who are professional and goal driven, and who fiercely advocate for their clients' well-being. The organisation actively strives to continually improve the field of counseling in its service to the profession and the Philippine society through research, meetings, and publications (Philippine Guidance and Counseling Association, Inc., 2017).

Philippine Association for Counselor Education, Research, and Supervision (PACERS). The organisation, PACERS, was established on 6 March 1976 as a way to promote the field of counselor education. Through their shared community, PACERS links counselors to researchers with the goal of exchanging expertise. With over 30 years of collaboration, and through supervision, professional training, and research, PACERS aims to take the lead in promoting counselor education (Philippine Association for Counselor Education, Research, and Supervision, n.d.). Members of PACERS are one of three categories, attesting to its academic stance: Regular/Associate (hold a Master's degree in Guidance and Counseling), Affiliate (in the process of completing a master's degree) and Life (sustained involvement as a member of the Board of Directors or a standing committee, nominated by the PACERS Board). PACERS is focused on the development of professionals who will contribute to the field of counseling, who promote discussion and high standards of ethical and professional competence, and who work to inspire counselors to contribute to training the next generation of counselors (Philippine Association for Counselor Education, Research, and Supervision, n.d.).

The Integrated Professional Counselors Association of the Philippines (IPCAP) was founded in 2006, in response to the Guidance and Counseling Act of 2004, to uphold the regulations outlined here. The IPCAP focuses on the development and professionalism of counselors, to increase networking, provide educational and counseling resources, and to enhance society though the competent practice of counseling. IPCAP is also an accredited provider for Continuing Professional Development (CPD) for Guidance Counselors (Integrated Professional Counselors Association of the Philippines, Inc., n.d.).

The following organisations, PACC and FPCAP, demonstrate the inherent value of faith and spirituality in Filipinos' lives (Dy-Liacco, Piedmont, Murray-Swank, Rodgerson, & Sherman, 2009), especially tapping into resources that are instrumental in counseling practice in the Philippines. What has evolved, therefore, is counseling that is rooted in the Philippine context and is therefore unique to the Philippines (Tanalega, 2004).

Philippine Association of Christian Counselors (PACC). The PACC was formed in 2000 after several different religious institutions met to create a group of Christian counselors dedicated to helping people reach emotional, relational, psychological, and spiritual wholeness while maintaining the highest standards for ethical practice in counseling. The PACC promotes the core values of authenticity, compassion, and competence. Unlike other professional organisations, the PACC does not require its members to hold specific academic degrees. Instead, prospective members must be active in the helping profession or with a fervent desire to serve through counseling in the future, abide by the PACC's code of ethics, and uphold the mission and vision of the PACC. The PACC has been approved by the Philippine Regulatory Commission Board for Guidance & Counseling as an accredited provider of CPD (Philippine Association of Christian Counselors, n.d.).

The Family and Pastoral Counseling Association of the Philippines (FPCAP www.fpcap. org/) was established in 2008 by 21 founding members, an organisation of pastoral and family counselors whose service is meant to serve, protect, and strengthen families. With the impetus of RA 9258, the FPCAP's mission is to dedicate itself to the development and welfare of professional practitioners who integrate counseling and spirituality. By combining psychotherapy and spirituality, counseling members of this organisation learn to promote relationship between families, God, and society. Members of FCAP are one of two categories: Regular (hold a Master's or doctoral degree in Counseling, Psychology, Family/Pastoral, or Theology and whose work centres around family/pastoral counseling) and Associate (students with at least 18 credits, practitioners, diploma certificate holders, or have been working in the field of family/pastoral counseling). FPCAP values high ethical standards of pastoral counseling, promotes integrity and service-orientation as well as continuous efforts to enrich lives through ministry (Family and Pastoral Counseling Association, n.d.).

Pathways to becoming a counselor in the Philippines

The most common way to become a practicing counselor in the Philippines is to study a Bachelor of Arts or Science in Psychology, Sociology, Theology or other related field, and then a Master's degree in Guidance Counseling, Counseling, Counseling Education, Pastoral Counseling, and so on. To practice as a counselor, after one's Master's degree, the next step is to register and be issued a valid Certificate of Registration and a valid Professional Identification Card, after having passed the licensure examination. A doctoral degree is not required to practice in the counseling profession, but a doctoral degree certainly predisposes someone to be in the leadership position of government or non-government organisations, as well as in academia or in research.

Supervision of counseling in the Philippines

Counseling supervision is usually provided through group/course supervision provided in the Practicum or Internship courses (usually two classes) in guidance and counseling Master's degrees. Students in Master's degree programmes usually and independently seek sites to practice counseling skills. In these placements, students gain experience in counseling practice, some are provided formal one-hour weekly supervision, some receive informal and irregular supervision, and some receive none. Other than group supervision provided in their classes, supervision is not systematic nor regulated, and is dependent on the supervisor or mentor the student works with. There is, however, a lot of mentoring and training happening outside the supervision hour, especially among peers.

Concluding remarks about counseling in the Philippines

Much like the diverse cultures inherent in the Philippines, counseling in the Philippines has developed with various names (guidance and counseling, counseling, pastoral/family counseling), but it has unified as a discipline and the practitioner's professional identity as a counselor has strengthened through the Guidance and Counseling Act of 2004. Because of the country's history (i.e., pre-colonial Philippines, Spanish colonisation, American occupation, the Marcos regime) (Roces & Roces, 1985) the roots of counseling straddle between indigenous (Enriquez, 1977) and religious/spiritual resources (Bulatao, 1992; Tanalega, 2004) and the societal problems that ensue from experiences of oppression. Competent counselors in the Philippines acknowledge the invaluable influences and resources in counseling that necessarily include the involvement of family, spirituality and/

or religiosity, and a powerful sense of hope and resilience (Tuason, Galang-Fernandez, Catipon, Dey, & Carandang, 2012).

The counseling practice in the Philippines needs to deeply respond to the protracted societal issues of widespread poverty, rampant violence, and trauma, frequent natural and human-made disasters, the inevitability of overseas working, countless street children and child labourers, prevalent graft and corruption in leadership positions, political unrest and senseless and unresolved deaths, and oppressive economic inequality, to be relevant advocates for well-being, mental health, and social justice (Tuason, 2008). In the Philippines, counseling has evolved into a recognised profession that is fundamental to increasing the wellbeing of individuals and essential to a movement of healing and nation building in society.

Final Note: Please address correspondence to Ma. Teresa Tuason, Department of Public Health, Bldg. 39, Rm 4067, University of North Florida, #1 UNF Drive, Jacksonville, FL 32224. Email: ttuason@unf.edu

References

Bulatao, J.C. (1992). *Phenomena and their interpretation: Landmark essays, 1957–1989.* Loyola Heights, Quezon City: Ateneo de Manila University Press.

Commission Higher Education https://ched.gov.ph/

Ching, G. S. (2012). Higher education accreditation in the Philippines: A literature review. *International Journal of Research Studies in Management*, 2, 63–74. doi:10.5861/ijrsm.2012.162

Commission of Higher Education. (2006). CHED Memorandum Order (CMO) No. 21, Series of 2006 'Guidelines on Student Affairs and Services Program'. Retrieved from https://ched.gov.ph/cmo-21-s-2006/

Commission on Higher Education. (2018, January 8). List of Higher Education Institutions. Retrieved from https://ched.gov.ph/list-higher-education-institutions/

Council for Accreditation of Counseling & Related Educational Programs (CACREP). (n.d.). Welcome to CACREP. Retrieved from www.cacrep.org

Department of Education. (2007). DM 424, Series of 2007 'Recognition of Guidance Counselors and Implementation of Career Guidance Programs in Public Secondary Schools'.

Dy-Liacco, G.S., Piedmont, R.L., Murray-Swank, N.A., Rodgerson, T.E., & Sherman, M.F. (2009). Spirituality and religiosity as cross-cultural aspects of human experience. *Psychology of Religion and Spirituality*, 1, 35–52. doi:10.1037/ a0014937

Enriquez, V.G. (1977). Filipino psychology in the third world. *Philippine Journal of Psychology*, 10(1), 3–18.

Family and Pastoral Counseling Association. (n.d.). Family and Pastoral Counseling Association, Inc. Retrieved from www.fpcap.org/home

Garabiles, M. (2010). Ang bagong ama: Predictors of wellbeing and involvement of Filipino fathers with migrant wives. Unpublished Master's thesis. Ateneo de Manila Quezon City, Philippines.

House Resolution No. 2057. (n.d.). A resolution on the Guidance and Counseling Act of 2004. Retrieved from http://congress. gov.ph/legisdocs/basic_16/HR02057.pdf

Nisperos, M. K. B. (1994). The world of the scavenger child: A phenomenological in-depth clinical study of scavenger children from Smokey Mountain. Unpublished Master's thesis. Ateneo de Manila University. Quezon City, Philippines.

Philippine Association of Christian Counselors. (n.d.). Retrieved from www.philacc.org/

Philippine Guidance and Counseling Association, Inc. (2017). Strengthening people helpers to care. Retrieved from www. pgca.com.ph/

Professional Regulatory Board of Guidance and Counseling. (2007). Implementing Rules and Regulations for the Guidance and Counseling Act of 2004 (RA 9258).

Professional Regulatory Board of Psychology. (2012). Implementing Rules and Regulations of Republic Act 10029, known as the 'Psychology Act of 2009'. Retrieved from https:// prc.gov. ph/sites/default/files/Board%20of%20Psychology%20 -%20Implementing%20Rules%20and%20 Regulation_0.pdf

Psychological Association of the Philippines. (n.d.). Psychological Association of the Philippines. Retrieved from www.pap. org.ph

Republic Act No. 9258. (n.d.). 'Guidance and Counseling Act of 2004'. Retrieved from www.lawp hil.net/statutes/repacts/ ra2004/ra_9258_2004.html

Republic Act No. 10029. (n.d.). 'Philippine Psychology Act of 2009'. Retrieved from www.lawphil. net/statutes/repacts/ ra2010/ra_10029_2010.html

Republic of the Philippines Regulation Commission. (n.d.). Professional Regulation Commission. Retrieved from https://prc. gov.ph

Roces, A., & Roces, G. (1985). *Philippines: Culture shock*. Singapore: Times Books Int'l.

Santamaria, J., & Watts, A. (2003). Public policies and career development: A framework for the design of career information, guidance and counseling services in developing and transition countries (Rep.). Retrieved from http://borbelytiborbors.extra. hu/GC/Philippines%20 Final%20Report.pdf

Tanalega, N.E. (2004). *Counseling Filipinos briefly*. Quezon City: Ugnayan at Tulong Para sa Maralitang Pamilya Foundation.

Tuason, M.T. (2008). Those who were born poor: A qualitative study of Philippine poverty. *Journal of Counseling Psychology*, 55, 158–171. doi:10.1037/00220167.55.2.158

Tuason, M.T., Galang-Fernandez, K.T., Catipon, M.A., Dey, M.L., & Carandang, M.L. (2012). Counseling in the Philippines: Past, present, future. *Journal of Counseling and Development*, 90(1), 373–377.

Valdez, D. (2018, 14 January). Lack of registered guidance counselors forces schools to keep unlicensed ones (Part 1). Retrieved from http://news.abs-cbn.com/focus/01/14/18/lackof-registered-guidance-counselors-forces-schools-to-keepunlicensed-ones-pa

31 The Professionalisation of Counselling Supervision in Singapore

Jeffrey Po

Introduction

As with most professionals providing services in the mental health field or who are part of the helping profession, counsellors and psychotherapists require supervision of their work. Until quite recently, practising counsellors and psychotherapists in Singapore (except those who were registered as specific allied health professionals or were registered with specific professional associations) have not generally been committed to engaging in supervision for counselling or psychotherapy practices. To many practitioners the practice of supervision appeared as some vague and unnecessary process and would have been considered by some as a nuisance that encroached into the professional lives of counsellors and psychotherapists. Hence professional supervision was lacking, and more often than not discharged superficially when applied, and often engage in with some sense of uncertainty.

While it is true that many courses and programmes in higher institutions of learning mention supervision and internship students often engage in supervision, many still view supervision as an unnecessary activity with little or no real purpose and just something they need to summarily complete to meet course requirements. Until recently, training schools in Singapore did not impress upon counselling students the necessity and significance of being supervised during their professional career. After graduation, many novice counsellors still hold hazy ideas about the concept of the practice and the usefulness of having their work supervised. The freshly graduated often catapult themselves into the clouds of high expectations and feel that through dedication, passion, and compassion they can save the world and ease suffering. Still many hold the belief that possession of a graduate qualification can ensure smooth navigation along their life journey as a counsellor or psychotherapist. A main culprit influencing this attitude could be the training institutions themselves that do not fully impart to students the meaningfulness of incorporating such a necessity as supervision into their career journey.

Fortunately, the stature and respectability of the professional practice of supervision is changing in Singapore. However, this change could be said to be slow. The counselling and psychotherapy profession is not legally regulated in Singapore (Pelling, 2013). Hence the role of gatekeeping to the industry and practitioner certification is very much self-regulatory and managed by registered associations and organisations, such as The Singapore Association for Counselling (SAC) and the Association of Psychotherapists and Counsellors (Singapore) – APACS.

DOI: 10.4324/9781003490067-38

Due to the voluntary nature of counselling regulation in Singapore, it is an incumbent responsibility of supervisors to provide guidance and advice on the following matters (Armstrong, 2017):

- The legal aspects of offering counselling and psychotherapy services
- Record keeping
- To protect supervisees against legal complaints
- To be familiar with some of the legal regulations and protective provisions of specific issues (e.g., family violence, child protection, adoption, etc.).
- To ensure supervisee's adherence to correct ethical, professional and workplace policies
- Ability to advise when workplace policies contradict Association's code of conduct.
- Occupational health safety issues
- Legislation on Mandatory reporting

New counsellors and therapists must be aided in their abilities in these areas. Unfortunately, the current author has found many supervisors in Singapore simply unaware of their legal and moral supervisory obligations. They seem oblivious to the fact that during supervision sessions they function as mentor, coach, facilitator, educator, and advisor. Instead, often the relationship is that of a counsellor and client. This is not appropriate. As stated by Haynes, Corey, and Moulton (2003) the role of professional supervision as providing growth and development through teaching; ensuring the protection of the client's welfare; monitoring and gatekeeping for the profession, and helping the supervisee to become independent and self-reflective as a professional. We aid clients by aiding the counsellors supporting clients. We need to honour the purpose of supervision in Singapore, develop our counselling workforce, and act ethically with both our supervisees and clients.

An example of supervision in Singapore: School counsellors

Within the Singaporean context, school counsellors have been grouped into four basic geographical regions: North, South, East and West. Each region is then divided into four or five clusters which each cluster comprising of about 15 to 20 counsellors. A lead counsellor, almost always a Master Counsellor level usually supervises the session that takes place once a month. For example, the career progression of a school counsellor often follows the path described below:

- School counsellor (approximately five to six years)
- Senior School counsellor (approximately four to five years
- Lead School counsellor (no time frame)
- Master counsellor

The 15 to 20 counsellors are required to participate in group supervision once a month and each session will run for approximately three hours. Normally it is pre-arranged that one or two participating counsellors will present a case with the aid of a 10-minute video clip of a counselling session that had taken place in the presenter's school. Transcripts are distributed to support the video presentation. Discussion will revolve around the scenario presented. In such a system, it means that one participant will probably be given a chance to present his/her case per year. Parental consent is usually obtained from students from the primary school while most often than not, no parental consent is obtained for students from the secondary school.

Most school counsellors find such a presentation practice useful to their work because of the sharing of experiences. The Master Counsellor, who is usually appointed by the Guidance branch of the Singapore Ministry of Education, facilitates the sessions. They may or may not get involved in providing mentoring, guidance, or psychoeducation. The sessions are often centred on the work of the counsellors. However, personal resolutions of issues are not discussed. If needed, a separate appointment would have to be made for the individual one-to-one session with the Master Counsellor. Nonetheless, few such requests are made because the Master Counsellor may be attached to a school that is some distance from the supervisee.

How might our Singaporean counselling workforce develop and further aid students if the supervisors were all not just experienced counsellors but trained in the various aspects and foci of professional supervision? How might the workforce benefit from supervision that is professional and covers various aspects and not just case presentations and clinical supervision? We will soon find out, as more and more supervisors gain professional supervision training and the focus of supervision broadens to areas including but not exclusive to clinical supervision and case management.

Accredited counselling supervisors in Singapore

In Singapore two organisations related to counselling and psychotherapy maintain a record of registered supervisors. Criteria for entry to these associations are diverse. This means that consistency is lacking in how supervisory activities are conceptualised and discharged. For instance, the Singapore Association for Counselling (SAC) webpage (2016) displays that applicants for being a Recognised Clinical Supervisor involves the following:

1. The individual must be an SAC Registered Counsellor with membership fees up-to-date.
2. The individual must have at least five years of experience as a Professional Counsellor at Clinical Level. This step will be fulfilled in the clinical experience section requested in the Application Form.
3. SAC Registered Counsellors wanting to be recognised as Clinical Supervisors must demonstrate competencies which benefit individual practitioners and training institutes that require supervision for their students and interns.

Similarly, the webpage for the Association of Psychotherapists and Counsellors Singapore (APACS) (2016) shows the following requirements:

1. Have successfully completed a formal training course in Professional Counselling Supervision approved and conducted by APACS appointed training provider;
2. Have completed a minimum of 500 hours of counselling practice;
3. Shows maturity in discharging counselling services;
4. Successful in a panel interview with senior members of APACS;
5. Submit a formal request to the Executive Committee for this upgrading of level.

Supervision training available in Singapore

Training of supervisors takes many varied forms and styles in Singapore. For instance, the *Co*unselling and Care Centre presently offers a Diploma in Clinical Supervision (DCS), which has been designed as a 150-hour part-time course designed to help senior social services and professionals develop their supervision practices in clinical work by equipping them with knowledge and skills essential for competent clinical supervision (Counselling and Care Centre, 2016). The course modules offered include the Concepts and Theories of Supervision, the Person of the Trainee Supervision and Issues of Supervision, and the Skills of Supervision Practices. The course is presented as enabling participants to:

• Grasp concepts and theories of supervision;
• Describe and demonstrate supervision skills;
• Utilise the systemic approach as a practice model of supervision;
• Understand how to work with supervisees and supervisory issues;
• Develop personally and professionally through developing self-reflectivity in clinical and supervisory practices;
• Enhance competency in supervision practice through a variety of supervision modalities and consultation of clinical work.

A second course offered is by **ACC School of Counselling and Psychology** and their webpage (2016) mentions that the programme has been designed for Senior counsellors/ social workers/psychologists who are supervising others and want to develop their skills in clinical supervision as well as Counsellors/social workers/psychologists who are going to supervise others and want to learn about skills and important issues in clinical supervision. This training programme has course modules comprising the context of clinical supervision, Professional and ethical issues, and Evaluation and Professional Practice as they relate to supervision.

Furthermore, there is the Graduate Diploma in Clinical Supervision offered by the **Executive Counselling & Training Academy (ECTA)** in collaboration with Swinburne University of Technology, Australia. This qualification meets the requirements of the Australian Qualification Framework (AQF) level 8. The associated web page (2016) indicates that the course focuses on the fundamentals of supervision and provides a comprehensive introduction to the theory and practices of clinical supervision. Generic key concepts, skills and approaches are explored for the application across different types of supervision required. It discusses the definitions, purposes and benefits of supervision. Using existing evidence to assist individuals in their role as supervisors, this course aims to provide students with the aptitude to supervise. The course modules comprise of the following:

• Introduction to clinical supervision
• Ethical and legal issues in supervision
• CBT modules in supervision
• Peer and group practical supervision assessment
• Developmental and psychodynamic module of supervision
• Integrative and postmodern models to supervision
• Systemic Model in Supervision and Group-Based Intervention
• Live supervision and placement

Association supervisory foci

It was previously mentioned that two main counselling associations in Singapore are SAC and APACS. The perspective taken by APACS towards the training of supervisors is two-pronged (APACS, 2016). First, the association seeks to offer a basic training in Professional Counselling Supervision to currently registered and practising counsellors who are members of APACS. This certification course will allow them some insights into the fundamental theories and various modalities of supervision. The course is evaluated on class attendance as well as written assignments. Competencies are also evaluated at the end of the course. Basic textbooks are part of the study curriculum. As mentioned above the attainment of this certification meets the professional requirements and standards as required by the APACS.

Second, upon successful completion students can further their educational path in Professional Counselling Supervision by enrolling via a vocational pathway to be awarded the Vocational Graduate Diploma in Counselling Supervision. The attainment of this level satisfies and meets the requirement of being in Level 8 of the Australian Qualification Framework (AQF). Students are given two years to complete the programme, and the study is self-paced. Lectures are held in Singapore.

Regarding training, APACS adopts the position of offering its current Level 4 registered and practising counsellors/psychotherapists the option to participate in a training course that involves the RISE UP (Relationship based Integrated Supervision and Education to Unlock Potential) Model of Professional Supervision developed by Armstrong (2017). Upon successful completion participants will be eligible to upgrade themselves to Level 4S (supervisor) and apply for membership into APACS Professional College of Supervisors.

APACS Professional College of Supervisors

APACS has a commitment to supervision and thus formed its own Professional College of Supervisors in the first half of 2016. Its final Manual of Procedures was endorsed during its Executive Committee meeting on 27 May 2016. Extracts from MOP – 28 are listed below (APACS, 2016):

1.0. Preamble:
1.1. This college shall be known as APACS Professional College of Supervisors.
1.2. This college is defined as a fraternity of all members of APACS, who have formally undergone an APACS approved supervision training course.
1.3. Those who are not members of APACS and who have undergone the formal course not approved and recognised by APACS can also apply for membership. Their application is however subjected to the approval of APACS Executive Committee. The application shall be considered on a case to case basis and shall not be taken as a precedent for others to join.

Upon approval, they shall join APACS as practising members.

2.0. Objectives of the College.
2.1. To keep a register of all those who have acquired the skills and training of Professional Counselling Supervision.

2.2. To offer platform for the members to meet occasional and to discuss the latest research and findings in the area of Professional Counselling Supervision

2.3. To ensure the members of the college discharge their services in the highest ethical and behavioural standards and conduct.

2.4. To implement and introduce new ideas, researches and findings that can upgrade the delivery skills of members of the college.

2.5. To disseminate knowledge and facilitate learning in this area to members of the general public so that they can understand the seriousness and meaning of those providing health care services to undergo and obtain supervision in their own field of expertise.

It is hoped that with the formation of the College, registered and practising supervisors can be made aware of the various components that make up the term Professional Supervision and the heavy social, moral and legal accountability and responsibilities that such a title carries. Thus, the professionalisation of counselling supervision in Singapore is well underway. No longer is supervision merely looking over the shoulders of someone and focusing upon clinical issue. Professional supervision is about caring, developing and moulding the supervisee towards care for themselves, as after all, workers who aspire to offer themselves to the service of others must invariably carry the personal objectives of firstly being aware of himself/herself and his/her own needs; possess the ability to deal with personality patterns within himself/herself and finally be free from limitations that they may place on their own abilities with clarity and honesty (Brill, 1993).

Conclusion

There appears the prevailing attitude by Singapore counsellors and therapists that counselling supervisors or any sort of supervision for that matter, seems only applicable and appropriate for trainees and the less experienced. Experienced counsellors and therapists feel somewhat demeaned when they are required to attend supervision sessions. Somehow, they fail to understand that on-going supervision is necessary because experienced counsellors as persons, do change over time. Being a counsellor facilitates change, and hence the need for continued self-monitoring and self-appraisal remains relevant throughout the lifetime of the practising counsellor (Bond, 1990). The professionalisation of counselling supervision will help change this attitude. The creation of a new attitude towards supervision ought to start with the institutions of higher learning, both from the private and public sector whereby students are instilled with the conviction that Professional supervision is part and parcel of the career journey of counsellors and our professional associations can support this important professionalisation of counselling supervision.

References

ACC School of Counselling and Psychology. (2016, 20 July). Retrieved from http://acc.edu.sg/e/index.php/

Armstrong, P. (2017). Conceptualising counselling supervision. In N.J. Pelling, & P. Armstrong (eds.) *The Practice of Clinical and Counselling Supervision*. Brisbane: Australian Academic Press.

Association of Psychotherapist and Counsellor Singapore (APACS). (2016, 20 July). Retrieved from http://apacs.org.sg/

Bond, T. (1990). Counselling–Supervision: Ethical issues. In S. Palmer, Dainow, & P. Milner (eds) *Counselling: The BAC Counselling Reader*. London: Sage Publications.

Brill, N. (1993). *Understanding Ourselves: Working with People*. Philadelphia: J. B. Lippincott & Co.

Counselling and Care Centre. (2016, 20 July). Retrieved from www.counsel.org.sg/

Executive Counselling & Training Academy. (2016, 20 July). Retrieved from www.ecta.edu.sg/

Haynes, R., Corey, G., & Moulton, P. (2003). *Clinical Supervision in the Helping Professions: A Practical Guide*. Pacific Grove, CA: Brookes/Cole Thomson Learning.

Pelling, N. (2013). Advertised psychologists and counsellors in Hong Kong and Singapore. *Asia Pacific Journal of Counselling and Psychotherapy*, 4(2), 185–199, DOI: 10.1080/21507686.2013.824907

Singapore Association for Counselling (SAC). (2016, 20 July). Retrieved from www.sac-counsel.org.sg/

32 Counseling Regulation, Education, and Representation in the United States of America

Janeé Steele and Tiffany Lee

In the United States, counseling is defined as 'a professional relationship that empowers diverse individuals, families, and groups to accomplish mental health, wellness, education, and career goals' (Kaplan et al., 2014, p. 368). The populations and settings in which this relationship occurs vary, yet, in this country, counseling at its core is a profession built on ethical and culturally relevant practices designed to promote wellness and optimal human development. As such, all licensed professional counselors in the United States must meet certain qualifications and are subjected to various levels of oversight. The sections in this chapter provide an overview of counseling regulation, education, and representation in the United States. Included in this overview is a discussion of pathways to becoming a counselor in the United States, as well as supervision requirements during and post-graduate-level training. The chapter concludes with final remarks concerning the outlook of the profession, focusing on current advocacy efforts to strengthen, unify, and build consensus within counseling.

Counseling regulation in the United States

Counseling in the United States is regulated through independent state licensure laws. The first counselor licensure laws were passed in the state of Virginia in 1976, while the last counselor licensure laws were adopted 33 years later by the state of California in 2009 (Lawson, 2016). These laws establish the profession's minimum education and training standards, and define the activities counselors are permitted to engage once licensed (American Counseling Association, https://archive.counseling.org/knowle dge-center/licensure-requirements). The typical scope of practice for a licensed counselor includes: (a) assessment, testing, and evaluation; (b) individual, family, and group counseling; (c) diagnosis and treatment planning for mental disorders; and (d) prevention, behaviour modification, and guidance to individuals, families, and organizations (Michigan Counseling Association Licensure Committee, 2010). Within this scope of practice, counselors are expected to adhere to a specified code of ethics, and are subject to oversight by a state board responsible for issuing licenses, enforcing regulations, and handling ethics complaints.

Because each state regulates counselor licensure independently, credential titles vary. The most common titles include licensed professional counselor (LPC), licensed mental health counselor (LMHC), licensed clinical professional counselor (LCPC), licensed professional clinical counselor of mental health (LPCC), licensed clinical mental health counselor (LCMHC), and licensed mental health practitioner (LMHP) (American Counseling Association [ACA], n.d.). The majority of states, 30 as of December 2020, have a

DOI: 10.4324/9781003490067-39

two-tiered licensure system that require applicants to meet certain education, examination, and supervised experience qualifications before full licensure is granted. Sixteen states have one tier, two states have three tiers, and two states have four tiers of licensure (ACA, n.d.). Once licensed, these counselors are permitted to practice independently, but may be required to complete periodic continuing education as part of the license renewal process subsequent to obtaining full licensure (ACA, n.d.).

Counseling education in the United States

For those individuals who wish to pursue a career in counseling, a minimum of a master's degree is required. After receiving a four-year bachelor's degree (most often in the behavioural health field), individuals may continue their education for typically two to three more years in order to obtain a master's degree in one of the following specialty areas: (a) addiction; (b) career; (c) clinical mental health; (d) clinical rehabilitation; (e) college counseling and student affairs; (f) marriage, couple, and family; or (g) school. The main accreditation is the Council for Accreditation of Counseling and Related Educational Programs (CACREP), which was formed in 1981. The organization is independent of the American Counseling Association (ACA) but influenced by the ACA through collaborations which maintain and update the standards used to obtain accreditation. Other accrediting bodies do exist (e.g., Masters in Psychology and Counseling Accreditation Council and National Addiction Studies Accreditation Commission). However, CACREP is the primary entity that students seek due to the alignment with their professional identity and the expectation that graduating from a CACREP will assist with state licensure requirements, as well as some national certifications. Currently, licensure in six states requires the applicant to have graduated from a CACREP accredited programme. A change for the counseling field worth noting here is that some accredited training programmes provide coursework online through distance learning (e.g., Capella University and Walden University). Institutions have the opportunity to obtain accreditation for fully online programmes, as well as a hybrid of face-to-face meetings and online content. If students choose to enroll in a hybrid distance learning programme, they may be required to travel and attend classes which can meet all day for several days in a row.

Most master's-level counseling programmes are 48 to 60 credit hours (3 or 4 credits per course). Education and training can vary slightly between specializations (e.g., school counseling and clinical mental health counseling); however, content for core courses tends to be guided by the CACREP core standards, and therefore, most institutions have a similar curriculum. For instance, all students will be expected to complete coursework in group dynamics, counseling techniques, multicultural counseling, professional ethics, research methods, etc. Counselors-in-training will also complete a practicum and field internship at the end of their education experience. Some programmes have the option of a thesis or capstone project as well and can be more research-focused in nature. Usually, the completion of such work would designate the difference in a master's of arts (MA) or a master's of science (MS) degree.

A PhD degree does not assist with advancing licensure, as full licensure is most often obtained within a few years after the master's degree. Individuals who desire advanced–level preparation in counseling and supervision complete the PhD in counselor education with the intention of teaching classes, engaging in research, and becoming a leader in the profession as a faculty member in higher education. On average, these programmes require between 60 and 70 credit hours (3 or 4 credits per course) after the master's degree is completed. Students usually finish and defend their dissertation research three to five years from initiating doctoral-level coursework.

Counseling representation in the United States

Founded in 1952, the ACA is a not-for-profit, professional, and educational organization, and is the largest association exclusively representing professional counselors in various practice settings. There are 56 chartered branches in Europe, Latin America, and the United States. The ACA has four regions, which serve members in those sections of the United States. ACA members also have the opportunity to belong to one or more of the 19 divisions that exist (e.g., Association for Multicultural Counseling and Development, International Association of Addictions and Offender Counselors, Association for Child and Adolescent Counseling). These divisions provide leadership, resources, and information unique to specialized areas and/or principles of counseling. In addition to the ACA, there are other national organizations, albeit smaller in membership numbers but are more specialized by profession, such as the American School Counselor Association and the American Association for Marriage and Family Therapists.

Pathways to becoming a counselor in the United States

Pathways to becoming a counselor in the United States are varied due to the profession's historical development. Counseling in America emerged early in the twentieth century, primarily as part of the educational and vocational guidance movements of the era. During this time, counseling in educational settings, first instituted by Jesse B. Davis in 1907, typically consisted of weekly guidance lessons for character building and prevention, while vocational guidance, established through the work of Frank Parsons in 1908 at Boston's Vocational Bureau, focused on preparing young adults to enter the workforce (Atkinson, 2002). These forms of counseling, vocational guidance in particular, continued to grow in the country as World War I and the Great Depression created a need to match returning servicepersons and unemployed workers with jobs. The focus on vocation in counseling continued until the 1940s, when increased psychological services for returning World War II veterans became available through the government's Veterans Administration, and counseling within the general population was extended beyond career into other areas of human development through the work of Carl Rogers (Atkinson, 2002). This extension of counseling to include a focus on general psychological and developmental concerns culminated in 1963 with the passage of the Community Mental Health Act (CMHA), which sought to relocate mental health treatment out of the hospital by establishing community based mental health centres throughout the United States (Lawson, 2016).

Until passage of the CMHA in 1963, counselors and psychologists regularly practiced in the same settings. Individuals with counseling or education degrees were even licensed as psychologists, as psychology was the only mental health profession licensed for independent practice at the time (Lawson, 2016). After passage of the CMHA, however, counselors began to be excluded from the profession through civil and criminal litigation, as well as changes that required individuals to hold psychology degrees in order to sit for the psychology exam. As a result, many counselors lost not only their jobs, but their careers as well. In response, counseling's primary professional organization, the American Personnel and Guidance (now known as the American Counseling Association), sought to have counseling recognized as a profession within its own right by lobbying for counselor licensure laws in every state. This effort was successful, but spanned three decades from 1975 until 2009, when California became the last of the 50 states to adopt counselor licensure laws (Lawson, 2016).

While counseling is now legally recognized as separate and distinct from other mental health professions, its shared history with related fields continues to be reflected in the various pathways to becoming a counselor in the United States. Many states, for example, allow graduates of programmes in fields related to counseling to obtain counselor licensure, provided the graduates have completed coursework in specific content areas (ACA, n.d.). Moreover, individuals licensed as counselors, psychologists, or even clinical social workers are often hired for the same positions in schools and community agencies, and are reimbursed for the same services by insurance companies when in private practice. This overlap among the professions is likely to continue given projections of future employment trends. According to the United States Department of Labor, the projected employment rate of mental health counselors (for years 2019–2029) is higher than many other occupations, including similar disciplines. More specifically, the rate is expected to grow 25 per cent during that time, compared to social workers (13%) and psychologists (3%) (Bureau of Labor Statistics, 2020).

Supervision of counseling in the United States

Supervision of counseling in the United States is required for individuals at both student and professional stages of their careers. Students enrolled in CACREP-accredited counselor education programmes must complete two levels of field experience. The first level is a supervised 100-hour counseling practicum that takes place over a minimum of ten weeks. The second level is a supervised 600-hour internship in the student's area of specialization, which is generally completed over one or two academic terms. According to the 2016 CACREP Standards, students at both levels of field experience must receive at least one hour per week of individual or triadic supervision by either a counselor education programme faculty member, a doctoral student supervisor who is under the supervision of a counselor education programme faculty member, or a site supervisor who collaborates with a counselor education programme faculty member in accordance with a supervision agreement. Site supervisors must have: (1) a minimum of a master's degree, preferably in counseling, or a related profession; (2) relevant certifications and/or licenses; (3) a minimum of two years of professional experience in the specialty area in which the student is enrolled; (4) knowledge of the programme's expectations, requirements, and evaluation procedures for students; and (5) relevant training in counselor supervision (www.cacrep.org/for-programs/2016-cacrep-standards/). In addition to individual supervision, practicum, and internship students must also participate in an average of 1.5 hours per week of group supervision throughout the practicum or internship experience. A counselor education programme faculty member or a student supervisor who is under the supervision of a counselor education programme faculty member must provide this form of supervision.

In order to obtain full licensure in the United States, counselors must complete a certain number of supervised post-master's-degree clinical hours, as well as pass a comprehensive examination on counseling. Thirty-six states and the District of Columbia require between 3,000 and 3,600 hours of supervised post-master's-degree experience for the highest level of licensure. These hours typically must be completed in no less than two years. States with more than two tiers of licensure generally require successively higher numbers of hours to obtain each level of licensure. Most states require supervision to take place face-to-face. Additionally, many states require supervisors to have specialized training in clinical supervision. This training may be obtained as part of doctoral-level counselor education, or through independent training providers. The content of clinical supervision training is focused in areas such as (a) roles and functions of clinical supervisors, (b) models of clinical supervision, (c) mental health–related professional development, (d) methods and techniques in clinical supervision, (e) supervisory relationship issues, (f) cultural issues in clinical supervision, (g) group supervision, (h) legal and ethical issues in clinical supervision, and (i) evaluation of supervisee competence and the supervision process (Center for Credentialing & Education, n.d.). Individuals who complete training in clinical supervision through an independent credentialing agency may earn certifications such as the approved clinical supervisor (ACS) credential, which is granted by an independent not-for-profit credentialing agency known as the Center for Credentialing and Education. To receive the ACS credential, counselors must: (a) have an earned master's degree or higher in a mental health field, (b) be licensed or certified as a mental health provider, (c) complete specialized training in supervision, (d) provide proof documenting at least 100 hours of supervision, (e) have at least 5 years and 4,000 hours of mental health counseling experience, and (f) develop a professional disclosure detailing supervision training and experience to be provided to all supervisees.

Concluding remarks about counseling in the United States

This chapter provided an overview of counseling regulation, education, and representation in the United States. As discussed, since its beginnings in the early twentieth century, counseling in this country has undergone a transition from a field focused primarily on educational and vocational guidance, to a profession of independently licensed mental health practitioners with specialized knowledge of psychological and human development principles (Atkinson, 2002). While counseling licensure laws have recently been obtained in all 50 states, the field's primary professional organizations continue to engage advocacy efforts aimed at strengthening, unifying, and building consensus within the profession. One of the most visible efforts has been the 20/20: A Vision for the Future of Counseling initiative, which is led by the American Counseling Association and 30 other participating organizations. This initiative focuses on advancing the profession by addressing several key issues in counseling, including outlining specific principles for strengthening and unifying the profession (Kaplan & Gladding, 2011); building a consensus definition of counseling (Kaplan et al., 2014); and developing a consensus licensure title and scope of practice as part of a larger scale counselor license portability project (Kaplan & Kraus, 2018). While several gains have been made, leaders within the field note much more work is needed in order to achieve even greater unification across the profession especially as it relates increased consistency and reciprocity in licensure laws from state to state. Accordingly, counseling in the United States continues to be in a state of growth and development. Nevertheless, given successes toward a more crystallized identity within the profession, as well as continued need for licensed counselors throughout the country, the outlook for counseling in the United States looks bright well into the twenty-first century.

Final Note: Please address correspondence to Dr Janeé Steele Walden University Email: janee.steele@mail.waldenu.edu and Dr Tiffany Lee Western Michigan University Email: tiffany.lee@wmich.edu

References

American Counseling Association (ACA). (n.d.). Licensure and certification – State professional counselor licensure boards. Retrieved from www.counseling.org/knowledge-center/ licensure-requirements/state-professional-counselor-licensureboards

Atkinson, D.R. (2002). Counseling in the 21st century: A mental health profession comes of age. In C.L. Juntunen, & D.R. Atkinson (Eds.), *Counseling across the lifespan: Prevention and treatment* (pp. 3–22). Thousand Oaks, CA: Sage Publications, Inc.

Bureau of Labor Statistics. (2020). Substance abuse, behavioral disorder, and mental health counselors: Summary. Retrieved from www.bls.gov/ooh/community-and-social-service/ substance-abuse-behavioral-disorder-and-mental-healthcounselors.htm

Center for Credentialing & Education (n.d.). Required training: Approved clinical supervisor. Retrieved from www.cceglobal.org/Credentialing/ACS/Training

Kaplan, D.M., & Gladding, S.T. (2011). A vision for the future of counseling: The 20/20 principles for unifying and strengthening the profession. *Journal of Counseling & Development*, 89(3), 367–372. doi:10.1002/j.1556-6678.2011.tb00101.x

Kaplan, D.M., & Kraus, K.L. (2018). Building blocks to portability: Culmination of the 20/20 initiative. *Journal of Counseling & Development*, 96(2), 223–228. doi:10.1002/jcad.12195

Kaplan, D.M., Tarvydas, V.M., & Gladding, S.T. (2014). 20/20: A vision for the future of counseling: The new consensus definition of counseling. *Journal of Counseling & Development*, 92(3), 366–372. doi:10.1002/j.1556-6676.2014.00164.x

Lawson, G. (2016). On being a profession: A historical perspective on counselor licensure and accreditation. *Journal of Counselor Leadership and Advocacy*, 3(2), 71–84. doi:10.1080/2326716X.2016.1169955

Michigan Counseling Association Licensure Committee. (2010). Licensed professional counselor quick fact sheet. Retrieved from www.michigancounselingassociation.com/ uploads/2/6/3/4/2634297/2010_lpc_quick_fact_sheet.pd

Appendix A
Contract for Professional Supervision

The following contract is between _____ (Professional Supervisor) and _ _____ (Supervisee).

1. Purpose, Goals, and Objectives of Professional Supervision:
   a. Monitor and promote welfare of clients seen by Supervisee;
   b. Promote development of Supervisee's professional identity and competence;
   c. Fulfil requirement for Supervisee certification and accreditation; and
   d. Fulfil professional (i.e., ACA or PACFA) membership requirement.
2. Context and Content of Professional supervision:
   a. Individual professional supervision at Professional Supervisor's office, via the phone, or on an as needed basis. In the case of a crisis, an appointment can be made as soon as possible outside this time;
   b. A variety of methods will be used within a multi-faceted framework.
3. Method of Evaluation:
   Feedback will be provided each session. Records will be limited to session details and major issues relevant to the professional supervision of the case. A formal evaluation will be conducted every six months. Professional supervision notes (if kept) may be shared with the Supervisee at the Professional Supervisor's discretion and upon request of the Supervisee. An unedited video/audio of a one-hour counselling session may be required if the Professional Supervisor needs to view a session to continue appropriate professional supervision. This will be discussed with the supervisee before a request is made. Written permission from the client will be required for same.
4. Duties and Responsibilities of Professional Supervisor–Supervisee:
   a. Professional supervisor:
      - Encourage on-going professional education.
      - Challenge Supervisee to validate approach and technique used.
      - Monitor basic microskills and advanced skills, including transference and counter-transferences.
      - Provide alternative approaches for the Supervisee.
      - Intervene where client welfare is at risk.
      - Ensure ethical guidelines and professional standards are maintained.
      - Provide consultation when necessary.
      - Discuss administrative procedures and marketing strategies.
   b. Supervisee:
      - Uphold ethical guidelines and professional standards.

- Discuss client cases with the aid of written case notes and video/audio tapes.
- Validate diagnoses made and approach and techniques used.
- Be open to change and alternative methods of practice.
- Consult Professional Supervisor or designated contact person in cases of emergency.
- Implement Professional supervisor directives in subsequent sessions.
- Maintain a commitment to supervise education and the counselling profession.

5. Procedural Considerations:
   a. Supervisee's written notes, diagnoses, action plans and videos may be reviewed in sessions;
   b. Issues related to the Supervisee's professional development will be discussed; and
   c. It is understood that important and seminal issues experienced in the counselling setting will be raised and addressed in professional supervision. Failure to raise such issues in a reasonable timeframe will be considered a breach of contract.

This contract is subject to revision at any time, upon request by either the Professional Supervisor or Supervisee. The contract will be reviewed each six months on the approval of both the Professional Supervisor and the Supervisee.

The price per one-hour session is $_____ (GST inclusive), which will be invoiced to you on occurrence/weekly/monthly. Payment to be made within _____ days by _____.

Cancellation policy No penalties exist if supervisee is to cancel a session with a minimum of 24/48 (circle one) hours' notice prior to the professional supervision session. Supervisees who do not keep to appointment times and have not cancelled the session with notice will incur a $_____ penalty. As a supervisee, there is an expectation by your Professional Supervisor to commit fully to the professional supervision process, and this includes keeping appointments. Unexpected emergencies can be discussed on an individual basis.

Contact outside of appointment times There may be occasions when you need to consult your professional supervisor outside of appointment times. This can be done by phone when necessary. Phone calls that are within a ten-minute time span will not attract any fees for service and will be considered part of the service, within reason. Phone calls that go over ten minutes will be considered as a professional supervision session, and a fee for service will be charged at the hourly rate.

Agreement We agree, to the best of our ability, to uphold the guidelines specified in the professional supervision contract and to manage the professional supervisory relationship process according to the ethical principles and Code of Conduct of _____ (i.e., an appropriate professional association such as the ACA or PACFA).

Please circle the frequency of professional supervision you require (weekly/fortnightly/monthly/as needed) and record the date from which you wish this contract to commence _____. Unless otherwise arranged supervision meetings will occur for _____ _____ minutes duration.

Indemnity: You are not an employee or an agent of your Professional Supervisor and thus you will indemnify your Professional Supervisor against any action arising from any client in relation to your activities. You affirm that you hold your own, or are covered by your agency's, professional indemnity and public liability insurance.

This supervision contract can be extended or cancelled by mutual agreement but is generally considered active for 6 months from the date of signing.

_____   _____

Professional Supervisor   Supervisee

Date: _____   Date_____

Consent Form

Private Information

As part of providing a professional supervision service to you, your supervisor, _____ _____, will need to collect and record personal information from you that is relevant to your current situation. This information will be a necessary part of the service provided.

Access

You may access the material recorded in your file upon request, subject to the exceptions in the National Privacy Act.

Confidentiality

All personal information and notes gathered by the supervisor during the provision of the supervision service will remain confidential and secure except when:

1. It is subpoenaed by a court, or
2. Failure to disclose the information would place you and/or another person at risk, or
3. Your prior approval has been obtained to
    a. Provide a written report to another professional or agency (e.g., a GP or a lawyer); or
    b. Discuss the material with another person (e.g., a parent or employer).

Fees

The cost of a one-hour consultation (usually around 55 minutes to allow for some paperwork completion following the meeting) is $_____ (GST incl), which is payable at the end of the session/week/month, by cash/cheque/bank deposit/credit card. Sessions that go over one hour will be charged at $_____ per quarter hour.

Cancellation policy

If, for some reason, you need to cancel or postpone the appointment, please give me at least 24/48 hours' notice. Otherwise, you will be charged a $_____ administration fee.

I, _____ (print name in Block Capitals), have read and understood the above Consent Form. I agree to these conditions for the service provided by __
_____.

Signature .... Date ....

Please Note: If, after reading this page, you are at all unsure of what is written, please ensure this is discussed between the supervisor and the supervisee.

Confidential

Please fill in and return this questionnaire to the Supervisor:

First Name_____Surname _____

Address_____

Contact number H _____ W _____Mobile_____

DOB _____ Gender: Male Female Other _____

Current profession _____

Current employer or self-employed _____

Qualifications or highest level of education _____

1. Please circle – currently: Married / Partnered / Single / Defacto
2. Have you been divorced? Yes / No Date _____
3. Are you currently separated? Yes / No Is your separation: permanent / trial?
4. Do you have any children? Yes / No Are you the biological parent? Yes / No
5. Do have any orders relevant to yourself in regard to the Family Law Court, Child Support Agency or police? Yes / No
6. Are you or have you ever been on medication for depression, anxiety, or any other psychological condition? Yes / No
7. Have you ever seen a supervisor, psychologist, or a psychiatrist before? Yes / No
8. Do you practice social drug taking? Yes / No
9. Have you ever been convicted of an offence by a court/professional body or been refused or had a professional membership cancelled or refused? Yes / No

Signature _____ Date _____

Appendix B
Sample Counselling Contract

Counselling services

As part of providing a counselling service to you, your counsellor _____ will need to collect and record personal information from you that is relevant to your current situation. This information will be a necessary part of the assessment and treatment that is conducted.

Access

You may access the material recorded in your file upon request in line with national privacy legislation. There may be instances where records collected for insurance purposes will be restricted.

Confidentiality

All personal information gathered by the counsellor during the provision of the counselling service will remain confidential and secure except when:

1. It is subpoenaed by a court of law or Government Department/Agency under the appropriate legislation, or
2. Failure to disclose the information would place you, and/or another person at risk, or
3. Your prior approval has been obtained to either provide a report to another professional or agency (e.g., physician, lawyer), or to discuss the clinical material with another person (e.g., parent, employer).

Consultation fee

The cost of a one hour therapy session (usually 50–55 minutes long to allow for administrative activities, such as making our next appointment/taking notes) is

$_____ (GST Included/Exempt), which is payable at the end of the session by cash/cheque/credit card/bank deposit).

Cancellation policy

If, for some reason you need to cancel or postpone the appointment, please give me at least 24/48 (circle one) hours' notice, otherwise you will be charged $_____.

Additional information

The attached _____ (i.e., Code of Ethics/Charter for Clients) explains your rights as a client of a counsellor and/or related privacy information.

I, (print name) _____ have read and understood this Counselling Contract. I agree to these conditions for the counselling service provided by

_____ (Counsellor's Name).

Signature: Date:

Please Note: If, after reading this contract you are unsure about any aspect, please feel free to discuss this with me.

Appendix C
Engagement with Your Family Violence Supervisor for Support and Guidance

Family Violence (FV) Counsellors should engage with their Supervisor when:

1. The client misses two sessions with the FV Counsellor without notifying reasons for the cancellation. Has the FV Counsellor investigated? Is this usual or a pattern?
2. The client expresses dissatisfaction with the FV Counsellor/or with the counselling strategies being offered.
3. A case conference needs to be called or the FV Counsellor has been invited to a case conference.
4. Is Trauma Informed Practice being used effectively by the FV Counsellor? Does the FV Counsellor have a good understanding of trauma and how to respond?
5. Child Inclusive Practice – is this being employed by the FV Counsellor? Who is the 'Child's Voice' in the room? What is the current effect of Family Violence on the Child?
6. Are children and/or adults exposed to Family Violence in danger of being abused emotionally, sexually, physically – is their conduct that needs to be reported to regulators?
7. Is it necessary for FV Counsellors to approach Police or other agencies to undertake a current welfare check on their client (e.g., Poverty, Homelessness, no social connectedness)?
8. Has the FV Counsellor noticed an unexpected change for the worst in the FV Client's physical wellbeing? Does the client see a Doctor or a Dentist? Take medication?
9. Has the FV Counsellor observed a significant change in the client's mood (e.g., Increased anxiety, increased depression, rumination, dichotomous thinking)?
10. How often is the FV Counsellor checking with the client regarding expressions of suicidal ideation? Threats to harm others? Threats to harm self?
11. Has the FV Counsellor completed a Family Violence Risk Assessment with the client? Do they understand the triggers for escalation of Family Violence?
12. Has the FV Counsellor gathered data or made observations that may suggest risk escalation towards others (e.g., Purchasing guns; intervention order breaches; increased substance use – even if the client denies these things)?
13. Does the FV Counsellor feel *stuck* in the session? What is the counselling plan or strategy moving forward?
14. Are there any suspected psychotic symptoms evident in the client (e.g., hallucinations, delusions)?. Is there any evidence that this might be drug induced?
15. Are there any noticeable changes in the alertness or moods of the client? Is there an observable pattern or trigger to these changes?
16. Is the client disengaging from the FV Counsellor? Or have they sought to access another service or agency?

17. If the FV Counsellor is closing with the client, has there been a review of the Family Violence Risks and Mitigating Strategies in Place?

18. Has the FV Counsellor offered the client a Resilience Plan and discussed what to do if desperate (e.g., suicidal) or feeling unsafe?

19. Does the client have a Safety Plan in place? (i.e., what to do, where to go, what to take, who to notify, what to do if in immediate danger)?

20. Does the FV Counsellor keep an up-to-date resource folder to enable secondary consultations or referrals to be effective? This can be jointly reviewed with the FV Counselling Supervisor

21. The FV Counsellor has a tense/taxing session with a client and needs to debrief.

22. Is the FV Counsellor practicing and regularly reviewing their own self-care? What strategies are in place to refresh and renew?

23. Is the FV Counsellor regularly demonstrating an ongoing commitment to professional development?

24. Does the FV Counsellor regularly test out their theories, modalities, hypotheses and ethical concerns with their FV Counselling Supervisor?

25. Does the FV Counsellor model and practice hope, compassion and justice with all clients regardless of whether they are recipients of, witnesses to, or perpetrators of Family Violence?

26. Does the FV Counsellor regularly check in with their supervisor about offering a professional service to all clients regardless of their own feelings about the client's attitudes and behaviours?

27. Does the FV Counsellor and their Supervisor discuss how many services are currently being received by the client and whether they need to withdraw from service provision?

28. Does the FV Counsellor have a clear understanding of the differences between a therapeutic response and a criminogenic response? Do they understand the role of Courts and the Justice system?

29. Even within a difficult Family Violence context, can the FV Counsellor develop a therapeutic alliance where clients feel safe to freely express feelings and emotions without judgement?

30. Does the FV Counsellor clearly understand the cultural dynamics of diverse groups and the impact on Family Violence (e.g., arranged marriages, sexual orientation, elder abuse, cultural norms, defined gender roles)?

Appendix D
Possible Answers to Educational Questions and Activities

Chapter 1

Educational questions & activities

1. Where and with whom did you experience supervision?
2. What were the stated and implicit aims?
3. What was the focus of the interaction?
4. What was the frequency, intensity, duration, and location of the supervision?
5. What format, style, or model did the supervisor use?
6. What material was discussed and how?
7. What was the fee and who paid for the sessions?
8. What were the beneficial aspects of the experience?
9. What were the unhelpful aspects of the experience?
10. What are some of the lasting effects of the encounters?
11. If you have never received supervision, what do you think you need for it to be additive to your personal and professional growth?

Answer: These educational questions & activities have no answers that can be marked as correct or incorrect.

Chapter 2

Educational questions & activities

1. True or False. Definitions of supervision have become more complex and multifaceted over time.

   Answer: True

2. According to the author supervision is a process in which all but the following can be discussed:
   a. Personal issues (where they impact on work)
   b. Professional or clinical issues
   c. Business and
   d. Industry/work related issues
   e. All of the above

   Answer: All of the above

3. Ponder and discuss in a group your feelings about having a male or female supervisor and how your past personal and professional have influenced your feelings about same.

Answer: This question/activity has no set answer.

Chapter 3

Educational questions & activities

1. List three types of insurance that may be needed for a private practitioner.

Answer:

a. Public Liability
b. Professional Indemnity
c. Product Liability

2. True or false? Providing coverage for Clinical Supervision is automatically covered in all Professional Liability insurance policies.

Answer: False. This is not an automatic inclusion in many policies and may have to be specifically requested.

3. Name two items that by law in Australia (or in your region) that must be included on an invoice for professional services.

Answer:

a. ABN or ACN
b. Whether the service is inclusive or exclusive of Goods and Services Tax.

4. In relation to keeping clinical notes and records, what is a major consideration in regard to keeping notes if your client base includes minors?

Answer: Minors may take legal action (criminal or civil) many years in the future. If any clients are in this group, the courts of law may expect you to still have copies of your notes (check legislation in your area for time periods).

Chapter 4

Educational questions & activities

1. What is the standard form of Supervision for MST?

Answer: Group Supervision

2. In Bernard and Goodyear's definition of clinical supervision what is made explicit?

Answer: The power differential between supervisor and supervisee.

3. Two themes were captured by supervisors from one Midwestern state in the United States who had provided sanctioned supervision to at least one counsellor in the past year. What were they?

Answer:

(1) sanctioned supervision is a different process than traditional supervision, and
(2) providing sanctioned supervision generates supervisor ambivalence.

4. What are the five ethical issues related to the supervision of EBP that are briefly discussed in this chapter?

Answer: (a) purpose of supervision, (b) managing multiple relationships and interpersonal dynamics, (c) format of supervision, (d) supervisor qualifications and competence, and (e) evaluation.

5. In EBP supervisors need skills beyond those of being a counsellor. The MST Supervisor Adherence Measure (SAM) measures three factors, what are these?

Answer:

(a) the extent to which supervision emphasized the primary underpinnings of MST,
(b) the extent to which the supervisor attempted to build the MST-related competencies of therapists, and
(c) the supervisor's knowledge and skill in MST and EBP intervention modalities

Chapter 5

Educational questions & activities

1. What are your thoughts about suicide and people who have suicidal thoughts or die by suicide? Do you notice any thoughts that reinforce suicide-related stigma?
2. Find a media story about a death by suicide and reframe the narrative of the cause of death using the biopsychosocial domains that caused overwhelming distress and the coping continuum.
3. Think of recent stressful events in your life. Using the coping continuum, identify all the healthy and unhealthy coping strategies you used to feel better.
4. Download the My Coping Plan app and enter your healthy coping strategies. Notice if having an explicit coping plan changes how you think about or what you do to feel better when you have unpleasant emotions.

Answer: The educational questions & activities provided for Chapter 5 have no answers that can be marked as correct or incorrect.

Chapter 6

1. What are the five general worst client case scenario categories outlined by Dr Pelling?

   Answer: Harm to client/client in great pain, difficult clients, danger to therapist, ethical responsibilities, and therapist competence.

2. Create a possible client scenario to go with each category and do either a literature search on the topic (knowledge), write your thoughts and feelings down about the topic (self/other awareness), or engage in an extended role place as client and then counsellor regarding the topic.

   Answer: There is no set answer to this question.

3. What is your favourite way of enhancing your knowledge on a topic?

   Answer: There is no set answer to this question.

4. What is your favourite way of developing your self/other awareness?

   Answer: There is no set answer to this question.

5. What is your favourite ways of developing your counselling skills?

   Answer: There is no set answer to this question.

6. What are your interest areas relevant to populations, settings, and issues/diagnoses?

   Answer: There is no set answer to this question.

Chapter 7

Educational questions & activities

1. In a neuro-scientific study, Decety and Yoder (2008) distinguish between empathic mimicry and true empathy. How do they explain true empathy?

   Answer: True empathy allows for an understanding that the emotions are external to the self, and derived from the other's experience of their environment and the meaning they make of that interaction.

2. What did a study of symptoms of somatic transference of 35 counsellors over a six-month period show?

   Answer: 70% experienced sleepiness, muscle tension, unexpected shift in the body, yawning, and tearfulness. Among some of the other effects experienced were headaches (54%), stomach disturbance (41%), loss of voice (32%), nausea (23%), and numbness (29%).

3. What does Rothschild strongly recommend when working with client's trauma stories?

Answer: A sense of calm detachment.

4. What is the key distinguishing characteristic of VT, what is its transformative nature?

Answer: Exposure to the trauma stories of clients can alter the perceptions of therapists, changing the way they view themselves, other people, and the world.

5. It has been suggested that using self-assessment tools periodically might assist in tracking changes in counsellors exposed to trauma stories. In 1996 Saakvitne and Pearlman developed a Self-Assessment Scale to aid workers in addressing their self-care needs. Name three other assessment tools used for this purpose?

Answer: Traumatic Stress Institute Belief Scale (Pearlman, 1996), Trauma and Attachment Belief Scale (Pearlman, 2003), and The Secondary Traumatic Stress Symptoms (Bride, Robinson, Yegidis, & Figley, 2004).

6. Empathy activates in the insular and anterior cingulate cortex. It is a 'self' related emotion producing negative feelings (stress) that over time leads to?

Answer: To poor health, withdrawal, and non-social behaviours.

Chapter 8

Educational questions & activities

1. When legal questions arise, what two behaviours does the FV Counselling Supervisor need to challenge in FV Counselling practice?

Answer:

   a. To ensure that FV Counsellors are NOT involved in questions of guilt or innocence (which are matters for the Courts); and
   b. To ensure FV Counsellors are NOT involved in moralizing behaviours or labelling, e.g., Victim; Perpetrator

2. If there are "grey" areas of FV Practice, how are these issues resolved?

Answer:

   a. Follow the Code of Ethics/Practice and associated guidelines for your registration/ membership body; and
   b. Clarification of any standards need to be referred to the ACA Ethics Committee

3. What protective mechanisms need to be in place to ensure the welfare of FV Counsellors?

   Answer:

   a. FV Counsellors need to be aware of the effects of vicarious trauma; and
   b. FV Counsellors must have an effective regime in place to monitor and practice self-care

4. To effectively understand the reasons for FV presentations, what three issues are often present?

   Answer:

   a. Client behaviours may be intergenerational and modelled on that provided by one or both parents, or result from the absence of parents
   b. There may have been poor communication practices and fractured relationships within the client's family of origin; and
   c. Basic life skills are often missing (e.g., where the client lacks basic literacy – has no reading, writing abilities, or comprehension)

Chapter 9

Educational questions & activities

1. In groups discuss the following:

   a. Define the key principles of psychodynamic, CBT, and IDM models of supervision.
   b. How do they differ in theoretical assumptions, processes and techniques?
   c. What is the contribution of each approach to supervisee skill development?
   d. Which approach do you like best and why?
   e. Can these approaches be integrated into your supervision practice? Provide a rationale?

   Answer: There are no set answers to these discussions.

2. What does a psychodynamic supervisor do in supervision?

   a. Teaches treatment planning skills and therapeutic techniques
   b. Develops a positive supervisory alliance with their supervisee
   c. Assesses supervisee skill and experience and structures the learning environment accordingly
   d. Helps the supervisee understand the interpersonal processes and intrapsychic issues that occur in therapy
   e. Both b and d

   Answer: e

3. Why do Psychodynamic, CBT, and IDM supervision prioritise the importance of a good working relationship between supervisor and supervisee?

a. All approaches assume that a positive working relationship will assist in achieving supervisory learning goals
b. Supervisors want their supervisee's to have a good experience working with them
c. It is important to feel good when in supervision
d. A good supervisory alliance makes it possible to give honest feedback to each other.

Answer: a

4. If your supervisee reports they are not making progress in therapy with a client what should you do from a CBT supervision perspective?

a. Revisit the treatment plan and provide more skilful techniques
b. Examine the interpersonal dynamics of the case
c. Decide how to address supervision session learning outcomes based on the developmental level of the supervisee
d. Examine how the supervisee really feels about working with their case

Answer: a

5. There is little evidence of efficacy for psychodynamic, CBT or IDM supervision. Consider the following:

a. What is the real value of supervision?
b. How do you know if supervision works?
c. How should supervision be evaluated?
d. Who is supervision ultimately for, the supervisee or the client?

Answer: There are no set answers for these items.

Chapter 10

Educational questions & activities

1. What are the key principles of TSAS?

a. Understanding therapeutic process from an alliance perspective
b. A focus on treatment techniques
c. Managing the working alliance with clients in therapy
d. Dealing with client resistance in therapy
e. a and c
f. All of the above

Answer: e

2. What does a TSAS orientated supervisor do in supervision?

a. Models TSAS skills for their supervisee
b. Develops a positive supervisory alliance with their supervisee
c. Teaches the TSAS model to supervisees

   d. Provides regular evaluation and feedback to supervisees

   e. a and c

   f. All of the above

Answer: f

3. Why might a focus on working alliance be more important than a focus on delivering the techniques of therapy in supervision?

   a. Working alliance between client and therapist predicts treatment outcome whereas therapy technique does not

   b. Working alliance as rated by clients mediates their response to therapy regardless of treatment approach

   c. Working alliance as rated by clients predicts engagement and retention in counselling

   d. All of the above

Answer: d

4. If your supervisee reports they are stuck in therapy with a client what should you do from a TSAS perspective?

   a. Revisit the treatment plan

   b. Confront the client about the impasse

   c. Provide more skilful techniques to address the impasse

   d. Examine the issues existing in the working relationship between therapist and client

Answer: d

5. What are the three components that constitute the TSAS model?

   a. Bond, task, goal; stages of alliance; managing strains and ruptures in the working alliance

   b. Education, learning goals, and experience level

   c. Understanding defences, transference and the unconscious processes in therapy

   d. Developing individualised treatment plans, teaching therapeutic skills and measuring symptom reduction

Answer: a

Chapter 11

Educational questions & activities

1. A historic consequence of seniority-based supervisory systems has been the establishment of hierarchical professional relationships and interactions between the supervisor and the supervisee (Wetchler, 1990). According to SFS theory, supervision structured on unequal power relationships characteristically forms what, and leads where?

Answer: Unclear relational boundaries that fluctuate between "closeness and distance" (Collins, 1993). This breeds uncertainty, and inhibits, discourages, and undermines supervisee self-confidence.

2. During SFS dialogue, the supervisor utilises narrativism to find out what?

Answer: The stories that the supervisee has developed, their contexts, what they inform about clients, and how the supervisee can shift the story and build a new one that creates satisfying outcomes (Skarp, 2012).

3. True or false? The focus is always placed on what is the correct situation, and not what seems to be working for a supervisee with a particular case. As supervisors take the stance of being curious about even the smallest exceptions which are successful, their supervisees are allowed to examine the solutions and their strengths.

Answer: False

4. What are three focuses of SFS?

Answer: SFS is present-focused, strengths-focussed, and goal-focussed.

Chapter 12

Educational questions & activities

1. Describe, using the contracting framework presented, your preferred supervisory working relationship. You may do this from either the perspective of a supervisor or supervisee.
   - What learning goals do you wish to emphasise?
   - What approach to learning suits you?
   - What type of relationship do you wish to have?
   - What management processes are important for you?

2. Identify two situations:
   - Where you felt that you received constructive feedback?
   - Where you felt that you received ineffective feedback?
     Can you identify:
   - What did you do that helped or hindered the feedback process?
   - What did others do that helped or hindered the feedback process?
   - How might your reflections be relevant to enhancing feedback processes in supervision?

3. Use the evidence-based protocol for giving developmental feedback to construct a feedback message to a supervisee.

4. Identify a critical incident or interaction and use the reflective practice cycle to critically review the choices you made.

5. Identify a critical incident or interaction and use the role play model to develop new responses or strategies.

Answer: There are no set answers for these questions.

Chapter 13

Educational questions & activities

1. As a Christian Supervisor how might you gain informed consent to incorporate Spiritual and Religious Interventions (SRIs) in supervision sessions?

Answer: It is advisable to gain prior written informed consent included in the signed supervision contract and verbal informed consent in sessions.

2. What might be some contextual situations where the use of SRIs may be considered appropriate in counselling as discussed in supervision?

Answer: Where the client presents with a declared faith and agrees to SRIs being included in sessions in both the signed intake agreement and more specifically with verbal informed consent during sessions.

3. Considering faith-based supervision practices, such as ministry supervision, how might this differ from supervising counsellors?

Answer: Contextually there is an expectation that faith-based practices, including discussions of SRIs, may be included in supervision sessions with ministry supervisees under agreement. This is not an expectation, and only offered by request and agreement, with other counsellors.

Chapter 14

Educational questions & activities

1. How does the AASW define supervision for social workers?

Answer: Supervision is a forum for reflection and learning...an interactive dialogue between at least two people, one of whom is a supervisor. This dialogue shapes a process of review, reflection, critique and replenishment for professional practitioners. Supervision is a professional activity in which practitioners are engaged throughout the duration of their careers regardless of experience or qualification. The participants are accountable to professional standards and defined competencies and to organisational policy and procedures.

2. What is the basis of the common question social workers have in supervision when in private practice?

Answer: In private practice the common question from social workers in supervision is rather based on the complex assessment of contracts and the contracts legal implications for their practice.

3. What does the author, Braid, believe that counsellors are reluctant to do in the assessment process and why?

Answer: Counsellors tend to include a wide range of variables in the assessment process yet are reluctant to ask about a client's religious or spiritual background lest they appear to be imposing their values on the client.

4. What does the author believe is pivotal in complex childhood trauma?

Answer: The addition of the concept of the administration of the supervisee in a complex childhood trauma issue for supervision is pivotal.

Chapter 15

Educational questions & activities

1. True or False: The three published workplace surveys of Australian counsellors show more similarities than differences.

Answer: True.

2. List one main difference found among the three discussed workplace surveys.

Answer: Theoretical orientation.

4. Is your favourite journal listed among the most popular for Australian counsellors?

Answer: No set correct answer.

4. Describe the general Australian counsellor in terms of demographic characteristics.

Answer: Generally speaking, Australian counsellors are women of middle-age. They tend to be married or in a partnered relationship, heterosexual, and living in urban environments. In terms of education, most counsellors tend to hold some type of baccalaureate degree.

Chapter 16

Educational questions & activities

1. *Classroom Discussion:* Discuss the implications of supervision of clinical supervision. When and how should supervisors seek supervision for casework related to supervisees? What would be the areas of consideration that would differ from the supervisor–supervisee relationship?

2. *Role Play:* Using the questions from the section *An Inventory of the Supervisory Relationship*, identify and role play scenarios where the selected questions can be answered in such a way that would strengthen the supervisory relationship.

   Answer: These questions have no set answers.

Chapter 17

1. What does the Supervisor Complexity Model have to say about supervisor development?

   Answer: That growth progresses through four different states and that during each stage supervisors have specific tasks to accomplish and responsibilities.

2. What are the SCM stages?

   Answer: Role Shock, Role Recovery and Transition, Role Consolidation, and Role Mastery.

3. List four influences on supervisory competence.

   Answer: Personal/relational variables, counselling experience, supervisory training, and supervisory experience.

4. Which of the four variables above do you see as most influential and why?

   Answer: No set answer.

Chapter 18

Educational questions & activities

1. Individual and Small Group Reflection Exercise

   The following reflection questions are intended to promote discussion about culture-infused supervision. Reflect about the way that you currently supervise students, or, if you are a student/supervisee, the way that you are supervised during your practicum or field placement.

a. How do you incorporate discussions about clients' cultural contents as an ongoing aspect of supervision?
b. How do introduce supervisor and supervisee cultural identities into supervision discussions?
c. What cultural influences in the relationship between supervisors and supervisees have you experienced?
d. What are some topics related to cultural contexts, cultural identities, and/or social justice that you would like to discuss with your supervisor/supervisee?
e. What barriers have you experienced in multicultural counselling supervision? How have you overcome those barriers?
f. What has helped you to build a strong working alliance with your supervisee/supervisor in which you discussed ideas about cultural contexts, cultural identities and/or social justice advocacy?

2. What does social justice advocacy mean to you? Give some examples of how counsellors can integrate advocacy roles into their practices.
3. Describe how you might approach intervention planning when a client's presenting issue is connected to a structural or social barrier?
4. What does the phrase, 'the professional is political' mean to you?

Answer: There are no set answers to these questions.

Chapter 19

Educational questions & activities

1. If the three domains of counselling mastery are the cognitive, the affective, and the relational (Jennings & Skovholt, 1999), how can we best evaluate if our program applicants are likely to be effective in these areas? In what ways can counsellor educators and supervisors assist potential students fairly in demonstrating their capacities to be worthy candidates for a postgraduate counselling program?

Answer: A combination of the following: Live panel interviews, Experiential group exercises, Referee reports, Academic transcripts, and possibly Other ways. This should not be a quick process; we should take time over this entry point, and faculty wide consultation should be part of the process. Well considered and comprehensive selection processes will save us time and resources later on in the program in dealing with students who lack competency.

2. Forrest and her colleagues (1999) summarised the ethical mandates incumbent upon trainers, educators and supervisors, in managing problematic student performance.

These include:

- Attending to the possibility that their trainees' personal problems might lead to harm of others
- Making sure that trainees are not harming clients or others under their care
- Attending to the possibility that trainees may misuse their influence

- Evaluating whether trainees are performing responsibly, competently, and ethically
- Articulating a clear set of professional standards
- Evaluating trainees based on these relevant and established requirements (cf. p.636).

Discuss how your program attends to these mandates effectively?

Answer: There are no set answers to these questions.

3. Discuss the significance of the language we use in defining and labelling certain behaviours and/or individuals who are problematic. What are the benefits and dangers in using the following terminology in regards to students? a) 'Incompetence'; b) 'impairment'; c) 'personal limitations'; d) 'inappropriateness'; e) 'unsuitability'; f) 'unfit to practice'; professional competence problems?

Answer: a)–e): The problem with these terms is that they: lack specificity and precision; blur behaviour and personality; mix-up cause and consequences. These terms can be seen as labels that are detrimental to the career future of the student, not only in the counselling profession. f). This term may cover the breadth and depth of the problems and concerns that counsellor educators and supervisors encounter in students who are not, for whatever reason, meeting professional standards of practice. Because it is behaviourally focussed, the term may lead to more attentive monitoring and evaluation of students, which will in turn lead "improved identification, remediation, and effective outcomes" (Elman & Forrest, 2007, p. 508).

4. Discuss how you can design, implement, and monitor remediation plans shaped to manage and address individual student's performance problems. Who should take responsibility for these plans in your program? Should the three tasks of design, implementation and monitoring be undertaken by different individuals on the faculty?

Answer: Forrest and her colleagues (1999) suggested that remediation plans should:

- Identify and describe deficiencies that are directly tied to the program's evaluation criteria,
- identify specific goals or changes that need to be made by the trainee,
- identify possible methods for meeting those goals,
- establish criteria for judging whether remediation has been successful, and
- determine a timeline for re-evaluation

Different decisions may be made regarding whose responsibility it is for such plans, implementation, and monitoring.

5. Discuss with your colleagues what behaviours, attitudes, and contexts demand the dismissal of a student from your program. What are our professional, ethical, and legal responsibilities as trainers and supervisors to this trainee, to the public, to the profession, and to our training institutes?

Answer: This is a demanding and difficult decision to come to for most counsellor educators. When remediation plans do not achieve positive outcomes for students, we need to face the fact that these students may need to be counselled off the program, or even dismissed from the program as being unsuitable for the profession, in that they never had or have not been able to achieve an adequate level of professional competence during the required time period. Some of the reasons for dismissal include continued poor academic performance, poor clinical performance, failed competency tests, ethical violations, psychopathology, emotional instability, personality disorder, unprofessional demeanour, poor interpersonal skills, sexual misconduct, and substance abuse (Forrest, et al., 1999).

Obviously due process needs to be followed according to the policies of the University or Training Institute, where students have been duly informed of professional competencies, standards and expectations, remedial plans that have not achieved sufficient change in the student's professional competency levels are recorded, extensive and detailed documentation is completed and placed in the student's file (Wilkerson, 2006).

Chapter 20

Educational questions & activities

1. Discuss how you define competence.

   Answer: There is no set answer to this question.

2. List two forms of assessment.

   Answer: Formative; summative

3. Who are some stakeholders who can assess competence?

   Answer: Trainers/supervisor; manager; external judge; self; peer; client.

Chapter 21

Educational questions & activities

1. Activity: Note-taking, Simulation, Self-Appraisal, Specific and General Discussion. Provide each student with a copy of the intake form (Figure 21.1) in this chapter. Prepare a comprehensive description of a complex clinical case.

   Step 1. Read the case to the class while students fill in the information on the intake form.
   Step 2. Allow students to ask you questions and ask you to repeat information they may have missed. (This allows students to be active and intentional in thinking about information they need from a client)
   Step 3. In pairs, have students compare and contrast their notes, while adding information to make this record more comprehensive.
   Step 4. Engage in an open-ended class discussion including the content of their record, what other information should be gathered initially, what could be gathered in later client sessions, and student reactions to the note-taking process.

2. Use Barletta's developmental model (Table 21.1) to discuss the concept of the growth of a helping professional, with particular attention to the student's current phase, individual plans to facilitate additional progress, and expectations of what the future phases might be like.

Answer: These questions have no set answers.

Chapter 22

1. What is the typical model used in psychology training?

Answer: Scientist-practitioner.

2. Why do some believe that clinicians should also be competent basic researchers?

Answer: So that the latest scholarly knowledge can influence applied work and so that clinicians can work in a self-reflective manner with clients.

3. What divide has historically existed among researchers?

Answer: One regarding methodology: quantitative versus qualitative methods.

4. What is the most popular type of scholarship in clinical supervision?

Answer: Discussion or reviews papers, including the presentation of models for use in supervision.

5. What country accounts for most of the publications found in the searches conducted?

Answer: The United States of America.

6. What does the author recommend regarding supervision scholarship?

Answer:
a. That more research and less editorialising be published.
b. That research supervision is a wide-open area for exploration.
c. That collaboration across countries and professional groups relating to supervision occur.

Chapter 23

Educational questions & activities

1. Why is the majority of psychotherapy research centred on European and American populations?

Answer: As noted in the chapter, the majority of the prominent counselling and psycho-therapeutic treatments in use today were developed by European or American psych-ologist and psychiatrists.

2. Has psychotherapy research focusing on East and Southeast Asian countries increased in the twenty-first century?

Answer: Yes, psychotherapy research has increased over the past two decades and has increased with the prevalence of psychological treatment in East and Southeast Asian countries.

3. What population does most East and Southeast Asian psychotherapy research focus upon?

Answer: Most psychotherapy research in East and Southeast Asia is focused upon the Chinese population (60% of articles) and adult treatment (39%).

4. How much of the East and Southeast Asian psychotherapy research focuses upon treating depressive disorders?

Answer: 18% of psychotherapy research in the East and Southeast Asian area focused upon treating depression.

5. What was the most popular treatment researched in East and Southeast Asian psycho-therapy Research?

Answer: Cognitive-behavioral therapy was the most popular treatment explored, accounting for 20% of articles.

Chapter 24

Educational questions & activities

1. What is the largest group of evidence-based treatment (EBT)?

Answer: The majority of EBTs in psychology relate to cognitive-behavioral therapy. These therapies help one change emotions by changing maladaptive thought processes or behaviours, often both.

2. If an evidence-based treatment (EBT) has a manualised version one must apply the treatment as per the manual exactly for effectiveness. Is this statement True or False?

Answer: False. It is important to remember that each client is unique and adaptations can be made to most effectively help a client.

3. Evidence-based treatments (EBTs) are effective in all cultures. Is this statement True or False?

Answer: Culture can act as a mediating variable and thus people from different cultures may respond differently to the exact same treatment. This is why the effectiveness of EBTs needs to be tested and verified amongst different people and cultures and ethnicities. While the therapeutic foundation needs to remain the same in EBTs (fidelity), adaptations may be made appropriately (flexibility).

4. Is the research on evidence-based practices used with Asian populations and coming out of Asian countries increasing, decreasing, or remaining steady?

Answer: Increasing.

Chapter 25

Educational questions & activities

1. As an individual, or a group, list all the possible benefits and drawbacks of being a member of a professional organisation.
2. Ask a trusted colleague or supervisor what they think the benefits and drawbacks of being a member of a professional organisation entail.
3. Look up one professional organisation in your practice area and in your home country and one in a country in which you are interested. What do the respective organisations say about your professional area in those countries?
4. How much does it cost for a student or a beginning professional to join the professional organisation most relevant to your work?

Answer: These questions have no set answers.

Chapters 26–32

Educational questions & activities with answers are not specifically provided for Chapters 26–32. Educators in the specific countries/regions included in this book are encouraged to create and provide answers for questions they deem most appropriate.